Bioequivalence Studies in Drug Development

Statistics in Practice

Statistics in Practice is an important international series of texts which provide detailed coverage of statistical concepts, methods and worked case studies in specific fields of investigation and study.

With sound motivation and many worked practical examples, the books show in down-to-earth terms how to select and use an appropriate range of statistical techniques in a particular practical field within each title's special topic area.

The books provide statistical support for professionals and research workers across a range of employment fields and research environments. Subject areas covered include medicine and pharmaceutics; industry, finance and commerce; public services; the earth and environmental sciences, and so on.

The books also provide support to students studying statistical courses applied to the above areas. The demand for graduates to be equipped for the work environment has led to such courses becoming increasingly prevalent at universities and colleges.

It is our aim to present judiciously chosen and well-written workbooks to meet everyday practical needs. Feedback of views from readers will be most valuable to monitor the success of this aim.

A complete list of titles in this series appears at the end of the volume.

Bioequivalence Studies in Drug Development

Methods and Applications

Dieter Hauschke

Department of Biometry
ALTANA Pharma, Germany

Volker Steinijans

Department of Biometry
ALTANA Pharma, Germany

Iris Pigeot

Bremen Institute for Prevention Research and Social Medicine,
University of Bremen, Germany

John Wiley & Sons, Ltd

Other Wiley Editorial Offices

John Wiley & Sons Inc., 111 River Street, Hoboken, NJ 07030, USA

Jossey-Bass, 989 Market Street, San Francisco, CA 94103-1741, USA

Wiley-VCH Verlag GmbH, Boschstr. 12, D-69469 Weinheim, Germany

John Wiley & Sons Australia Ltd, 42 McDougall Street, Milton, Queensland 4064, Australia

John Wiley & Sons (Asia) Pte Ltd, 2 Clementi Loop #02-01, Jin Xing Distripark, Singapore 129809

John Wiley & Sons Canada Ltd, 22 Worcester Road, Etobicoke, Ontario, Canada M9W 1L1

Wiley also publishes its books in a variety of electronic formats. Some content that appears in print may not
be available in electronic books.

Library of Congress Cataloging in Publication Data

Hauschke, Dieter.
   Bioequivalence studies in drug development : methods and applications / Dieter Hauschke,
   Volker Steinijans, Iris Pigeot.
       p.   ;   cm.
   Includes bibliographical references and indexes.
   ISBN-13: 978-0-470-09475-4 (HB : alk. paper)
   ISBN-10: 0-470-09475-3 (HB : alk. paper)
   1. Drugs—Therapeutic equivalency.   I. Steinijans, Volker.   II. Pigeot, Iris.   III. Title.   [DNLM:
   1. Therapeutic Equivalency.   2. Clinical Trials—methods.   3. Drug Design.   QV 38 H376b 2007]
   RM301.45.H38 2007
   615′.19—dc22
                                                                              2006029953

British Library Cataloguing in Publication Data

A catalogue record for this book is available from the British Library

ISBN-13: 978-0-470-09475-4 (HB)
ISBN-10: 0-470-09475-3 (HB : alk. paper)

Typeset in 10/12pt Times by Integra Software Services Pvt. Ltd, Pondicherry, India
Printed and bound in Great Britain by TJ International, Padstow, Cornwall
This book is printed on acid-free paper responsibly manufactured from sustainable forestry in which at least
two trees are planted for each one used for paper production.

The book is for

- *my family, for their encouragement: Carmen, Simon, Andreas, Eva and Andi (Dieter Hauschke)*

- *Helga, Eva and Uwe (Volker Steinijans)*

- *my husband Jürgen and the BIPS, for their neverending patience (Iris Pigeot)*

Contents

Preface

The design, performance, and evaluation of bioavailability and bioequivalence studies have received major attention from academia, the pharmaceutical industry and health authorities over the last couple of decades. Hence, the focus of the book is to provide an up-to-date overview of available methods, adopting a practical approach via numerous examples using real data. We also include recent methodology, most notably on the concepts of population and individual bioequivalence.

This book is a useful reference for clinical pharmacologists, biopharmaceutical scientists, reviewers from regulatory affairs, and biometricians working in the pharmaceutical industry. In addition, the presented material provides a springboard for all scientists from academia who are conducting research in this area of biopharmaceutics and clinical pharmacokinetics.

The book consists of 10 chapters, which cover planning, conduct, analysis, and reporting of bioequivalence studies according to current regulatory requirements. The methods are illustrated by a large number of real datasets. Moreover, the corresponding SAS® code is provided to assist the reader in implementing the analysis.

We are grateful to our colleagues Anton Drollmann, Christian Gartner, Kai Grosch, Dietrich Knoerzer, Olaf Michel, Rüdiger Nave, and Stephen Senn for comments on individual chapters, Martin Burke, Edgar Diletti, and Marc Suling for contributing SAS® code and generating the figures. We are also grateful for editorial help to Regine Albrecht, Elena Gamp, Beate Riedlinger, Rita Sauter, and Birgit Schroeder. At Wiley & Sons, we thank Wendy Hunter for providing continuous support during the production process.

Finally, we take responsibility for any errors in the book. Comments are most welcome for the preparation of further editions.

Dieter Hauschke
Volker Steinijans
Iris Pigeot

1

Introduction

Comparison of therapeutic performance of two medicinal products containing the same active substance is critical for assessing the possibility of supplanting an innovator with any essentially similar medicinal product. In practice, demonstration of bioequivalence is generally the most appropriate method of substantiating therapeutic equivalence between medicinal products. Assuming that, in the same subject, similar plasma concentration-time courses will result in similar concentrations at the site of action and thus in similar effects, pharmacokinetic data instead of therapeutic results may be used to demonstrate bioequivalence as an established surrogate marker for therapeutic equivalence.

The design, performance and evaluation of bioequivalence studies have received major attention from academia, the pharmaceutical industry and health authorities over the last couple of decades. Since 2003 there has been international consensus and current regulatory guidelines (Committee for Proprietary Medicinal Products (CPMP), 2001; Food and Drug Administration (FDA), 2003) require the demonstration of average bioequivalence between a test and a reference formulation, which means equivalence with regard to the population means.

The purpose of this chapter is to provide some essential features of bioequivalence trials. In particular we shall

- give the underlying definitions;

- explain when bioequivalence studies are performed;

- refer to the design and conduct of these studies.

1.1 Definitions

Although the beginning of the search for bioequivalence standards dates back to the early 1970s, there is no International Conference on Harmonization (ICH) Guidance on bioavailability and bioequivalence. Thus, the definitions given in the following primarily reflect the current guidelines of the US Food and Drug Administration and the European Committee for Proprietary Medicinal Products (FDA, 2003; CPMP, 2001). However, in order to illustrate how these concepts developed, other definitions are also cited.

1.1.1 Bioavailability

In the 2003 FDA guidance,

> 'Bioavailability is defined as the rate and extent to which the active ingredient or active moiety is absorbed from a drug product and becomes available at the site of action. For drug products that are not intended to be absorbed into the bloodstream, bioavailability may be assessed by measurements intended to reflect the rate and extent to which the active ingredient or active moiety becomes available at the site of action.'

This definition focuses on the processes by which the active ingredients or moieties are released from an oral dosage form and move to the site of action. Such processes may also be influenced by drug properties such as permeability and the influences of presystemic enzymes and/or active transporters (e.g., p-glycoprotein).

To avoid an inconsistent use of the term 'absorption', Chiou (2001) suggested that absorption be defined as movement of drug across the outer mucosal membranes of the GI tract, while bioavailability be defined as availability of drug to the general circulation or site of pharmacological actions.

1.1.2 Bioequivalence

One of the operationally most feasible definitions of bioequivalence was given at the BIO-International '94 Conference in Munich (Skelly, 1995),

> 'Two pharmaceutical products are considered to be equivalent when their concentration vs. time profiles, from the same molar dose, are so similar that they are unlikely to produce clinically relevant differences in therapeutic and/or adverse effects.'

It is this definition that comes closest to the operational procedure of comparing concentration-time profiles, or suitable metrics characterizing such profiles, in order to assess bioequivalence.

However, this practical definition was not adopted in the 2001 CPMP guidance on bioavailability and bioequivalence, which hardly changed its previous 1991 definition (CPMP, 2001),

> 'Two medicinal products are bioequivalent if they are pharmaceutically equivalent or pharmaceutical alternatives and if their bioavailabilities after administration in the same molar dose are similar to such a degree that their effects, with respect to both efficacy and safety, will be essentially the same.'

The definition of pharmaceutical equivalents and alternatives is given as,

> 'Medicinal products are pharmaceutically equivalent if they contain the same amount of the same active substance(s) in the same dosage forms that meet

the same or comparable standards. They are pharmaceutical alternatives if they contain the same active moiety but differ in chemical form (salt, ester, etc.) of that moiety, or in the dosage form or strength. It is well known that pharmaceutical equivalence does not necessarily imply bioequivalence as differences in the excipients and/or the manufacturing process can lead to faster or slower dissolution and/or absorption.'

Although the 2001 CPMP definition of bioequivalence addresses both similar efficacy, and similar safety, it should be noted that it is virtually impossible to conclude similar safety on the basis of a bioequivalence study with its limited number of subjects and limited exposure time. The conjecture appears to be that similarity of the concentration-time profiles, in particular similarity of the maximum concentrations, may serve as a surrogate marker for the similarity of the adverse event profiles to be anticipated.

In the 2003 FDA guidance,

'Bioequivalence is defined as the absence of a significant difference in the rate and extent to which the active ingredient or active moiety in pharmaceutical equivalents or pharmaceutical alternatives becomes available at the site of drug action when administered at the same molar dose under similar conditions in an appropriately designed study.'

The FDA definition explicitly mentions rate and extent of drug availability as the two primary characteristics of the concentration-time profile. It is this concept of similarity in rate and extent of drug absorption which continues to define the bioequivalence metrics for rate and extent, and thereby the basis of the bioequivalence assessment.

It is interesting to note that there were various attempts to move away from this initial concept of rate and extent of drug absorption, particularly as some of the traditional rate characteristics such as C_{max} were identified as rather indirect, and frequently poor, measures of the true absorption rate. Steinijans *et al.* (1995a, 1996) proposed that bioequivalence assessment should focus on shape analysis of the concentration-time curves rather than on absorption rates. Chen *et al.* (2001) presented the concept of early, peak and total exposure, which at that time was under examination by the FDA. However, none of these alternative concepts were directly reflected in the corresponding guidelines.

1.1.3 Therapeutic equivalence

The 2001 CPMP guidance on bioavailability and bioequivalence also addresses the concept of therapeutic equivalence,

'A medicinal product is therapeutically equivalent with another product if it contains the same active substance or therapeutic moiety and, clinically, shows the same efficacy and safety as that product, whose efficacy and safety has been established. In practice, demonstration of bioequivalence is generally the most appropriate method of substantiating therapeutic equivalence between medicinal products, which are pharmaceutically equivalent or pharmaceutical alternatives, provided they contain excipients generally recognized as not having an influence on safety and efficacy and comply with labeling requirements with respect to excipients. However, in some cases where similar extent of absorption but different rates of absorption are observed the products can still be judged therapeutically equivalent if those differences are not of therapeutic relevance. A clinical study to prove that differences in absorption rate are not therapeutically relevant will probably be necessary.'

1.2   When are bioequivalence studies performed

1.2.1   Applications for products containing new active substances

During the development of a new active substance (new chemical entity) intended for systemic action, bioequivalence studies are necessary as bridging studies between (i) pivotal and early clinical trial formulations; (ii) pivotal clinical trial formulations, especially those used in the dose finding studies, and the to-be-marketed medicinal product.

1.2.2   Applications for products containing approved active substances

In vivo bioequivalence studies are needed when there is a risk that possible differences in bioavailability may result in therapeutic inequivalence. The CPMP guidance (2001) devotes an entire section to the necessity of bioequivalence studies for various dosage forms, taking into consideration the concepts underlying the Biopharmaceutics Classification System (Amidon *et al.*, 1995), i.e., high solubility, high permeability for the active substance, and high dissolution rate for the medicinal product. This section also addresses special topics such as

- Exemptions from bioequivalence studies in the case of oral immediate release forms (*in vitro* dissolution data as part of a bioequivalence waiver).

- Post approval changes.

- Dose proportionality of immediate release oral dosage forms (bioequivalence assessment for only one dose strength).

- Suprabioavailability (which necessitates reformulation to a lower dosage strength, otherwise the suprabioavailable product may be considered as new medicinal product, the efficacy and safety of which have to be supported by clinical studies).

1.2.3   Applications for modified release forms essentially similar to a marketed modified release form

The requirements for modified release forms are stated in the CPMP Note for Guidance on Modified Release Oral and Transdermal Dosage Forms (1999), which differentiates between prolonged, delayed and transdermal release forms.

Prolonged release formulations can be assessed as bioequivalent on the basis of single-dose and multiple-dose studies, which are designed to demonstrate that

- The test formulation exhibits the claimed prolonged release characteristics of the reference.

- The active drug substance is not released unexpectedly from the test formulation (dose dumping).

- Performance of the test and reference formulation is equivalent after single dose and at steady state.

- The effect of food on the *in vivo* performance is comparable for both formulations when a single-dose study is conducted comparing equal doses of the test formulation with those of the reference formulation administered immediately after a predefined high fat meal. This study should be conducted with the same strength(s) as those of the pivotal bioequivalence studies.

In the case of prolonged release single unit formulations with multiple strengths, a single-dose study under fasting conditions is required for each strength. Studies at steady state may be conducted with the highest strength only, if certain criteria for extrapolating bioequivalence studies (linear pharmacokinetics, same qualitative composition, etc.) are fulfilled. For multiple unit formulations of a medicinal product showing linear pharmacokinetics with multiple strengths, a single-dose study under fasting conditions on the highest strength is sufficient, provided that the compositions of the lower strengths are proportional to that of the highest strength, the formulations contain identical beads or pellets, and the dissolution profiles are acceptable.

For delayed release formulations, postprandial bioequivalence studies are necessary as food can influence the absorption of an active substance administered in an enteric-coated formulation.

The bioequivalence of a transdermal drug delivery system (TDDS) in comparison to the innovator's product should usually be assessed after single dose as well as after multiple dose administration. When marketing authorization of multiple strengths is required, the bioequivalence study can be performed with the highest dosage strength provided that exact proportionality in the formulation is given, i.e., the composition is the same, and the strength is proportional to the effective surface area of the patch, and that there is an acceptable *in vitro* release test (CPMP, 1999).

1.3 Design and conduct of bioequivalence studies

1.3.1 Crossover design and alternatives

A bioequivalence study should be designed in such a way that the formulation effect can be distinguished from other effects. In the standard situation of comparing a test formulation (T) with a reference formulation (R), the two-period, two-sequence crossover design is the RT/TR design. Subjects are randomly allocated to two treatment sequences; in sequence 1, subjects receive the reference formulation and test formulation in periods

Table 1.1 The RT/TR design.

Sequence	Period 1	Washout	Period 2
1	R		T
2	T		R

1 and 2, respectively, while in sequence 2, subjects receive the formulations in reverse order. Between period 1 and period 2 is a washout period, which has to be sufficiently long to ensure that the effect of the preceding formulation has been eliminated (see Table 1.1).

Under certain circumstances and provided that the study design and the statistical analyses are scientifically sound, alternative designs could be considered such as a parallel group design for substances with a very long half-life and replicate designs for substances with highly variable disposition.

1.3.2 Single- vs. multiple-dose studies

In general, single-dose studies will suffice, but steady-state studies may be required in the case of dose- or time-dependent pharmacokinetics. Moreover, in case of some modified release products (prolonged release formulations and transdermal drug delivery systems), steady-state studies are required in addition to the single-dose investigations (CPMP, 1999). Steady-state studies can be considered, e.g., if problems of sensitivity preclude sufficiently precise plasma concentration measurements after single dose administration. In steady-state studies washout of the previous treatment's last dose can overlap with the build-up of the second treatment, provided the build-up period is sufficiently long (at least three times the terminal half-life). When differences between morning and evening dosing are known, e.g., due to circadian rhythms influencing drug absorption, sampling should be carried out over a full 24-hour dosing cycle.

1.3.3 Pharmacokinetic characteristics

In most cases evaluation of bioequivalence will be based upon measured concentrations of the parent compound. Bioequivalence determinations based on metabolites should be justified in each case. If metabolites significantly contribute to the net activity of an active substance and the pharmacokinetic system is nonlinear, it is necessary to measure both parent drug and active metabolite plasma concentrations and to evaluate them separately.

According to the CPMP guidance (2001), $AUC(0-t)$ (area under the plasma concentration curve from administration to last observed concentration at time t), $AUC(0-\infty)$ (area under the curve extrapolated to infinite time), C_{max} (maximum plasma concentration), t_{max} (time from administration to maximum plasma concentration), $Ae(0-t)$ (cumulative urinary excretion from administration until time t), and $Ae(0-\infty)$ (cumulative urinary excretion extrapolated to infinite time) are appropriate bioavailability characteristics. Pharmacokinetic principles imply that the area under concentration-time curve from zero to infinity, $AUC(0-\infty)$, and not a partial area up to a certain time point, serves as characteristic of the extent of absorption in single-dose studies. This becomes evident from the fundamental pharmacokinetic relationship

$$f \cdot dose = clearance \cdot AUC(0-\infty), 0 < f \leq 1,$$

which states that the fraction, f, of the dose that is ultimately absorbed is proportional to $AUC(0-\infty)$, clearance being the proportionality factor. The sampling schedule should allow adequate estimation of the primary pharmacokinetic characteristics for rate and extent of absorption. The latter will be achieved if the AUC derived from measurements is at least 80 % of the AUC extrapolated to infinity. Standard techniques for AUC extrapolation to infinity have been described by Sauter *et al.* (1992). For drugs with a long half-life, relative bioavailability can be adequately estimated by using a truncated AUC as long as the total collection period is justified. For additional information $t_{1/2}$ (plasma concentration half-life) and MRT (mean residence time) can be estimated. For studies at steady state, the following characteristics should be calculated during one dosing interval or cycle, τ, at steady state: $AUC(0-\tau)$; C_{max}; C_{min}; and peak-trough fluctuation, $PTF = (C_{max} - C_{min})/C_{av}$, where $C_{av} = AUC(0-\tau)/\tau$ denotes the average steady-state concentration. For confirmative bioequivalence assessment, primary characteristics for rate and extent of absorption should be stipulated prospectively in the study protocol.

Adequate choice of the pharmacokinetic characteristics is discussed in Chapter 2 'Metrics to characterize concentration-time profiles in single- and multiple-dose bioequivalence studies'.

1.3.4 Subjects

The subject population for bioequivalence studies should be selected with the aim of minimizing variability and permitting detection of differences between pharmaceutical products. Therefore, the studies should normally be performed with healthy volunteers. Subjects could belong to either sex; however, the risk to women of childbearing potential should be considered on an individual basis. In general, subjects should be between 18–55 years old, of weight within the normal range, preferably nonsmokers, and without a history of alcohol or drug abuse. They should undergo a routine screening of clinical laboratory tests and a comprehensive medical examination.

If the investigated active substance is known to have adverse effects and the pharmacological effects or risks are considered unacceptable for healthy volunteers, it may be necessary to use patients instead, under suitable precautions and supervision.

Phenotyping and/or genotyping of subjects should be considered for exploratory bioavailability studies and all studies using parallel group design. If the metabolism of a drug is known to be affected by a major genetic polymorphism, studies could be performed in panels of subjects of known phenotype or genotype for the polymorphism in question.

1.3.5 Statistical models

The statistical models described in the regulatory guidelines (CPMP, 2001; FDA, 2001) are generally defined on the logarithmic scale (e.g., natural logarithms are taken). In the case of average bioequivalence (ABE), the model refers to the classical unscaled criterion for the difference in treatment means. For population bioequivalence (PBE) and individual bioequivalence (IBE), aggregate criteria are proposed which, apart from the mean difference, include a component for the difference in variances, and for IBE, an additional component to reflect subject-by-treatment interaction. The aggregate criteria are generally scaled, either by the variance of the reference formulation or by a constant value. The exact definitions are summarized below.

1.3.5.1 Average bioequivalence

Based upon the two-period, two-sequence crossover design (see Table 1.1), average bioequivalence is concluded if the two-sided 90 % confidence interval for the test/reference ratio of population means is within the appropriate bioequivalence acceptance range, for example (0.80, 1.25) for AUC. More precisely, if μ_T and μ_R denote the population means for test and reference on the logarithmic scale, and $\exp(\mu_T)/\exp(\mu_R) = \exp(\mu_T - \mu_R)$ denotes, in case of variance homogeneity, the respective ratio of the population means on the original scale, the average bioequivalence criterion on the original scale,

$$H_0^{ABE} : \exp(\mu_T - \mu_R) \le 0.80 \ \text{ or } \ \exp(\mu_T - \mu_R) \ge 1.25$$

vs.

$$H_1^{ABE} : 0.80 < \exp(\mu_T - \mu_R) < 1.25,$$

corresponds to

$$H_0^{ABE} : \mu_T - \mu_R \le \ln 0.80 \ \text{ or } \ \mu_T - \mu_R \ge \ln 1.25$$

vs.

$$H_1^{ABE} : \ln 0.80 < \mu_T - \mu_R < \ln 1.25$$

on the logarithmic scale. Hence, for ABE the test problem on the additive scale after logarithmic transformation has a natural counterpart on the original (untransformed) scale. It should be noted that the inference on ABE is always correct for the ratio of population medians, but only in the case of equal variances is it also correct for the ratio of population means, because only for homogeneous variances does the ratio of medians equal the ratio of means.

Testing this two-sided bioequivalence problem is equivalent to simultaneous testing of the following two one-sided hypotheses

$$H_{01}^{ABE} : \mu_T - \mu_R \le \ln 0.80 \ \text{ vs. } \ H_{11}^{ABE} : \mu_T - \mu_R > \ln 0.80$$

and

$$H_{02}^{ABE} : \mu_T - \mu_R \ge \ln 1.25 \ \text{ vs. } \ H_{12}^{ABE} : \mu_T - \mu_R < \ln 1.25,$$

Table 1.2 Point estimate and 90 % confidence interval for the ratio of expected means $\exp(\mu_T)/\exp(\mu_R)$ in the dose equivalence study (see Chapter 4). Reference: $2 \cdot 200$ mg $+ 2 \cdot 300$ mg theophylline, Test: $2 \cdot 500$ mg theophylline.

		Point estimate	Confidence limits		Level of confidence
Statistical method			Lower	Upper	
Parametric analysis	Two one-sided t-tests	1.00	0.925	1.085	0.90
Nonparametric analysis	Two one-sided Wilcoxon tests	1.03	0.942	1.097	0.9061

by means of two independent t-tests (Schuirmann, 1987) or Wilcoxon tests (Hauschke *et al.*, 1990), each at the 5 % level.

It is well known that rejection of the two one-sided null hypotheses at the 5 % level is equivalent to the inclusion of the 90 % confidence interval in the acceptance range (0.80, 1.25). Therefore, in practice the statistical method for demonstrating average bioequivalence is based on the 90 % confidence interval for the ratio of population means (test/reference) and its inclusion in the prospectively stipulated bioequivalence acceptance range. For example, in Table 1.2 the parametric and nonparametric point estimates and the corresponding 90 % confidence intervals for the ratio of expected means $\exp(\mu_T)/ \exp(\mu_R)$ are given for the dose equivalence study examined in Chapter 4, which compares pellet formulations at the same daily dose, but administered at different dosage strengths. The results reveal that, with respect to the extent of absorption, equivalence can be concluded.

The bioequivalence acceptance range for the *AUC* ratio is generally (0.80, 1.25). In specific cases of a narrow therapeutic range the acceptance interval may need to be tightened. In rare cases a wider acceptance range may be acceptable if it is based on sound clinical justification. The 90 % confidence interval for the C_{max} ratio should lie within the (0.80, 1.25) acceptance range. As with the *AUC* ratio, the acceptance interval for the C_{max} ratio may need to be tightened in specific cases of narrow therapeutic range. In certain cases a wider interval may be acceptable. The bioequivalence acceptance range must be prospectively defined, e.g., (0.75, 1.333), and justified, addressing in particular any safety or efficacy concerns for patients switched between formulations. Statistical evaluation of t_{max} makes sense only if there is a clinically relevant claim for rapid release or action, or signs related to adverse effects. In these cases, a nonparametric analysis (Hauschke *et al.*, 1990) is recommended for untransformed t_{max} data.

In Chapter 4 'Assessment of average bioequivalence in the *RT/TR* design', not only the adequate analysis of variance is discussed, but also details are presented for performing a parametric and a nonparametric analysis.

1.3.5.2 Population bioequivalence

Population bioequivalence encompasses equivalence of the entire distributions of the respective metric between test and reference. Since the lognormal distribution is fully described by the median and the variance, population bioequivalence is commonly restricted to the equivalence of population medians and variances for test and reference. Hence, the conventional *RT/TR* crossover design may be used to assess bioequivalence in a stepwise approach. Starting with average bioequivalence, population equivalence will be considered only if average equivalence is approved (Vuorinen and Turunen, 1996).

Figure 1.1 shows the sequence-by-period plot for the extent characteristic $AUC(0 - \infty)$ for the dose equivalence study. This presentation enables a simultaneous graphical assessment of the medians and the underlying variability. The results are given separately for each sequence in each period as geometric mean and the range corresponding to ± 1 standard deviation in the logarithmically transformed domain. Figure 1.1 reveals that the variability of test is similar to that of the reference.

Further graphical methods for illustrating differences in variability are presented in Chapter 6 'Presentation of bioequivalence studies'.

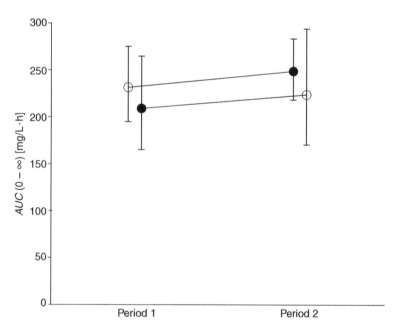

Figure 1.1 Sequence-by-period plot for the primary extent characteristic $AUC(0 - \infty)$ in the dose equivalence study (see Chapter 4). The results are given separately for each sequence in each period as geometric mean and the range corresponding to ± 1 standard deviation (sd) in the logarithmically transformed domain, i.e., [exp(mean(ln AUC) $-$ sd(ln AUC)), exp (mean(ln AUC) + sd (ln AUC))], ($\circ =$ Reference, $\bullet =$ Test; Reference: $2 \cdot 200$ mg + $2 \cdot 300$ mg theophylline, Test: $2 \cdot 500$ mg theophylline).

According to the FDA guidance (2001), the following scaled moment-based aggregate criterion was suggested for population equivalence assessment

$$H_0^{PBE} : \frac{(\mu_T - \mu_R)^2 + \sigma_T^2 - \sigma_R^2}{\sigma_*^2} \geq \frac{(\ln 1.25)^2 + 0.02}{0.04}$$

vs.

$$H_1^{PBE} : \frac{(\mu_T - \mu_R)^2 + \sigma_T^2 - \sigma_R^2}{\sigma_*^2} < \frac{(\ln 1.25)^2 + 0.02}{0.04},$$

where $\sigma_*^2 = \max(\sigma_R^2, 0.04)$ switches between reference and constant scaled, and σ_T^2 and σ_R^2 denote the total variances for test and reference, respectively.

Population bioequivalence can be concluded at the $\alpha = 0.05$ significance level if the upper limit of the one-sided 95 % confidence interval for $\left((\mu_T - \mu_R)^2 + \sigma_T^2 - \sigma_R^2\right) / \sigma_*^2$ is less than $\left((\ln 1.25)^2 + 0.02\right) / 0.04$. For calculation of the confidence interval a parametric approach was recommended by the FDA (2001), which is based on the method of moments estimation with a Cornish-Fisher expansion.

A detailed overview of this concept for bioequivalence assessment is provided in Section 9.4 'Population bioequivalence'.

1.3.5.3 Individual bioequivalence

The primary objective for introducing individual bioequivalence is to account for subject-by-formulation interaction, and to use the comparison of the reference formulation to itself as the basis for the comparison of test and reference. In contrast to average and population bioequivalence, individual bioequivalence compares within-subject distributions of the respective bioavailability metrics, and thus, needs at least replication of the reference formulation.

The subject-by-formulation interaction is a measure of the extent to which the between-formulation differences vary among the individuals. As an example, a graphical illustration of this parameter is given in Figure 1.2 for the data of the dose equivalence study (see Chapter 4). Although displaying a certain within-subject variability, the plot does not reveal a systematic subject-by-formulation interaction.

For individual bioequivalence, the following scaled aggregate criterion was proposed in the FDA guidance (2001):

$$H_0^{IBE} : \frac{(\mu_T - \mu_R)^2 + \sigma_D^2 + \sigma_{WT}^2 - \sigma_{WR}^2}{\sigma_*^2} \geq \frac{(\ln 1.25)^2 + 0.05}{0.04}$$

vs.

$$H_1^{IBE} : \frac{(\mu_T - \mu_R)^2 + \sigma_D^2 + \sigma_{WT}^2 - \sigma_{WR}^2}{\sigma_*^2} < \frac{(\ln 1.25)^2 + 0.05}{0.04},$$

where $\sigma_*^2 = \max(\sigma_{WR}^2, 0.04)$ switches between reference and constant scaled, σ_D^2 is the variance component for the subject-by-formulation interaction, and σ_{WT}^2 and σ_{WR}^2 denote the within-subject variances for test and reference, respectively.

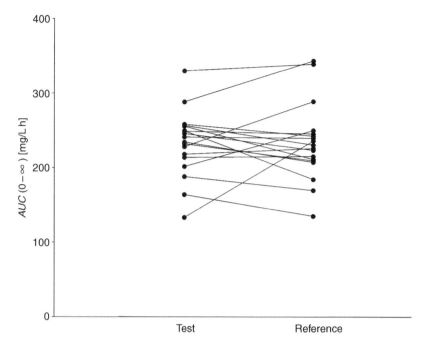

Figure 1.2 Graphical representation of the subject-by-formulation interaction for the 18 subjects in the dose equivalence study (see Chapter 4). Reference: $2 \cdot 200$ mg $+ 2 \cdot 300$ mg theophylline, Test: $2 \cdot 500$ mg theophylline.

Individual bioequivalence can be concluded at the $\alpha = 0.05$ significance level, if the upper limit of the one-sided 95% confidence interval for $\left((\mu_T - \mu_R)^2 + \sigma_D^2 + \sigma_{WT}^2 - \sigma_{WR}^2 \right) / \sigma_*^2$ is less than $\left((\ln 1.25)^2 + 0.05 \right) / 0.04$. In analogy to the population bioequivalence approach, calculation of the confidence interval is based on the method of moments estimation with a Cornish-Fisher expansion (FDA, 2001).

In contrast to the FDA Guidance for Industry: Statistical Approaches to Establishing Bioequivalence (2001), the FDA Guidance for Industry: Bioavailability and Bioequivalence Studies for Orally Administered Drug Products - General Considerations (2003) states that the recommended method of analysis of nonreplicate and replicate studies to establish bioequivalence is average bioequivalence. This is in line with the CPMP guidance (2001), which gives no specific recommendation on population and individual bioequivalence. It is argued that, to date, most bioequivalence studies are designed to evaluate average bioequivalence and that experience with population and individual bioequivalence is limited.

The above and further issues are discussed in detail in Section 9.5 'Individual bioequivalence'.

1.3.6 Sample size

The sample size, i.e., the number of subjects required to obtain an *a priori* stipulated power of correctly concluding bioequivalence, is a function of the bioequivalence acceptance range, e.g., (0.80, 1.25); the type I error (i.e., the consumer risk of incorrectly concluding bioequivalence); the expected deviation of the test from the reference formulation, which obviously has to be within the bioequivalence acceptance range; and the coefficient of variation associated with the primary characteristic. The latter can be obtained from a pilot experiment, from previous studies or from published data (Steinijans *et al.*, 1995b). Algorithms, power charts and tables for sample size planning have been provided by Diletti *et al.* (1991, 1992).

For example, Figure 1.3 gives an illustration of the attained power for commonly used sample sizes. The power curves are given for sample sizes of $n = 12$, 16, 18, assuming the within-subject coefficient of variation $CV_W = 20\%$, a type I error of $\alpha = 0.05$, and the bioequivalence range of (0.80, 1.25). As expected, the power is highest if $\theta = \exp(\mu_T)/\exp(\mu_R) = 1$, the point of equality. As the ratio approaches the limits of the bioequivalence range, the power decreases dramatically.

It should be noted that, notwithstanding appropriate sample size planning, the CPMP guidance (2001) states that the minimum number of subjects should not be smaller than 12, unless justified.

In Chapter 5 'Power and sample size determination for testing average bioequivalence in the *RT/TR* design', the methodology for determining the required sample size is given.

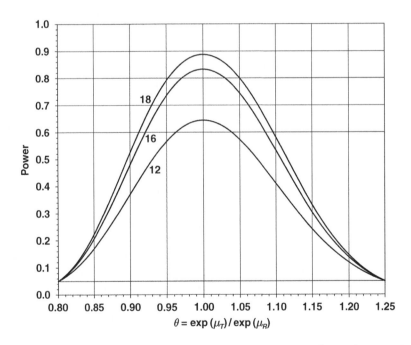

Figure 1.3 Probability of correctly concluding equivalence (power) as a function of the ratio $\theta = \exp(\mu_T)/\exp(\mu_R)$ calculated over the acceptance range (0.8, 1.25); power curves refer to a total sample size of $n = 12$, 16, 18 subjects, $\alpha = 0.05$ and $CV_W = 20\%$.

1.4 Aims and structure of the book

The focus of this book is on the planning, conduct, analysis and reporting of bioequivalence studies and covers all features required by regulatory authorities. The book targets three groups of readers. The first is the biometrician working in the pharmaceutical industry, who wishes to obtain information on the pharmacokinetic background and medical rationale of these types of clinical studies in phase I. The second is the clinical pharmacologist or biopharmaceutical scientist who performs bioequivalence studies and wishes to understand the basic principles of statistical planning and analysis of these studies. The third is the reviewer from regulatory affairs who wants to assess these studies from a regulatory point of view. Therefore, emphasis is laid on illustration of the statistical methods and the underlying pharmacokinetic background by real-world examples, avoiding topics that are only of academic interest.

An overview and an assessment of the characteristics of rate and extent of absorption for immediate and modified release products in single- and multiple-dose studies are given in Chapter 2.

The main statistical methods used in bioequivalence trials are described in Chapters 3–5. Starting in Chapter 3 with the basic statistical methodology, Chapter 4 provides the underlying methodology for adequate statistical analysis of average bioequivalence according to regulatory guidelines. Planning a bioequivalence study and its statistical analysis are closely linked. In accordance with regulatory requirements, sample size determination should be based on the methods developed for this type of study. Hence, the focus of Chapter 5 is power and sample size calculation for the commonly used two-period, two-sequence crossover design.

For successful regulatory submission of a bioequivalence study, the outcomes must be presented in an adequate manner. Therefore, Chapter 6 deals with the appropriate presentation of results from single- and multiple-dose trials.

Chapter 7 provides the corresponding techniques for analyzing bioequivalence studies with more than two formulations. Also addressed is the ensuing problem of multiplicity.

Pharmacokinetic interaction or, more precisely, lack-of-interaction studies are part of the clinical investigation of a new drug. While in drug-drug interaction studies the focus is on demonstrating that concomitant administration of the investigational drug has no clinically relevant influence on another concomitantly administered drug, food-drug interaction studies are performed to investigate the food effect on release and absorption of the investigational drug. These interaction studies are discussed in detail in Chapter 8.

New approaches to population and individual bioequivalence have been motivated by the limitations of average bioequivalence to handle unequal variances and subject-by-treatment interaction. Thus, it is the purpose of Chapter 9 to discuss and highlight the conceptual issues of population and individual bioequivalence.

In the chapters described so far, bioequivalence is evaluated based on the underlying pharmacokinetic characteristics that are determined from the plasma concentration-time curves. However, for drugs with no systemic availability, other clinical endpoints have to be investigated. The corresponding methodology for planning and analyzing this type of clinical study is given in Chapter 10.

References

Amidon, G.L., Lennernäs, H., Shah, V.P. and Crison, J.R. (1995) A theoretical basis for a biopharmaceutics drug classification: the correlation of *in vitro* drug product dissolution and *in vivo* bioavailability. *Pharmaceutical Research* **12**, 413–20.

Chen, M.L., Lesko, L. and Williams, R.L. (2001) Measures of exposure versus measures of rate and extent of absorption. *Clinical Pharmacokinetics* **40**, 565–72.

Chiou, W.L. (2001) The rate and extent of oral bioavailability versus the rate and extent of oral absorption: clarification and recommendation of terminology. *Journal of Pharmacokinetics and Pharmacodynamics* **28**, 3–6.

Committee for Proprietary Medicinal Products (1991) *Note for guidance: investigation of bioavailability and bioequivalence*, EMEA, London.

Committee for Proprietary Medicinal Products (1999) *Note for guidance on modified release oral and transdermal dosage forms: section II (pharmacokinetic and clinical evaluation)*, EMEA, London.

Committee for Proprietary Medicinal Products (2001) *Note for guidance on the investigation of bioavailability and bioequivalence*, EMEA, London.

Diletti, E., Hauschke, D. and Steinijans, V.W. (1991) Sample size determination for bioequivalence assessment by means of confidence intervals. *International Journal of Clinical Pharmacology, Therapy and Toxicology* **29**, 1–8.

Diletti, E., Hauschke, D. and Steinijans, V.W. (1992) Sample size determination: extended tables for the multiplicative model and bioequivalence ranges of 0.9 to 1.11 and 0.7 to 1.43. *International Journal of Clinical Pharmacology, Therapy and Toxicology* **30**, 287–90.

Food and Drug Administration (2001) *Guidance for industry: statistical approaches to establishing bioequivalence*, Center for Drug Evaluation and Research, Rockville, MD.

Food and Drug Administration (2003) *Guidance for Industry: bioavailability and bioequivalence studies for orally administered drug product – general considerations*, Center for Drug Evaluation and Research, Rockville, MD.

Hauschke, D., Steinijans, V.W. and Diletti, E. (1990) A distribution-free procedure for the statistical analysis of bioequivalence studies. *International Journal of Clinical Pharmacology, Therapy and Toxicology* **28**, 72–8.

Sauter, R., Steinijans, V.W., Böhm, A., Diletti, E. and Schulz, H.-U. (1992) Presentation of results from bioequivalence studies. *International Journal of Clinical Pharmacology, Therapy and Toxicology* **30**, 233–56.

Schuirmann, D.J. (1987) A comparison of the two one-sided tests procedure and the power approach for assessing the equivalence of average bioavailability. *Journal of Pharmacokinetics and Biopharmaceutics* **15**, 657–80.

Skelly, J.P. (1995) Session I: bioequivalence: quality control and therapeutic surrogate? In: Midha, K.K. and Blume, H.H. (eds) *Bio-International II: bioavailability, bioequivalence and pharmacokinetic studies, International conference of F.I.P. "Bio-International '94", Munich, Germany*, 16–17, Medpharm Scientific Publishers, Stuttgart.

Steinijans, V.W., Sauter, R. and Diletti, E. (1995a) Shape analysis in single- and multiple-dose studies of modified-release products. In: Midha, K.K. and Blume, H.H. (eds) *Bio-International II: bioavailability, bioequivalence and pharmacokinetic studies, International conference of F.I.P. "Bio-International '94", Munich, Germany*, 193–206, Medpharm Scientific Publishers, Stuttgart.

Steinijans, V.W., Sauter, R., Diletti, E. and Hauschke, D. (1996) Overview: shape analysis versus rate measures. In: Midha, K.K. and Nagai, T. (eds) *Bioavailability, bioequivalence and pharmacokinetic studies. International conference of F.I.P. "Bio-International '96", Tokyo, Japan*, 163–7, Business Center of Academic Societies Japan, Tokyo.

Steinijans, V.W., Sauter, R., Hauschke, D., Diletti, E., Schall, R., Luus, H.G., Elze, M., Blume, H., Hoffmann, C., Franke, G. and Siegmund, W. (1995b) Reference tables for the intra-subject coefficient of variation in bioequivalence studies. *International Journal of Clinical Pharmacology and Therapeutics* **33**, 427–30.

Vuorinen, J. and Turunen, J.A. (1996) A simple three-step procedure for assessing bioequivalence in the general mixed model framework. *Statistics in Medicine* **15**, 2635–55.

2

Metrics to characterize concentration-time profiles in single- and multiple-dose bioequivalence studies

2.1 Introduction

In bioequivalence assessment, pharmacokinetic characteristics of concentration-time curves have traditionally been associated with rate and extent of drug absorption. As the availability of drug to the general circulation is of primary interest, the term bioavailability would be more appropriate than absorption, because the term absorption – in the strict sense – is reserved for the movement of drug across the outer mucosal membranes of the GI tract (Chiou, 2001). Thus 'rate and extent of bioavailability' are of interest. In line with common technical language we will also use the terminology 'rate and extent of absorption'. The area under the concentration-time curve (AUC) is universally accepted as characteristic of the extent of drug absorption, that is, of total drug exposure. However, the choice of an appropriate rate characteristic has been discussed with great controversy (Bois *et al.*, 1994; Elze *et al.*, 1995; Endrenyi *et al.*, 1991–1998; Lacey *et al.*, 1994, 1995; Reppas *et al.*, 1995; Schall *et al.*, 1994; Steinijans, 1989b, Steinijans *et al.*, 1995a, b). This is not surprising since the time course of absorption is a fairly complex process, particularly in the case of modified release formulations.

Rate of drug absorption may be determined using either direct or indirect metrics. Direct metrics for the rate of absorption include model-based rate constants or rate-time profiles generated by deconvolution. Peak plasma or serum drug concentration (C_{max}),

Bioequivalence Studies in Drug Development: Methods and Applications   D. Hauschke, V. Steinijans and I. Pigeot
© 2007 John Wiley & Sons, Ltd

mean residence time (MRT) and mean absorption time (MAT) are indirect measures (Chen *et al.*, 2001).

Information on the absorption process may be retrieved fairly completely in a deconvoluted absorption profile. However, the absorption profile can only be retrieved once the disposition kinetics (distribution and elimination) are known. A further drawback of using deconvolution for bioequivalence assessment is that appropriate statistical methods allow the comparison of single characteristics such as C_{max}, but not of entire rate profiles. The disposition kinetics are usually derived from an additional study period with intravenous administration in the same subject. If for reasons of feasibility the intravenous reference is replaced by an oral solution, the deconvoluted input function does not any more reflect all input steps but primarily the rate of drug release from the solid oral formulation and the solution of the drug substance.

Deconvolution methods reconstruct the so-called 'input function' from the 'response function', which, for example, is the concentration-time curve after oral administration, and the 'weighting function', which, for example, is the concentration-time curve after intravenous administration. The input function can be considered as a cumulative distribution function of intravenous microboli, the superposition of which results in the concentration-time curve after oral administration. The calculation of the response function from the input and weighting functions is mathematically denoted as convolution, the recovery of the input function from the response and weighting functions as deconvolution (Langenbucher, 1982). Apart from the classical mass-balance methods according to Wagner and Nelson (1963) for the one-compartment model, and according to Loo and Riegelman (1968) for the two-compartment model, so-called numerical deconvolution methods have been used (Langenbucher, 1982; Tucker, 1983; Vaughan and Dennis, 1978). Numerical deconvolution methods do not assume a specific compartmental model but merely linearity and time invariance of the disposition kinetics.

Linearity of the disposition kinetics means that distribution and elimination, and hence clearance, are not dependent on the dose administered.

Time invariance of the disposition kinetics means that the clearance does not change over time. Auto- and hetero-induction represent classical examples of time dependency in pharmacokinetics. The autoinduction of carbamazepine clearance (Pitlick and Levy, 1977) may serve as an example for time-dependent disposition kinetics. Mathematical equations to describe the resulting time course of drug concentrations have been derived by Levy *et al.* 1979, under the assumption that the metabolic clearance increases exponentially to a maximum value and that the rate of this increase is governed by the degradation rate constant of the induced enzyme.

An example of a numerical deconvolution is presented in Figure 2.1.

Another way of characterizing the rate of absorption would be some integral metric such as the mean absorption time (MAT). As with the deconvolution methods, an additional study period with an intravenous administration is needed. This separate period is usually not included in the design of bioequivalence studies, and the mean residence time (MRT) for the formulations to be compared is chosen as a surrogate metric for the mean absorption time. For drugs with a long elimination half-life, however, the half-life will dominate the MRT, which thereby becomes of rather limited use for characterizing the rate of absorption.

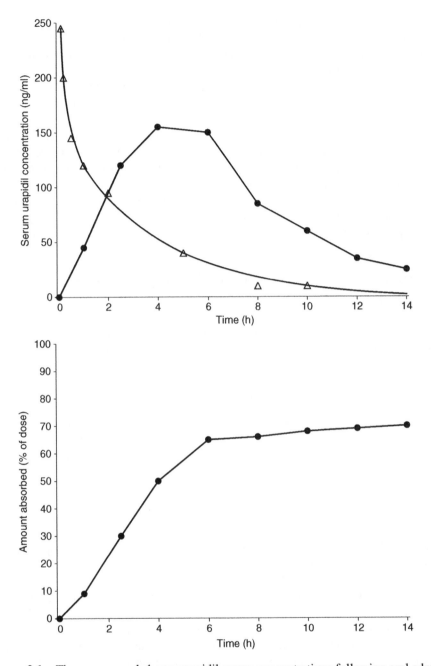

Figure 2.1   The upper panel shows urapidil serum concentrations following oral administration of 30 mg urapidil as controlled release capsule and 10 mg urapidil as intravenous
bolus injection in the same subject; the lower panel shows the *in vivo* absorption profile
calculated by means of the point-area deconvolution method (Vaughan and Dennis, 1978).
It should be noted that urapidil has a first-pass effect of 20–25 % (Zech *et al.*, 1982).

The maximum concentration, C_{max}, and the time of its occurrence, t_{max}, have traditionally been and are still requested as rate characteristics (CPMP, 2001; FDA, 2003). In some cases, the use of C_{max} was motivated by its inverse relationship to the frequency and/or intensity of certain adverse events of a drug or drug formulation. Both, t_{max} and C_{max} are strongly dependent on the discrete sampling scheme, and both are of rather limited value for the discrimination of modified release formulations with their flat, and sometimes multiple, peaks.

Various working groups have contrasted the performance of conventional rate characteristics such as t_{max} and C_{max} to that of more sophisticated absorption metrics such as C_{max}/AUC and partial areas in single-dose studies, and to various peak-trough characteristics and plateau times after multiple dosing.

A survey of the most common pharmacokinetic characteristics (metrics) to assess the shape of concentration-time curves is given in the following sections, classified by single- and multiple-dose studies and metrics for immediate and modified release formulations.

2.2   Pharmacokinetic characteristics (metrics) for single-dose studies

Figure 2.2 depicts two typical concentration-time courses after a single dose, the steep one for an immediate release formulation, the flatter one for a prolonged release formulation.

2.2.1   Extent of bioavailability

Pharmacokinetic principles imply that the area under the concentration-time curve from zero to infinity, $AUC(0 - \infty)$, and not a partial area up to a certain time point, serves as characteristic of the extent of absorption in single-dose studies. This becomes evident from the fundamental pharmacokinetic relationship

$$f \cdot dose = clearance \cdot AUC\,(0 - \infty), \ 0 < f \leq 1,$$

which states that the fraction, f, of the dose that is ultimately absorbed is proportional to $AUC(0 - \infty)$, clearance being the proportionality factor.

Clearance can be viewed as the volume of blood from which all drug would appear to be removed per unit time (Rowland and Tozer, 1995). The units of clearance, like those of flow, are volume per unit time. For example, if at a concentration of 1 mg/liter, the rate of drug elimination is 1 mg/hour, then the clearance is 1 liter/hour.

The fundamental pharmacokinetic relationship given above and the within-subject invariance of the clearance are the cornerstones of bioequivalence assessment. Only if the intra-individual clearance is constant for the test and the reference period, will this cancel out in the formula below, so that the intra-individual ratios of $AUCs$ for test (T) and reference (R) can be used as a measure for relative bioavailability of test versus reference:

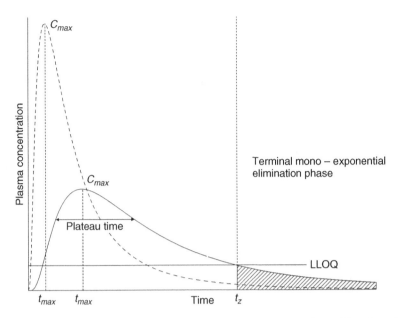

Figure 2.2 Typical concentration-time profile after a single dose. The dotted curve refers to an immediate release formulation, the flatter solid curve to a prolonged release formulation. C_{max} denotes the maximum concentration. Let t_z be the sampling time of the last concentration observed above the lower limit of quantification (LLOQ), which will be denoted by C_z. As explained in Section 2.2.1, bioequivalence assessment is based on the total AUC from zero to infinity, which is the sum of the AUC up to t_z, and the extrapolated fraction beyond t_z (see Section 2.2.1): $AUC(0 - \infty) = AUC(0 - t_z) + \hat{C}_z / \hat{\lambda}_z$.

$$\frac{AUC_T}{AUC_R} = \frac{f_T \cdot dose_T \cdot clearance_R}{f_R \cdot dose_R \cdot clearance_T} = \frac{f_T}{f_R}$$

$$= \text{ratio of absorbed dose fractions for test and reference}$$

$$= \text{relative bioavailability of test versus reference.}$$

Another straightforward assumption in the cascade above is that equal doses were administered for test and reference. If this is not the case, but linear kinetics can be assumed, then the ratio of dose adjusted $AUCs$, rather than that of $AUCs$, serves as a measure for relative bioavailability, i.e.,

$$\frac{AUC_T / dose_T}{AUC_R / dose_R} = \frac{f_T}{f_R}.$$

In a single-dose study, the $AUC(0 - \infty)$ is usually calculated in two steps: trapezoidal formula, plus extrapolation to infinity (APV, 1987; Sauter *et al.*, 1992). More precisely, linear regression, of the natural logarithms of the observed concentrations during the terminal mono exponential phase versus time, is used to estimate the terminal rate constant λ_z. Let (t_z, C_z) denote the last sampling point above the limit of quantitation that is used in this log-linear regression, and let $\hat{\lambda}_z$ denote the estimate of the terminal rate constant and $\hat{C}_z$ the concentration estimated at time t_z. In order to avoid a discontinuity between the measured concentration-time curve until t_z and the fitted mono-exponential phase used from t_z onwards, the estimate $\hat{C}_z$ is used instead of the observed value C_z in the calculation of $AUC(0 - t_z)$ by linear (or logarithmic linear) trapezoidal formula up to $(t_z, \hat{C}_z)$.

Extrapolation to infinity is done by means of $AUC(t_z - \infty) = \hat{C}_z/\hat{\lambda}_z$. Thus $AUC(0 - \infty) = AUC(0 - t_z) + \hat{C}_z/\hat{\lambda}_z$. This formula also applies if $\hat{\lambda}_z$ has been obtained by iterative nonlinear regression techniques instead of simple log-linear regression. The latter has the advantage of easy and exact reproducibility by using explicit formulae, and is independent of the tuning parameters of iterative procedures. It is important that the interval for the calculation of $\hat{\lambda}_z$ is documented for each subject in each period (see Section 6.2, Tables 6.2a and 6.2b). The percentage ratio $100\ AUC(0 - t_z)/AUC(0 - \infty)$ should exceed 80 % in each subject. In other words, the extrapolated fraction should not exceed 20 % of the total AUC (CPMP, 2001).

The example given in Figure 2.3 illustrates the frequently arising difficulty in estimating the terminal half-life from a log-linear plot of the measured concentration-time curve. Depending on the interval selected for the estimation of the terminal half-life, estimates ranging between 37.8 hours and 100.7 hours will be obtained (see Table 2.1).

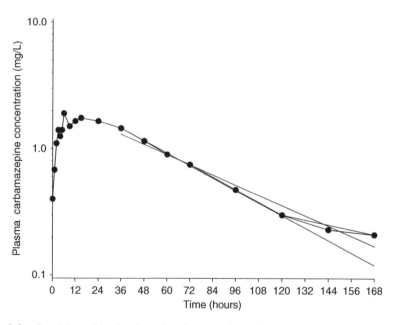

Figure 2.3 Semi-logarithmic plot of carbamazepine plasma concentration-time profile in a healthy subject (28 years, 83 kg, 176 cm) after a single dose of 300 mg carbamazepine as controlled release tablet.

Table 2.1   Effect of selecting various time intervals for the estimation of the terminal half-life, on the half-life itself, on $AUC(0-\infty)$, $AUMC(0-\infty)$ and on the mean residence time $MRT(0-\infty)$ (for concentration-time profile see Figure 2.3). In addition to the estimates using extrapolation to infinity, information is also provided on the corresponding estimates utilizing only the data up to the respective last concentration. Finally, the estimate using only data up to the last concentration in the selected time interval is expressed as a percentage of the estimate using extrapolation.

Characteristics	Range for estimation of λ_z (hours)		
	36–120	36–168	120–168
Apparent half-life (hours)	37.8	45.8	100.7
C_z (measured)	0.320	0.230	0.230
C_z (fitted)	0.320	0.186	0.224
$AUC(0-t_z)$ $(mg/L \cdot h)$	123.7	135.8	136.2
$AUC(0-\infty)$ $(mg/L \cdot h)$	141.2	148.1	168.8
%	88	92	81
$AUMC(0-t_z)(mg/L \cdot h^2)$	7513.5	9181.3	12660.3
$AUMC(0-\infty)(mg/L \cdot h^2)$	8464.1	9993.7	17388.7
%	89	92	73
$MRT(0-t_z)(h)$	60.7	67.6	92.9
$MRT(0-\infty)(h)$	60.0	67.5	103.0
%	101	100	90

The selection of the most suitable time interval cannot be left to a programmed algorithm based on mathematical criteria, but necessitates scientific judgment by both the clinical pharmacokineticist and the person who determined the concentrations and knows about their reliability. In the example given, a half-life of more than 100 hours would result when utilizing only the last 3 concentrations at 120, 144 and 168 hours. The clinical pharmacologist would tell us that such a long half-life is unlikely in a healthy volunteer in whom a half-life of about 27 hours would be expected (Klotz, 1984).

Figure 2.3 and Table 2.1 illustrate the difficulties in the correct calculation of the terminal half-life and its impact on the AUC and even more so on the mean residence time, $MRT = AUMC/AUC$, where $AUMC = \int tC(t)dt$ denotes the area under the first moment curve. Apart from AUC extrapolation, the MRT calculation also involves the extrapolation of $AUMC$, $AUMC(0-\infty) = AUMC(0-t_z) + t_z\hat{C}_z/\hat{\lambda}_z + \hat{C}_z/\hat{\lambda}_z^2$ (Steinijans, 1989b). It should be borne in mind that an AUC extrapolation of 20 % or less does not necessarily imply an $AUMC$ extrapolation of 20 % or less. Consequently, adequate calculation of mean residence time may require an even more extended sampling scheme than that for adequate calculation of AUC.

2.2.2   Rate of bioavailability

Even though C_{max} has become a standard regulatory measure of rate of absorption, it has several drawbacks (Chen *et al.*, 2001)

- C_{max} is not a pure measure of absorption rate, but is confounded with the distribution and, in turn, the extent of absorption of the drug.

- C_{max} is generally insensitive to changes in rate of input using an absorption rate constant as an index.

- C_{max} contains little information about the absorption process of a drug.

- As a single-point determination, the value of C_{max} depends substantially on the sampling schedule.

- The use of C_{max} alone cannot discern differences in t_{max} or lag-time between formulations.

- C_{max} is poorly estimated in cases where multiple peaks or flat profiles occur after drug administration.

Endrenyi and co-workers (1991, 1993) were the first to show that C_{max}/AUC is a better characteristic of the absorption rate than C_{max} itself. They showed that the ratio C_{max}/AUC is independent of both within-subject variations and possible differences in the extent of absorption and – in the case of a one-compartment body model with first-order absorption – reflects only the contrast between the absorption and disposition rate constants, k_a/k_{el}. Lacey *et al.* (1994) considered simulated and real experiments and came up with the conclusion that C_{max}/AUC is a more powerful metric than C_{max} in establishing bioequivalence when formulations are truly bioequivalent, and that C_{max}/AUC is more sensitive than C_{max} at detecting differences in rate of absorption when they exist. Schall and co-workers (1994) showed that under fairly general conditions t_{max} and C_{max}/AUC are equivalent characteristics of the absorption rate. C_{max}/AUC can be observed with higher precision, and is easier to handle statistically than t_{max}. On the basis of data from 20 bioequivalence studies they came up with the rather subtle recommendation that for drugs with short (<5 hours) elimination half-lives or fastest disposition half-lives in the case of higher compartmental models, C_{max}/AUC is the best rate characteristic, but that for drugs with long elimination or fastest disposition half-lives, t_{max} can be superior to C_{max}/AUC.

With regard to partial areas, the following two concepts are of interest. The partial area under the curve from zero to t_{max} of the reference formulation is denoted by AUC_R; the partial area from zero to t_{max} of the test or reference formulation, whichever occurs earliest, is denoted by AUC_e. Obviously, partial *AUCs* are confounded by the extent of absorption. The normalized metrics AUC_R/AUC and AUC_e/AUC do not contain this confounding and should be more sensitive than C_{max} and the unnormalized partial *AUCs* at detecting true differences in rate of absorption. The performance of AUC_e/AUC when used with real data was poor, which may imply that it has little practical value: on the other hand, the performance of AUC_R/AUC was good. C_{max}/AUC is more precisely estimated than AUC_R/AUC or AUC_e/AUC and should, therefore, be a superior metric at demonstrating bioequivalence in terms of rate of absorption when formulations are truly bioequivalent (Lacey *et al.*, 1995).

These findings were confirmed at least in part by Elze *et al.* (1995) in their database analysis of three drugs (ibuprofen, glibenclamide, and verapamil). They confirmed that AUC_e and the corresponding normalized characteristic AUC_e/AUC had the highest within-subject coefficient of variation (87 %) among the investigated metrics, and therefore, cannot be recommended. They also expressed concern about the variability of AUC_R/AUC, which, however, reflected the rate of absorption best in case of nonrandom lag-times. In general, they found that the residual coefficients of variation for C_{max} and C_{max}/AUC were much lower than those for the partial areas. Although Elze *et al.* (1995) found C_{max}/AUC superior to C_{max} in the majority of cases, they could not come up with a clear recommendation like Lacey and co-workers (1995), who stated that C_{max} and t_{max} should be discontinued as metrics of rate of drug absorption in relative bioavailability studies involving immediate-release dosage forms.

Even less definitive were the simulation results by Bois *et al.* (1994), who concluded that there is no universal measure of drug absorption. Solely on the basis of Monte Carlo simulations they showed that neither C_{max}, C_{max}/AUC, nor partial areas were able to reflect a 25 % change in the modeled first-order rate constant k_a. This, however, is neither surprising nor critical, because in the context of bioequivalence assessment the similarity of the shapes of the concentration-time profiles is relevant rather than the similarity of the apparent first-order absorption rate constants.

Chen *et al.* (2001) summarized the above concepts and coined the terms early, peak and total exposure, with partial $AUCs$, C_{max} and AUC being the respective metrics. Their recommendation to add partial areas as a further metric for early exposure did not result in a statutory change in general, and C_{max} and AUC remained the two regulatory metrics to assess bioequivalence (CPMP, 2001; FDA, 2003). However, the 2003 FDA guidance acknowledges the usefulness of partial areas in special situations, e.g., if the focus is on the rapid onset of an analgesic effect or the avoidance of an initially excessive hypotensive action of an antihypertensive drug.

The pros and cons described above largely hold for both immediate and modified release formulation. Modified release formulations include two essentially different types of modification, so-called 'prolonged release' formulations and 'delayed release' formulations.

Delayed release formulations are characterized by the fact that drug release is intentionally delayed, for example by an enteric coating, in order to prevent drug release in the acidic environment of the stomach. The concentration-time curves of such enteric-coated formulations frequently show concentrations below the lower limit of quantification at early time points of measurement, and thus can be characterized by a lag-time of drug release, which – incorrectly – is sometimes denoted as lag-time of absorption (t_{lag}). It is obvious that in this case t_{max} itself has little meaning as a rate characteristic, and only $t_{max} - t_{lag}$ may provide a meaningful metric. In contrast to t_{max}, the maximum concentration C_{max} may not be affected by the delayed release.

Prolonged release formulations are characterized by the fact that the release of the drug from the formulation becomes the rate-controlling step for the appearance of the drug in the systemic circulation. Such formulations are developed in case of an unfavorable ratio between elimination half-life and envisaged dosing interval. Depending on the technology used the resulting concentration-time profiles may display rather flat, and even multiple, peaks. Hence, t_{max} and C_{max} are of limited value for discrimination of prolonged release formulations. In this case, the mean absorption time and the so-called 'plateau time' may be more suitable characteristics (Steinijans *et al.*, 1995a, b). The plateau time is defined as the duration, during which the plasma or serum concentration deviates from the maximum concentration by less than a clinically specified difference or percentage. In the case of a 50 % deviation from the maximum, the plateau time corresponds to the half-value duration (*HVD*) introduced by Meier *et al.* (1974). The concept of the plateau time will be discussed in greater detail in the following section on multiple-dose studies.

2.3   Pharmacokinetic rate and extent characteristics (metrics) for multiple-dose studies

Figure 2.4 depicts the build-up of the concentration-time profiles after a single dose and subsequent multiple doses for a constant dosing interval. Figure 2.5 shows a corresponding profile from a combined single- and multiple-dose study with the refinement that the build-up of the steady state started only after 48 hours, which corresponds to two 24-hour

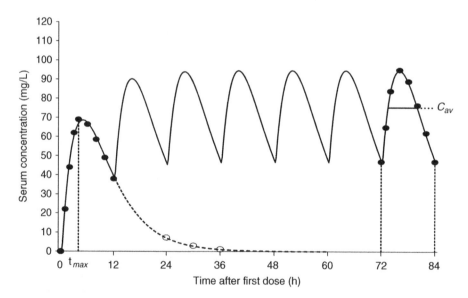

Figure 2.4   Serum concentration-time profile after single and multiple doses with a constant dosing interval of $\tau = 12$ hours. The closed dots indicate observed concentrations after the first dose and during a 12-hour dosing interval in steady state. C_{av} denotes the time-averaged steady-state concentration based on the *AUC* during this 12-hour dosing interval.

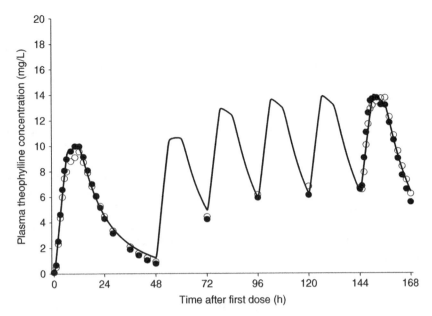

Figure 2.5   Plasma theophylline concentration-time profiles after single and multiple doses. The dots (○ = Reference, ● = Test) indicate observed mean concentrations after the first dose, which was followed up for 48 hours, and during a 24-hour dosing interval at steady state. Prior to each dose, the so-called trough values were measured in order to verify steady-state conditions between 144 and 168 hours after the first dose (Steinijans *et al.*, 1989a).

dosing intervals. This approach had been chosen to cover at least 80 % of the total *AUC* after the first dose by measured concentrations, and to allow the estimation of the apparent half-life, which was needed for steady-state simulations.

Before dwelling on various steady-state characteristics that may serve as metrics in multiple-dose studies, it is worthwhile to recall the requirements for multiple dose studies in the two most prominent guidelines on bioavailability and bioequivalence (CPMP, 2001; FDA, 2003).

The FDA Guidance for Industry: Bioavailability and Bioequivalence Studies for Orally Administered Drug Product (FDA, 2003) generally recommends single-dose pharmacokinetic studies for both immediate and modified release drug products to demonstrate bioequivalence because they are generally more sensitive in assessing release of the drug substance from the drug product into the systemic circulation. It is recommended that if a multiple-dose study design is important, appropriate dosage administration and sampling be carried out to document attainment of steady state.

The CPMP Note for Guidance: Investigation of Bioavailability and Bioequivalence (CPMP, 2001) states that in general, single-dose studies will suffice, but steady-state studies may be required in the case of dose- or time-dependent pharmacokinetics. Moreover, in case of certain modified release products (prolonged release formulations and transdermal drug delivery systems), steady-state studies are required in addition to the single-dose investigations. Steady-state studies can be considered, e.g., if problems of sensitivity preclude sufficiently precise plasma concentration measurements after single-dose administration. They can also be considered if the intra-individual variability, which would render a single-dose study infeasible due to the required sample size, is markedly reduced at steady state. This phenomenon has been discussed for certain highly variable drugs (Blume *et al.*, 1992).

In contrast to single-dose studies, where the two treatment periods have to be separated by a sufficiently long washout period without any treatment, such a washout period can be skipped in favor of a direct switch at steady state after the first treatment period. Thus, in steady-state studies, the washout of the last dose of the treatment given in period 1 can overlap with the build-up of the treatment given in period 2, provided the build-up period is sufficiently long (at least three times the terminal half-life).

When differences between morning and evening dosing are known, e.g., due to circadian rhythms influencing drug absorption, sampling should be carried out over a full 24-hour cycle.

In multiple-dose studies, steady-state characteristics may either refer to one dosing interval, for example, 12 hours in the case of twice daily (b.i.d.) dosing; or to one dosing cycle, usually 24 hours with, probably, unequal dosing intervals, for example, 6, 6 and 12 hours. For the sake of brevity, the term dosing interval will generally be used.

Based on the requirements of the current European and US guidelines on bioavailability and bioequivalence (CPMP, 2001; FDA, 2003), the discussion of steady-state characteristics can be restricted to modified release formulations.

Although the FDA primarily requires single-dose studies, the guidance explicitly recommends the following pharmacokinetic information for steady-state studies:

$$C_{min}, \text{ concentration at the end of the dosing interval,}$$

$$C_{av}, \text{ average concentration during the dosing interval,}$$

$$degree \ of \ fluctuation = (C_{max} - C_{min})/C_{av},$$

and

$$swing = (C_{max} - C_{min})/C_{min}.$$

It should be noted that in the FDA guidance the characteristic C_{min} has been associated with the concentration at the end of the dosing interval, the so-called pre-dose or trough value. However, for prolonged release formulations which exhibit an apparent lag-time of absorption, the true minimum (trough) concentration may be observed some time after the next dosing, but not necessarily at the end of the previous dosing interval.

The CPMP guidance also mentions that for studies in steady state, AUC_{τ} (AUC over one dosing interval, τ), C_{max}, C_{min} and fluctuation should be provided.

Figure 2.7 shows for a panel of 12 subjects the individual values of C_{max}, C_{min} and $C_{av} = AUC_{\tau}/\tau$ for the test and the reference formulation. These steady-state characteristics were derived from the 12 individual concentration-time curves after multiple once-daily

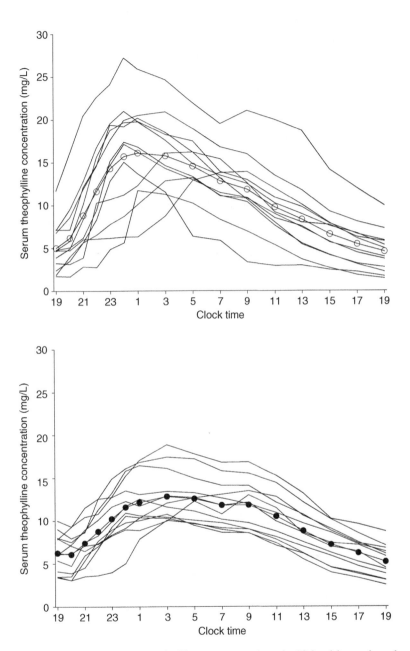

Figure 2.6 Individual serum theophylline concentrations in 12 healthy male volunteers, and mean-value curve (○ = Reference,● = Test) on trial day 7 after repeated once-daily dosing of 800 mg theophylline at 7 p.m.

doses of 800 mg theophylline, which together with the respective mean value curves, are depicted in Figure 2.6 for the test and the reference formulation (Steinijans *et al.*, 1986).

The presentation in Figure 2.7 has the advantage that, on an individual basis, it simultaneously displays the extent characteristic, C_{av}, and the rate characteristic C_{max} – C_{min}, the peak-trough difference at steady state. As this difference may be confounded by the extent of absorption, it is adjusted to the average steady-state concentration, and this improved rate characteristic is the so-called peak-trough fluctuation (PTF),

$$peak\text{-}trough\ fluctuation = (C_{max} - C_{min})/C_{av},$$

which in the FDA guidance (2003) is denoted by 'degree of fluctuation'.

It is worthwhile to point out that the characteristic *PTF* after multiple dosing is the analogue of the characteristic C_{max}/AUC after a single dose. When the concentration at the end of the dosing interval is much less than the maximum concentration, then *PTF* will be approximately equal to $\tau \cdot C_{max}/AUC_\tau$.

It is common to multiply *PTF* by 100 and thereby express the steady-state difference as a fraction of the average steady-state concentration, the so-called % peak-trough fluctuation (*%PTF*),

$$\%peak\text{-}trough\ fluctuation = 100(C_{max} - C_{min})/C_{av}.$$

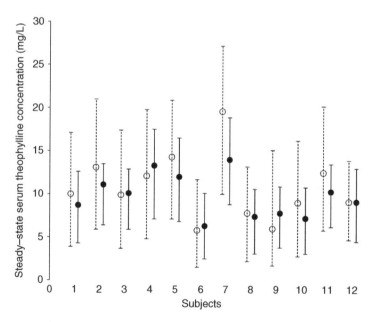

Figure 2.7 Individual 24-hour concentration-time average, C_{av}, (o = Reference, ● = Test), peak and trough concentrations, on trial day 7 after repeated once-daily dosing of 800 mg theophylline at 7 p.m.

Reppas *et al.* (1995) evaluated different metrics (C_{max}, C_{max}/AUC, %*PTF* and *AUC*-normalized partial areas) as indirect measures of rate of drug absorption from prolonged release dosage forms at steady state. Based on simulation studies, they came to the conclusion that all metrics, with the exception of %*PTF*, resulted in much smaller increases than the 50 % increase (test versus reference) in the modeled absorption rate, k_a. None of the metrics provided reliable information about the changes in the underlying rate of absorption from the prolonged release dosage forms. However, as pointed out earlier, in the context of bioequivalence assessment the similarity of the shapes of the concentration-time profiles is more relevant than the similarity of the absorption rate constants.

In summary, the % peak-trough fluctuation is considered the steady-state characteristic of choice by regulatory authorities (CPMP, 2001; FDA, 2003). It is more robust than the so-called swing which relates the peak-trough difference $C_{max} - C_{min}$ to the trough concentration C_{min},

$$swing = (C_{max} - C_{min})/C_{min};$$

the corresponding definition of the % swing is:

$$\% \, swing = 100(C_{max} - C_{min})/C_{min}.$$

Another steady-state characteristic is the so-called

$$\% \, AUC \, fluctuation = 100(AUC \, between \, C(t) \, and \, C_{av})/AUC_\tau.$$

This characteristic relates the area between the measured and linearly interpolated concentration-time curve $C(t)$ and the horizontal line C_{av}, which represents the average steady-state concentration, to the total AUC during one dosing interval, τ, at steady state. It turned out that the % AUC fluctuation has a low sensitivity to discriminate between different formulations.

Notwithstanding the merits of the peak-trough fluctuation, there are situations where this metric is not able to detect relevant differences in concentration-time profiles: a pertinent example was presented by Steinijans *et al.* (1995b).

The mean value curves at steady state are depicted in Figure 2.8. Whereas the reference formulation shows a distinct peak in the middle of the 24-hour dosing interval (a 'Matter-horn' profile), the test formulation shows a sustained plateau ('Table Mountain' profile) during the entire nocturnal period between 2 a.m. and 6 a.m. Such differences may not only be reflected in the tolerability of the two formulations. In view of the pronounced circadian rhythm of asthma and related respiratory diseases (so-called 'morning dip' in lung function), this difference in concentration-time profiles may also affect clinical efficacy. For theophylline sustained release formulations the plateau time is defined as the time during which the steady-state concentration exceeds at least 75 % of the maximum concentration (Steinijans *et al.*, 1987). Therefore, it is denoted by $T75\%C_{max}$.

Geometric mean and 90 % confidence limits for the test/reference ratio are shown in Table 2.2 for the pertinent pharmacokinetic characteristics AUC, %*PTF* and plateau

Table 2.2 Geometric means with 90% confidence intervals for the test/reference ratios of pertinent pharmacokinetic steady-state characteristics; the within-subject coefficient of variation is also displayed.

Characteristic (day 8/9)	Within-subject CV (%)	Test/Reference Geometric mean (n = 18) 90% confidence limits
AUC	11.6	0.92 [0.86, 0.98]
%PTF	20.6	0.95 [0.85, 1.07]
Plateau time	20.4	1.23 [1.10, 1.39]

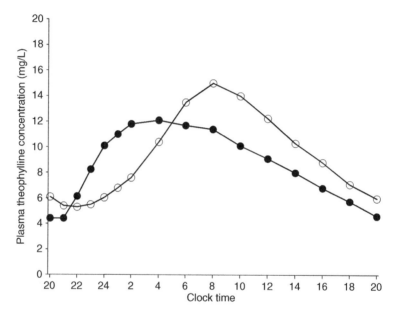

Figure 2.8 Geometric mean value curves (n = 18) of plasma theophylline concentrations following individualized once-daily evening doses of 800 (600–1200) mg (○ = Reference, ● = Test).

time. Equivalence with respect to the extent of absorption can be concluded as the 90 % confidence interval for the *AUC* is entirely in the bioequivalence range of 0.80 to 1.25. This is also the case for the % peak-trough fluctuation, from which equivalence also with regard to the rate of absorption would be concluded. However, the analysis of the plateau time picks up the pronounced and clinically relevant differences in the concentration-time profiles.

Steinijans *et al.* (1995b) proposed the following criteria for the selection of an appropriate steady-state characteristic:

- it should be able to differentiate obviously distinct concentration-time profiles ('Table Mountain' versus 'Matterhorn');

- it should be sensitive enough to detect major *in vitro* modifications;

- it should have a small within-subject coefficient of variation.

When applying these criteria, the plateau time proves to be a useful and clinically interpretable criterion, to be used in addition to, or in lieu of the peak-trough fluctuation.

In conclusion, there is no optimum metric for differentiating steady-state profiles. The above example demonstrates that the % fluctuation metric favored by health authorities may not necessarily be the most sensitive one. In view of this situation, it should be 'good biostatistical practice' to stipulate the primary characteristics for rate and extent of bioavailability prospectively in the study protocol and/or the statistical analysis plan (SAP).

An overview of the most common pharmacokinetic characteristics (metrics) to assess the shape of concentration-time curves, which directly or indirectly reflect the rate of absorption in single- and multiple-dose bioequivalence studies, was presented by Steinijans *et al.* (1995a) and is given in Table 2.3.

Table 2.3 Overview of the most common pharmacokinetic characteristics (metrics) to assess the shape of concentration-time curves, which directly or indirectly reflect the rate of absorption in single- and multiple-dose bioequivalence studies. Differentiated for immediate and controlled (prolonged) release formulations, square brackets indicate limited suitability in the respective situation.

Formulation: immediate release (IR) or controlled release (CR)	Metric (shape characteristics)	
	Single-dose studies	Multiple-dose studies (steady state)
IR, [CR]	t_{max}	$[t_{max}]$
IR, [CR]	C_{max}	C_{max}
IR, [CR]	C_{max}/AUC	C_{max}/AUC_τ
[IR, CR]	AUC_R	
IR, [CR]	AUC_R/AUC	
[IR, CR]	AUC_e	
[IR, CR]	AUC_e/AUC	
IR, CR	MAT	
[IR, CR]	MRT	
[IR], CR	Plateau time (HVD, $T75\%C_{max}$)	Plateau time (HVD, $T75\%C_{max}$)
[IR], CR	$[T$ above $C_{av}]$	T above C_{av}
IR, CR		$\%PTF$
[IR], CR		$\%swing$
IR, CR		$\%AUC$ fluctuation

2.4   Conclusions

The area under the concentration-time curve (*AUC*) is universally accepted as characteristic of the extent of drug absorption, that is, of total drug exposure. With regard to rate characteristics, regulatory authorities favor C_{max} in single-dose studies and the % peak-trough fluctuation in multiple-dose studies. Scrutiny of the literature indicates that C_{max}/AUC may be a better rate characteristic in single-dose studies, and that the plateau time may be a particularly suitable shape characteristic in multiple-dose studies of controlled (prolonged) release formulations.

References

APV (1987) Studies on bioavailability and bioequivalence (APV guideline). *Drugs Made in Germany* **30**, 161–6.

Blume, H.H., Scheidel, B. and Siewert, M. (1992) Application of single-dose vs multiple-dose studies. In: Midha, K.K. and Blume, H.H. (eds) *Bio-International: bioavailability, bioequivalence and pharmacokinetics*, 37–52, Medpharm Scientific Publishers, Stuttgart.

Bois, F.Y., Tozer, T.N., Hauck, W.W., Chen, M.L., Patnaik, R. and Williams, R.L. (1994) Bioequivalence: performance of several measures of rate of absorption. *Pharmaceutical Research* **11**, 966–74.

Chen, M.L., Lesko, L. and Williams, R.L. (2001) Measures of exposure versus measures of rate and extent of absorption. *Clinical Pharmacokinetics* **40**, 565–72.

Chiou, W.L. (2001) The rate and extent of oral bioavailability versus the rate and extent of oral absorption: clarification and recommendation of terminology. *Journal of Pharmacokinetics and Pharmacodynamics* **28**, 3–6.

Committee for Proprietary Medicinal Products, London (2001) Note for guidance: investigation of bioavailability and bioequivalence, EMEA, London.

Elze, M., Potthast, H. and Blume, H.H. (1995) Metrics of absorption: data base analysis. In: Blume, H.H. and Midha, K.K. (eds) *Bio-International 2: bioavailability, bioequivalence and pharmacokinetic studies*, 61–71, Medpharm Scientific Publishers, Stuttgart.

Endrenyi, L., Fritsch, S. and Yan, W. (1991) Cmax/AUC is a clearer measure than Cmax for absorption rates in investigations of bioequivalence. *International Journal of Clinical Pharmacology, Therapy and Toxicology* **29**, 394–9.

Endrenyi, L. and Yan, W. (1993) Variation of Cmax and Cmax/AUC in investigations of bioequivalence. *International Journal of Clinical Pharmacology, Therapy and Toxicology* **31**, 184–9.

Endrenyi, L., Tothfalusi, L. and Zha, J. (1994) Metrics assessing absorption rates: principles, and determination of bioequivalence in the steady state. In: Blume, H.H. and Midha, K.K. (eds) (1995) *Bio-International 2: bioavailability, bioequivalence and pharmacokinetic studies*, 77–85, Medpharm Scientific Publishers, Stuttgart.

Endrenyi, L., Csizmadia, F., Tothfalusi, L., Balch, A.H. and Chen, M-L. (1998) Metrics comparing simulated early concentration profiles for the determination of bioequivalence. *Pharmaceutical Research* **15**, 1292–9.

Endrenyi, L., Csizmadia, F., Tothfalusi, L., Balch, A.H. and Chen, M-L. (1998) The duration of measuring partial AUCs for the assessment of bioequivalence. *Pharmaceutical Research* **15**, 399–404.

Food and Drug Administration (2003) Guidance for industry: bioavailability and bioequivalence studies for orally administered drug product - general considerations, Rockville, MD.

Klotz, U. (1984) *Klinische Pharmakokinetik*, 2nd edition, Fischer Verlag, Stuttgart, New York.

Lacey, L.F., Keene, O.N., Duquesnoy, C. and Bye, A. (1994) Evaluation of different indirect measures of rate of drug absorption in comparative pharmacokinetic studies. *Journal of Pharmaceutical Sciences* **83**, 212–15.

Lacey, L.F., Bye, A. and Keene, O.N. (1995) Glaxo's experience of different absorption rate metrics of immediate release and extended release dosage forms. *Drug Information Journal* **29**, 821–40.

Langenbucher, F. (1982) Numerical convolution/deconvolution as a tool for correlating *in vitro* with *in vivo* drug availability. *Die Pharmazeutische Industrie* **44**, 1166–72.

Levy, R.H., Dumain, M.S. and Cook, J.L. (1979) Time-dependent kinetics. V: time course of drug levels during enzyme induction (one-compartment model). *Journal of Pharmacokinetics and Biopharmaceutics* **7**, 557–78.

Loo, J.C.K. and Riegelman, S. (1968) New method for calculating the intrinsic absorption rate of drugs. *Journal of Pharmaceutical Sciences* **57**, 918–28.

Meier, J., Nüesch, E. and Schmidt, R. (1974) Pharmacokinetic criteria for the evaluation of retard formulations. *European Journal of Clinical Pharmacology* **7**, 429–32.

Pitlick, W.H. and Levy, R.H. (1977) Time-dependent kinetics. I: exponential auto-induction of carbamazepine in monkeys. *Journal of Pharmaceutical Sciences* **66**, 647–9.

Reppas, C., Lacey, L.F., Keene, O.N., Macheras, P. and Bye, A. (1995) Evaluation of different metrics as indirect measures of rate of drug absorption from extended release dosage forms at steady-state. *Pharmaceutical Research* **12**, 103–7.

Rowland, M. and Tozer, T.N. (1995) *Clinical pharmacokinetics – concepts and applications* (3rd edition), Lippincott Williams and Wilkins, Philadelphia.

Sauter, R., Steinijans, V.W., Diletti, E., Böhm, A. and Schulz, H.-U. (1992) Presentation of results from bioequivalence studies. *International Journal of Clinical Pharmacology, Therapy and Toxicology* **30**, 233–56.

Schall, R., Luus, H.G., Steinijans, V.W. and Hauschke, D. (1994) Choice of characteristics and their bioequivalence ranges for the comparison of absorption rates of immediate-release drug formulations. *International Journal of Clinical Pharmacology and Therapeutics* **32**, 323–8.

Steinijans, V.W. (1989b) Pharmacokinetic characteristics of controlled release products and their biostatistical analysis. In: Gundert-Remy, U. and Moeller, H. (eds) *Oral controlled release products – therapeutic and biopharmaceutic assessment*, 99–115, APV Band 22, Wissenschaftliche Verlagsgesellschaft mbH, Stuttgart.

Steinijans, V.W., Sauter, R. and Diletti, E. (1995b) Shape analysis in single- and multiple-dose studies of modified-release products. In: Midha, K.K. and Blume, H.H. (eds) *Bio-International II: bioavailability, bioequivalence and pharmacokinetic studies. International conference of F.I.P. "Bio-International '94", Munich, Germany*, 193–206, Medpharm Scientific Publishers, Stuttgart.

Steinijans, V.W., Sauter, R., Hauschke, D. and Elze, M. (1995a) Metrics to characterize concentration-time profiles in single- and multiple-dose bioequivalence studies. *Drug Information Journal* **29**, 981–7.

Steinijans V.W., Sauter R., Jonkman, J.H.G., Schulz, H.U., Stricker, H. and Blume, H.H. (1989a) Bioequivalence studies: single vs multiple dose. *International Journal of Clinical Pharmacology, Therapy and Toxicology* **27**, 261–6.

Steinijans, V.W., Schulz, H.U., Beier, W. and Radtke, H.W. (1986) Once daily theophylline: multiple-dose comparison of an encapsulated micro-osmotic system (Euphylong) with a tablet (Uniphyllin). *International Journal of Clinical Pharmacology, Therapy and Toxicology* **24**, 438–47.

Steinijans, V.W., Trautmann, H., Johnson, E. and Beier, W. (1987) Theophylline steady-state pharmacokinetics: recent concepts and their application in chronotherapy of reactive airway diseases. *Chronobiology International* **4**, 331–47.

Tucker, G.T. (1983) The determination of the *in vivo* drug absorption rate. *Acta Pharmaceutica Technologica* **29**, 159–64.

Vaughan, D.P. and Dennis, M. (1978) Mathematical basis of point-area deconvolution method for determining *in vivo* input functions. *Journal of Pharmaceutical Sciences* **67**, 663–5.

Wagner, J.G. and Nelson, E. (1963) Per cent absorbed time plots derived from blood level and/or urinary excretion data. *Journal of Pharmaceutical Sciences* **52**, 610–11.

Zech, K., Sturm, E. and Steinijans, V.W. (1982) Pharmakokinetik und metabolismus von urapidil (ebrantil) bei Tier und Mensch. In: Kaufmann, W. and Bruckschen, E.G. (eds) *Urapidil, Darstellung einer neuen antihypertensiven Substanz*, 50–64, Excerpta Medica, Amsterdam.

3

Basic statistical considerations

3.1 Introduction

Regulatory acceptance of a bioequivalence study requires that appropriate statistical analyses be performed, as illustrated by the following excerpts from the relevant European Committee for Proprietary Medicinal Products (CPMP, 2001) and Food and Drug Administration guidance (FDA, 1992).

On performing the statistical analysis, the note for guidance on the investigation of bioavailability and bioequivalence, published by the CPMP (2001), states:

> 'The statistical method for testing relative bioavailability (e.g., bioequivalence) is based upon the 90 % confidence interval for the ratio of the population means (test/reference), for the parameters under consideration. This method is equivalent to the corresponding two one-sided tests procedure with the null hypothesis of bioinequivalence at the 5 % significance level. The statistical analysis (e.g., ANOVA) should take into account sources of variation that can be reasonably assumed to have an effect on the response variable. A statistically significant sequence effect should be handled appropriately. Pharmacokinetic parameters derived from measures of concentration, e.g., AUC, C_{max} should be analyzed using ANOVA. The data should be transformed prior to analysis using a logarithmic transformation. If appropriate to the evaluation the analysis technique for t_{max} should be nonparametric and should be applied to untransformed data. For all pharmacokinetic parameters of interest in addition to the appropriate 90 % confidence intervals for the comparison of two formulations, summary statistics such as median, minimum and maximum should be given.'

Bioequivalence Studies in Drug Development: Methods and Applications   D. Hauschke, V. Steinijans and I. Pigeot
© 2007 John Wiley & Sons, Ltd

On presenting adequate summary statistics, the FDA guidance (1992) on statistical procedures for bioequivalence using a standard two-treatment crossover design states:

> 'Standard statistical methodology based on the null hypothesis (*that is of no difference*) is not appropriate to assess bioequivalence. The Division of Bioequivalence has therefore employed a testing procedure termed the two one-sided tests procedure to determine whether average values for pharmacokinetic parameters measured after administration of the test and reference products are comparable. This procedure involves the calculation of a confidence interval for the ratio (or difference) between the test and reference product pharmacokinetic variable averages.'

It is the purpose of this chapter to provide the basic statistical methodology necessary for adequate analyses of bioequivalence studies.

3.2   Additive and multiplicative model

The emphasis in bioequivalence assessment is on inference about the ratio of mean extent or rate of bioavailability of two formulations of the same drug substance. The fundamental pharmacokinetic equation

$$AUC = \frac{f \cdot dose}{clearance},$$

where f denotes the fraction absorbed, describes a multiplicative relationship with formulation effect f and subject effect clearance. With regard to the statistical analysis, this suggests the assumption of a lognormal distribution of the underlying extent characteristic, AUC.

Logarithmic transformation of the above equation results in

$$\ln AUC = -\ln clearance + \ln f + \ln dose$$

and thus in an additive relationship. This then leads to an additive model under the normality assumption of the logarithmically transformed characteristic AUC. As the normal and lognormal distributions play a central role in bioequivalence assessment, their fundamental properties will be recalled in the following.

3.2.1   The normal distribution

The normal distribution, sometimes called the Gaussian distribution, is of major importance in bioequivalence assessment. An outcome, Y_T, is normally distributed with expected mean μ_T and variance σ_T^2, denoted by $Y_T \sim N(\mu_T, \sigma_T^2)$, if the probability density function is given by

$$f(y) = \frac{1}{\sqrt{2\pi}\sigma_T} \exp\left(-\frac{(y-\mu_T)^2}{2\sigma_T^2}\right), \quad -\infty < y < \infty.$$

For the normal distribution, this function is determined by the two parameters, expected mean $E(Y_T) = \mu_T$ and variance $Var(Y_T) = \sigma_T^2$. It should be noted that in practice the expected mean and variance are also called population mean and variance. They describe the unknown location and variability of the underlying variable in the entire population of interest.

In Figure 3.1 the density functions are given for two normally distributed variables, Y_T and Y_R, with identical expected means $\mu_T = \mu_R = 3$ but different standard deviations: the square roots of the variances, $\sigma_T = \sqrt{\sigma_T^2} = 1$ (solid line) and $\sigma_R = \sqrt{\sigma_R^2} = 0.5$ (dotted line).

An important measure of dispersion is the coefficient of variation because it describes the variation in the population relative to the expected mean:

$$CV(Y_T) = \frac{\sigma_T}{\mu_T}.$$

The median of a random variable, Y_T, is a value ζ_T (i.e., $M(Y_T) = \zeta_T$), such that the probabilities of the random variable Y_T being equal to or less than ζ_T, and of it being equal to or greater than ζ_T, are 0.5; that is $P(Y_T \leq \zeta_T) = P(Y_T \geq \zeta_T) = 0.5$. Obviously, for the normal distribution the median and the expected mean coincide, that is,

$$E(Y_T) = M(Y_T) = \mu_T = \zeta_T.$$

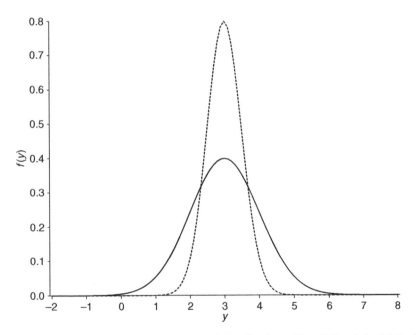

Figure 3.1   Density functions for two normal distributions, $Y_T \sim N(3, 1)$ (solid line) and $Y_R \sim N(3, 0.25)$ (dotted line).

To estimate the unknown population mean and variance, a random sample $Y_{T1}, \ldots, Y_{Tn}$ is drawn from the population with underlying normal distribution and expected mean μ_T and variance σ_T^2, i.e., $Y_{Tj} \sim N(\mu_T, \sigma_T^2)$, $j = 1, \ldots, n$. The intuitive estimators

$$\hat{\mu}_T = \overline{Y}_T = \frac{1}{n} \sum_{j=1}^{n} Y_{Tj}$$

and

$$\hat{\sigma}_T^2 = \frac{1}{n-1} \sum_{j=1}^{n} (Y_{Tj} - \overline{Y}_T)^2$$

are unbiased estimators of the population mean and variance, respectively; that is $E(\hat{\mu}_T) = \mu_T$ and $E(\hat{\sigma}_T^2) = \sigma_T^2$. Please note the distinction between an estimator and an estimate. An estimator is a function of the random sample, for example the mean, while an estimate is the observed value of the estimator in a specific study population.

Useful measures to describe the strength of a relationship between two random variables are the covariance and correlation. Let $Y_T \sim N(\mu_T, \sigma_T^2)$ and $Y_R \sim N(\mu_R, \sigma_R^2)$ be two dependent variables. Then, the covariance is defined as

$$Cov(Y_T, Y_R) = E(Y_T Y_R) - E(Y_T)E(Y_R) = \sigma_{TR},$$

and the correlation is the standardized covariance, with

$$Corr(Y_T, Y_R) = \frac{Cov(Y_T, Y_R)}{\sqrt{Var(Y_T)Var(Y_R)}}.$$

A positive correlation implies that if the random variable Y_R increases, so does the other variable Y_T; a negative correlation means that if one variable increases the other decreases. While the covariance can take values from $-\infty$ to ∞, the correlation is restricted from -1 to 1 due to the standardization.

An important feature of the normal distribution is that the distributions of linear combinations such as sums and differences of normally distributed variables are also normally distributed, i.e.,

$$Y_T + Y_R \sim N(\mu_T + \mu_R, \sigma_T^2 + \sigma_R^2 + 2\sigma_{TR})$$
$$Y_T - Y_R \sim N(\mu_T - \mu_R, \sigma_T^2 + \sigma_R^2 - 2\sigma_{TR}).$$

The presentation of point estimates should be always accompanied by corresponding $(1 - \alpha)100\,\%$ confidence intervals, which give the coverage probability of $(1 - \alpha)$ of capturing the parameter of interest. Hence, let $Y_{T1}, \ldots, Y_{Tn_1}$ and $Y_{R1}, \ldots, Y_{Rn_2}$ be random samples from normal distributions with expected means μ_T and μ_R, respectively. For the two-sample situation it is assumed that these random variables are independent from each other and have a common but unknown variance $\sigma_T^2 = \sigma_R^2 = \sigma^2$, while the covariance is assumed to be zero, i.e., $\sigma_{TR} = 0$. A two-sided $(1 - \alpha)100\%$ confidence interval for the difference in the expected means, $\mu_T - \mu_R$, can be calculated as follows

$$\left[\overline{Y}_T - \overline{Y}_R - t_{1-\alpha/2,n_1+n_2-2}\, \hat{\sigma} \sqrt{\frac{1}{n_1} + \frac{1}{n_2}},\, \overline{Y}_T - \overline{Y}_R + t_{1-\alpha/2,n_1+n_2-2}\, \hat{\sigma} \sqrt{\frac{1}{n_1} + \frac{1}{n_2}} \right],$$

where $t_{1-\alpha/2,n_1+n_2-2}$ is the $(1 - \alpha/2)$ quantile of the central Student's t-distribution with $n_1 + n_2 - 2$ degrees of freedom, $\overline{Y}_T = \hat{\mu}_T$ and $\overline{Y}_R = \hat{\mu}_R$ denote the corresponding sample means and

$$\hat{\sigma}^2 = \frac{1}{n_1 + n_2 - 2} \left(\sum_{j=1}^{n_1} (Y_{Tj} - \overline{Y}_T)^2 + \sum_{j=1}^{n_2} (Y_{Rj} - \overline{Y}_R)^2 \right)$$

is the pooled estimator of σ^2.

The above $(1 - \alpha)100\%$ confidence interval results from the fact that a normally distributed random variable Y with expected mean 0, standardized with an estimated variance that is χ^2 distributed with ν degrees of freedom and independent of Y, follows a central Student's t-distribution with ν degrees of freedom. In Table 3.1, the $(1 - \alpha/2) = 0.975$ quantiles are tabulated. For increasing degrees of freedom, the $(1 - \alpha/2)$ quantiles of the central t-distribution converge to the $(1 - \alpha/2)$ quantiles of the standard normal distribution, e.g., the $(1 - \alpha/2) = 0.975$ quantiles converge for increasing degrees of freedom to 1.960.

3.2.2   The lognormal distribution

Many pharmacokinetic characteristics follow a lognormal distribution rather than a normal distribution. For example, the distributions of concentration-related characteristics like

Table 3.1   0.975 quantiles of the central t-distribution for different degrees of freedom, df.

df	$t_{0.975,df}$	df	$t_{0.975,df}$	df	$t_{0.975,df}$	df	$t_{0.975,df}$
10	2.2281	21	2.0796	32	2.0369	43	2.0167
11	2.2010	22	2.0739	33	2.0345	44	2.0154
12	2.1788	23	2.0687	34	2.0322	45	2.0141
13	2.1604	24	2.0639	35	2.0301	46	2.0129
14	2.1448	25	2.0595	36	2.0281	47	2.0117
15	2.1314	26	2.0555	37	2.0262	48	2.0106
16	2.1199	27	2.0518	38	2.0244	49	2.0096
17	2.1098	28	2.0484	39	2.0227	50	2.0086
18	2.1009	29	2.0452	40	2.0211	100	1.9840
19	2.0930	30	2.0423	41	2.0195	1000	1.9620
20	2.0860	31	2.0395	42	2.0181	∞	1.9600

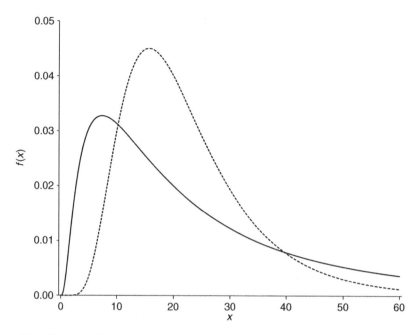

Figure 3.2 Density functions for two lognormal distributions, $X_T = \exp(Y_T)$, $Y_T \sim N(3, 1)$ (solid line), and $X_R = \exp(Y_R)$, $Y_R \sim N(3, 0.25)$ (dotted line).

AUC and C_{max} tend to be skewed and the underlying variances increase with the expected means.

A positive-valued random variable X_T follows a lognormal distribution when the logarithm of X_T is normally distributed, that is $Y_T = \ln X_T \sim N(\mu_T, \sigma_T^2)$. For $Y_T = \ln X_T \sim N(3, 1)$ and $Y_R = \ln X_R \sim N(3, 0.25)$ the density functions for $X_T = \exp(Y_T)$ and $X_R = \exp(Y_R)$ are given in Figure 3.2.

The population mean, median and variance of a lognormally distributed random variable, X_T, are

$$E(X_T) = \exp\left(\mu_T + \frac{\sigma_T^2}{2}\right)$$

$$M(X_T) = \exp(\mu_T)$$

$$Var(X_T) = \exp(2\mu_T + \sigma_T^2)(\exp(\sigma_T^2) - 1).$$

In contrast to the normal distribution, the coefficient of variation of a lognormally distributed variable X_T only depends on the variance on the logtransformed scale:

$$CV(X_T) = \frac{\sqrt{Var(X_T)}}{E(X_T)} = \frac{\sqrt{\exp(2\mu_T + \sigma_T^2)(\exp(\sigma_T^2) - 1)}}{\exp\left(\mu_T + \frac{\sigma_T^2}{2}\right)}$$

$$= \sqrt{\frac{\exp(2\mu_T + \sigma_T^2)(\exp(\sigma_T^2) - 1)}{\left(\exp\left(\mu_T + \frac{\sigma_T^2}{2}\right)\right)^2}} = \sqrt{\frac{\exp(2\mu_T + \sigma_T^2)(\exp(\sigma_T^2) - 1)}{\exp(2\mu_T + \sigma_T^2)}},$$

and therefore

$$CV(X_T) = \sqrt{\exp(\sigma_T^2) - 1}.$$

This corresponds to $\sigma_T^2 = \ln(1 + (CV(X_T))^2)$. Whenever the square of the coefficient of variation is small, $\ln(1 + (CV(X_T))^2) \approx (CV(X_T))^2$ holds. Hence, in this case the coefficient of variation can be directly approximated by the standard deviation σ_T.

The product and the ratio of two lognormally distributed variables are also lognormally distributed. Let $Y_T = \ln X_T \sim N(\mu_T, \sigma_T^2)$, $Y_R = \ln X_R \sim N(\mu_R, \sigma_R^2)$ and $Cov(Y_T, Y_R) = \sigma_{TR}$. It follows directly that

$$Y_T + Y_R = \ln X_T + \ln X_R = \ln(X_T X_R) \sim N(\mu_T + \mu_R, \sigma_T^2 + \sigma_R^2 + 2\sigma_{TR})$$

$$Y_T - Y_R = \ln X_T - \ln X_R = \ln\left(\frac{X_T}{X_R}\right) \sim N(\mu_T - \mu_R, \sigma_T^2 + \sigma_R^2 - 2\sigma_{TR}).$$

To estimate the unknown population mean of the lognormal distribution, a random sample, $X_{T1}, \ldots, X_{Tn}$, is drawn from a lognormal distribution with corresponding expected mean μ_T and variance σ_T^2 on the transformed scale, i.e., $Y_{Tj} = \ln X_{Tj} \sim N(\mu_T, \sigma_T^2)$, $j = 1, \ldots, n$. The arithmetic mean $\overline{Y}_T$ on the logtransformed scale is the point estimator of μ_T. Exponential transformation of this estimator results in the geometric mean of the untransformed variables

$$\exp(\overline{Y}_T) = \exp\left(\frac{1}{n}\sum_{j=1}^{n} Y_{Tj}\right) = \exp\left(\frac{1}{n}\sum_{j=1}^{n} \ln X_{Tj}\right) = \sqrt[n]{\prod_{j=1}^{n} X_{Tj}}.$$

The geometric mean is not an unbiased estimator of the population mean on the original scale:

$$E(\exp(\overline{Y}_T)) = E\left(\sqrt[n]{\prod_{j=1}^{n} X_{Tj}}\right) = \exp\left(\mu_T + \frac{\sigma_T^2}{2n}\right)$$

$$= \exp\left(\mu_T + \frac{\sigma_T^2}{2}\right)\exp\left(-\frac{\sigma_T^2}{2}\left(1 - \frac{1}{n}\right)\right)$$

$$= E(X_T)\exp\left(-\frac{\sigma_T^2}{2}\left(1 - \frac{1}{n}\right)\right) < E(X_T),$$

because $\exp\left(-\sigma_T^2(1 - 1/n)/2\right)$ is always smaller than 1 for $\sigma_T^2 > 0$. Hence, for large sample sizes, that is for $1/n \approx 0$, the geometric mean is an approximately unbiased estimator of the median rather than of the expected mean:

$$E(\exp(\overline{Y}_T)) = E\left(\sqrt[n]{\prod_{j=1}^{n} X_{Tj}}\right) = \exp\left(\mu_T + \frac{\sigma_T^2}{2n}\right) \approx \exp(\mu_T) = M(X_T).$$

In the following, the focus is on the estimation of the ratio of expected medians of two lognormal distributions. Let $X_{T1}, \ldots, X_{Tn_1}, X_{R1}, \ldots, X_{Rn_2}$ be two independent samples from two lognormal distributions with unknown but identical variances $\sigma_T^2 = \sigma_R^2 = \sigma^2$ on the logarithmically transformed scale, that is $Y_{Tj} = \ln X_{Tj} \sim N(\mu_T, \sigma^2)$, $j = 1, \ldots, n_1$, and $Y_{Rj} = \ln X_{Rj} \sim N(\mu_R, \sigma^2)$, $j = 1, \ldots, n_2$, respectively. In the case of equal variances, the ratio of expected medians coincides with the ratio of means,

$$\frac{M(X_T)}{M(X_R)} = \frac{\exp(\mu_T)}{\exp(\mu_R)} = \frac{\exp\left(\mu_T + \frac{\sigma^2}{2}\right)}{\exp\left(\mu_R + \frac{\sigma^2}{2}\right)} = \frac{E(X_T)}{E(X_R)}.$$

A two-sided $(1-\alpha)100\%$ confidence interval for

$$\frac{M(X_T)}{M(X_R)} = \frac{E(X_T)}{E(X_R)} = \frac{\exp(\mu_T)}{\exp(\mu_R)}$$

can be calculated by exponential transformation of the two-sided $(1-\alpha)100\%$ confidence interval for the difference $\mu_T - \mu_R$,

$$\left[\exp\left(\overline{Y}_T - \overline{Y}_R - t_{1-\alpha/2, n_1+n_2-2}\hat{\sigma}\sqrt{\frac{1}{n_1} + \frac{1}{n_2}} \right), \exp\left(\overline{Y}_T - \overline{Y}_R + t_{1-\alpha/2, n_1+n_2-2}\hat{\sigma}\sqrt{\frac{1}{n_1} + \frac{1}{n_2}} \right) \right].$$

It should be noted that for heterogeneous variances $\sigma_T^2 \neq \sigma_R^2$, the ratios of expected means and medians are no longer equal:

$$\frac{M(X_T)}{M(X_R)} = \frac{\exp(\mu_T)}{\exp(\mu_R)} \neq \frac{\exp\left(\mu_T + \frac{\sigma_T^2}{2}\right)}{\exp\left(\mu_R + \frac{\sigma_R^2}{2}\right)} = \frac{E(X_T)}{E(X_R)}$$

and the above two-sided $(1-\alpha)100\%$ confidence interval is only valid for the ratio of medians.

In summary, the homogeneity of the variances on the transformed scale, that is $\sigma_T^2 = \sigma_R^2 = \sigma^2$, is a fundamental assumption to guarantee equality of the ratios of population means and of medians. For heterogeneous variances, the classical $(1-\alpha)100\%$ confidence interval only refers to the ratio of medians.

3.3 Hypotheses testing

3.3.1 Consumer and producer risk

Hypotheses are statements about population parameters, for example about the means of distributions. Based on samples from the corresponding populations, the goal of a hypothesis test is to decide which of two complementary hypotheses is more likely to

Table 3.2 Type I and type II errors in a hypothesis test.

	The null hypothesis is	
	True	False
Fail to reject the null hypothesis	Correct decision	Type II error β
Reject the null hypothesis	Type I error α	Correct decision

be true. These two hypotheses are called the null hypothesis and alternative hypothesis and are denoted by H_0 and H_1, respectively. A testing procedure is a decision rule that specifies for which sample values to reject, or fail to reject, the null hypothesis H_0.

The procedure of testing H_0 versus H_1 is associated with two types of error. If the null hypothesis H_0 is true, but the procedure erroneously rejects H_0 in favor of the alternative H_1, then a type I error occurs. The probability of committing a type I error will be limited by the prespecified significance level α. On the other hand, if the null hypothesis H_0 is false, and the test procedure fails to reject H_0, a type II error, β, occurs. These types of error are shown in Table 3.2.

For the sake of illustration, suppose that bioequivalence of a test and a reference formulation is investigated in a clinical trial, and the test problem would indirectly be formulated as follows

$$H_0 : \text{bioequivalence vs. } H_1 : \text{bioinequivalence.}$$

Failure to reject the above null hypothesis by a statistical test at level α might lead to the conclusion of bioequivalence. The major pitfall of this indirect approach is that the probability of erroneously concluding bioinequivalence is controlled, and thereby the producer risk, but not the consumer risk (see Table 3.3). Therefore, the indirect approach is not accepted by regulatory authorities.

However, the primary regulatory concern is the control of the consumer risk, that is, limiting the probability of erroneously concluding bioequivalence. One reason for this logical difficulty is described by Fisher (1935):

Table 3.3 Type I and type II errors for indirect bioequivalence testing.

	The null hypothesis of bioequivalence is	
	True	False
Fail to reject the null hypothesis of bioequivalence	Correct decision	Consumer risk β
Reject the null hypothesis of bioequivalence	Producer risk α	Correct decision

Table 3.4 Type I and type II errors for direct bioequivalence testing.

	The null hypothesis of bioinequivalence is	
	True	False
Fail to reject the null hypothesis of bioinequivalence	Correct decision	Producer risk β
Reject the null hypothesis of bioinequivalence	Consumer risk α	Correct decision

'The null hypothesis is never proved or established, but is possibly disproved in the course of experimentation. Every experiment may be said to exist only in order to give the facts a chance of disproving the null hypothesis.'

Thus, the adequate test problem has to be formulated by transposing the null hypothesis and the alternative of the indirect approach. This direct approach is generally requested by regulatory authorities (CPMP, 2001; FDA, 2001):

$$H_0 : \text{bioinequivalence vs. } H_1 : \text{bioequivalence.}$$

The consumer and producer risks for the direct approach for bioequivalence assessment are illustrated in Table 3.4.

Obviously, a decision rule is optimal if it limits the actual consumer risk, which is usually set to 5 %, and, in addition, minimizes the producer risk. It should be noted that $1 - \beta$ is called the power of the decision rule. The power is the probability of correctly concluding bioequivalence.

3.3.2 Types of hypotheses

For the sake of completeness, the following section presents tests for difference, superiority, noninferiority, and equivalence in a systematic manner. To illustrate the different types of hypotheses, consider the two-sample situation, test versus reference with n_1 and n_2 subjects and independent normally distributed outcomes Y_T and Y_R for the test and reference formulation, respectively, with

$$Y_{Tj} \sim N(\mu_T, \sigma^2), \ j = 1, \ldots, n_1, \ \text{and} \ Y_{Rj} \sim N(\mu_R, \sigma^2), \ j = 1, \ldots, n_2,$$

with common but unknown variance σ^2. Without loss of generality, it is assumed that higher values of the outcome refer to greater effects.

3.3.2.1 Test for difference

The traditional two-sided test problem of difference is formulated as

$$H_0 : \mu_T - \mu_R = 0 \text{ vs. } H_1 : \mu_T - \mu_R \neq 0$$

and the graphical presentation of the test problem is shown in Figure 3.3.

The null hypothesis H_0 of equality is rejected by Student's t-test at a significance level α, if

$$T = \frac{|\overline{Y}_T - \overline{Y}_R|}{\hat{\sigma} \sqrt{\dfrac{1}{n_1} + \dfrac{1}{n_2}}} > t_{1-\alpha/2, n_1 + n_2 - 2},$$

where $|y|$ denotes the absolute value of y, $\overline{Y}_T$ and $\overline{Y}_R$ the sample means of the test and reference group and $\hat{\sigma}^2$ the pooled estimator of σ^2.

Due to the duality of the test procedure and the corresponding confidence interval, rejection of H_0 by the two-sided t-test is equivalent to the exclusion of zero from the two-sided $(1 - \alpha)100\%$ confidence interval for $\mu_T - \mu_R$:

$$0 \notin \left[\overline{Y}_T - \overline{Y}_R - t_{1-\alpha/2, n_1 + n_2 - 2}\, \hat{\sigma} \sqrt{\frac{1}{n_1} + \frac{1}{n_2}},\, \overline{Y}_T - \overline{Y}_R + t_{1-\alpha/2, n_1 + n_2 - 2}\, \hat{\sigma} \sqrt{\frac{1}{n_1} + \frac{1}{n_2}} \right].$$

3.3.2.2 Test for superiority

In many practical situations it is not sufficient to demonstrate that there is a difference between test and reference. The primary aim of the comparison is to show that test is better than reference and hence, for this type of comparison the one-sided test problem of superiority is indicated:

$$H_0 : \mu_T \leq \mu_R \text{ vs. } H_1 : \mu_T > \mu_R.$$

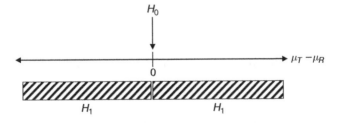

Figure 3.3 Graphical illustration of the two-sided test problem for difference. The hashed bars indicate the range of $\mu_T - \mu_R$ values belonging to the alternative hypothesis H_1.

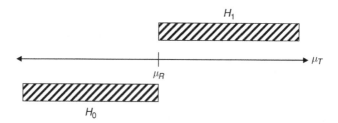

Figure 3.4 Graphical illustration of the one-sided test problem for superiority. The upper hashed bar indicates the range of μ_T values belonging to the alternative hypothesis H_1.

The graphical presentation of the test problem is shown in Figure 3.4.

The null hypothesis, H_0, is rejected at a significance level α, if

$$T = \frac{\overline{Y}_T - \overline{Y}_R}{\hat{\sigma}\sqrt{\dfrac{1}{n_1} + \dfrac{1}{n_2}}} > t_{1-\alpha, n_1+n_2-2},$$

which is equivalent to

$$\overline{Y}_T - \overline{Y}_R - t_{1-\alpha, n_1+n_2-2}\,\hat{\sigma}\sqrt{\frac{1}{n_1} + \frac{1}{n_2}} > 0,$$

that is, the lower limit of the two-sided $(1 - 2\alpha)100\%$ confidence interval for $\mu_T - \mu_R$ must be greater than zero.

3.3.2.3 Test for noninferiority

When a new test formulation has certain advantages over the reference, such as fewer side effects or no pharmacokinetic interactions, to prove overall superiority it may be sufficient to show, for the primary endpoint, that test is not relevantly inferior to reference. Such studies are called noninferiority trials, and the test problem can be described as follows:

$$H_0: \mu_T - \mu_R \leq \delta \text{ vs. } H_1: \mu_T - \mu_R > \delta,$$

or reformulated as

$$H_0: \mu_T \leq \mu_R + \delta \text{ vs. } H_1: \mu_T > \mu_R + \delta,$$

where δ denotes the maximum irrelevant threshold value, with $\delta < 0$. The test problem is illustrated in Figure 3.5.

The null hypothesis, H_0, is rejected at a significance level α, if

$$T_\delta = \frac{\overline{Y}_T - \overline{Y}_R - \delta}{\hat{\sigma}\sqrt{\dfrac{1}{n_1} + \dfrac{1}{n_2}}} > t_{1-\alpha, n_1+n_2-2},$$

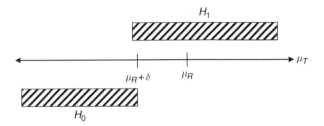

Figure 3.5 Graphical illustration of the one-sided test problem for noninferiority. The upper hashed bar indicates the range of μ_T values belonging to the alternative hypothesis H_1. Note that $\delta < 0$, so that $\mu_R + \delta < \mu_R$.

which is equivalent to

$$\overline{Y}_T - \overline{Y}_R - t_{1-\alpha, n_1+n_2-2}\, \hat{\sigma} \sqrt{\frac{1}{n_1} + \frac{1}{n_2}} > \delta,$$

that is, the lower limit of the two-sided $(1-2\alpha)100\%$ confidence interval for $\mu_T - \mu_R$ must be greater than δ.

3.3.2.4 Test for equivalence

Some clinical trials aim to demonstrate that two formulations do not differ by more than a prespecified irrelevant amount. Let the interval (δ_1, δ_2), with $\delta_1 < 0 < \delta_2$, denote the equivalence range, then the test problem for equivalence is formulated as follows:

$$H_0: \mu_T - \mu_R \leq \delta_1 \text{ or } \mu_T - \mu_R \geq \delta_2$$

vs.

$$H_1: \delta_1 < \mu_T - \mu_R < \delta_2.$$

The test problem for equivalence is shown in Figure 3.6.

A split of the above two-sided test problem into two one-sided test problems (Schuirmann, 1987) results in

$$H_{01}: \mu_T - \mu_R \leq \delta_1 \text{ vs. } H_{11}: \mu_T - \mu_R > \delta_1$$

and

$$H_{02}: \mu_T - \mu_R \geq \delta_2 \text{ vs. } H_{12}: \mu_T - \mu_R < \delta_2.$$

In the literature this decomposition is referred to as the TOST (two one-sided tests) procedure. From the graphical presentation in Figure 3.7 it can be seen that

$$H_0 = H_{01} \cup H_{02} \text{ vs. } H_1 = H_{11} \cap H_{12}.$$

According to the intersection-union principle (Berger and Hsu, 1996), H_0 is rejected at significance level α in favor of H_1 if both hypotheses H_{01} and H_{02} are rejected at significance level α:

$$T_{\delta_1} = \frac{\overline{Y}_T - \overline{Y}_R - \delta_1}{\hat{\sigma}\sqrt{\dfrac{1}{n_1} + \dfrac{1}{n_2}}} > t_{1-\alpha, n_1+n_2-2}$$

and

$$T_{\delta_2} = \frac{\overline{Y}_T - \overline{Y}_R - \delta_2}{\hat{\sigma}\sqrt{\dfrac{1}{n_1} + \dfrac{1}{n_2}}} < -t_{1-\alpha, n_1+n_2-2}.$$

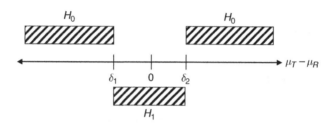

Figure 3.6 Graphical illustration of the two-sided test problem for equivalence. The lower hashed bar indicates the range of $\mu_T - \mu_R$ values belonging to the alternative hypothesis H_1.

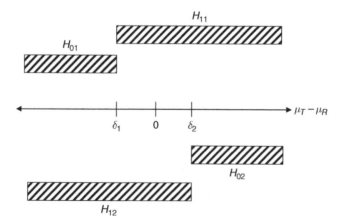

Figure 3.7 Graphical illustration of the decomposition of the two-sided test problem for equivalence.

This is equivalent to

$$\overline{Y}_T - \overline{Y}_R - t_{1-\alpha,n_1+n_2-2}\,\hat{\sigma}\sqrt{\frac{1}{n_1}+\frac{1}{n_2}} > \delta_1$$

and

$$\overline{Y}_T - \overline{Y}_R + t_{1-\alpha,n_1+n_2-2}\,\hat{\sigma}\sqrt{\frac{1}{n_1}+\frac{1}{n_2}} < \delta_2,$$

and hence to the inclusion of the two-sided $(1-2\alpha)100\,\%$ confidence interval for $\mu_T-\mu_R$ in the equivalence range:

$$\left[\overline{Y}_T - \overline{Y}_R - t_{1-\alpha,n_1+n_2-2}\,\hat{\sigma}\sqrt{\frac{1}{n_1}+\frac{1}{n_2}},\ \overline{Y}_T - \overline{Y}_R + t_{1-\alpha,n_1+n_2-2}\,\hat{\sigma}\sqrt{\frac{1}{n_1}+\frac{1}{n_2}}\right] \subset (\delta_1,\delta_2).$$

3.3.3 Difference versus ratio of expected means

3.3.3.1 The normal distribution

The inherent problem in noninferiority or equivalence studies is the definition of what constitutes an irrelevant difference. To test the problem

$$H_0: \mu_T - \mu_R \leq \delta_1 \text{ or } \mu_T - \mu_R \geq \delta_2$$

vs.

$$H_1: \delta_1 < \mu_T - \mu_R < \delta_2,$$

it has to be assumed that the equivalence limits δ_1 and δ_2 are known. However, a more common situation in practice is that the maximum irrelevant differences in $\mu_T - \mu_R$ are expressed as proportions of the unknown reference mean $\mu_R \neq 0$, that is $\delta_1 = f_1\mu_R$ and $\delta_2 = f_2\mu_R$, $-1 < f_1 < 0 < f_2$. The above test problem can then be formulated as

$$H_0: \mu_T - \mu_R \leq f_1\mu_R \text{ or } \mu_T - \mu_R \geq f_2\mu_R$$

vs.

$$H_1: f_1\mu_R < \mu_T - \mu_R < f_2\mu_R.$$

A reformulation of the equivalence problem results in:

$$H_0: \mu_T \leq (1+f_1)\mu_R \text{ or } \mu_T \geq (1+f_2)\mu_R$$

vs.

$$H_1: (1+f_1)\mu_R < \mu_T < (1+f_2)\mu_R,$$

which, for $\mu_R \neq 0$, can be restated as

$$H_0: \frac{\mu_T}{\mu_R} \leq \theta_1 \text{ or } \frac{\mu_T}{\mu_R} \geq \theta_2$$

vs.

$$H_1: \theta_1 < \frac{\mu_T}{\mu_R} < \theta_2,$$

where (θ_1, θ_2), $\theta_1 = 1 + f_1$, $\theta_2 = 1 + f_2$, $0 < \theta_1 < 1 < \theta_2$, is the corresponding equivalence interval for the ratio of the expected means μ_T / μ_R. Testing equivalence of two formulations is equivalent to simultaneous testing of the following two one-sided hypotheses

$$H_{01}: \frac{\mu_T}{\mu_R} \leq \theta_1 \text{ vs. } H_{11}: \frac{\mu_T}{\mu_R} > \theta_1$$

and

$$H_{02}: \frac{\mu_T}{\mu_R} \geq \theta_2 \text{ vs. } H_{12}: \frac{\mu_T}{\mu_R} < \theta_2.$$

Berger and Hsu (1996) demonstrated that H_0 is rejected at significance level α in favor of H_1 if both hypotheses H_{01} and H_{02} are rejected at significance level α, that is

$$T_{\theta_1} = \frac{\overline{Y}_T - \theta_1 \overline{Y}_R}{\hat{\sigma} \sqrt{\dfrac{1}{n_1} + \dfrac{\theta_1^2}{n_2}}} > t_{1-\alpha, n_1 + n_2 - 2}$$

and

$$T_{\theta_2} = \frac{\overline{Y}_T - \theta_2 \overline{Y}_R}{\hat{\sigma} \sqrt{\dfrac{1}{n_1} + \dfrac{\theta_2^2}{n_2}}} < -t_{1-\alpha, n_1 + n_2 - 2}.$$

Hauschke *et al.* (1999) have shown that rejection is equivalent to the inclusion of the $100(1 - 2\alpha)$ % confidence interval for μ_T / μ_R, given by Fieller (1954), in the equivalence range (θ_1, θ_2):

$$\left[\frac{\overline{Y}_T \overline{Y}_R - \sqrt{a_R \overline{Y}_T^2 + a_T \overline{Y}_R^2 - a_T a_R}}{\overline{Y}_R^2 - a_R}, \frac{\overline{Y}_T \overline{Y}_R + \sqrt{a_R \overline{Y}_T^2 + a_T \overline{Y}_R^2 - a_T a_R}}{\overline{Y}_R^2 - a_R} \right] \subset (\theta_1, \theta_2)$$

with $\overline{Y}_R^2 > a_R$, where $a_T = \dfrac{\hat{\sigma}^2}{n_1} t_{1-\alpha, n_1 + n_2 - 2}^2$, $a_R = \dfrac{\hat{\sigma}^2}{n_2} t_{1-\alpha, n_1 + n_2 - 2}^2$.

3.3.3.2 The lognormal distribution

Up to this point it has been assumed that the outcomes are normally distributed. However, as mentioned earlier, many concentration-related characteristics follow a lognormal distribution. Hence, in the following the outcomes are assumed to be independent samples from two lognormal distributions

$$Y_{Tj} = \ln X_{Tj} \sim N(\mu_T, \sigma_T^2), \ j = 1, \ldots, n_1, \text{ and } Y_{Rj} = \ln X_{Rj} \sim N(\mu_R, \sigma_R^2), \ j = 1, \ldots, n_2.$$

The parameter of interest is the ratio of the population means for test and reference and the test problem concerns equivalence:

$$H_0: \frac{E(X_T)}{E(X_R)} \leq \theta_1 \text{ or } \frac{E(X_T)}{E(X_R)} \geq \theta_2$$

vs.

$$H_1: \theta_1 < \frac{E(X_T)}{E(X_R)} < \theta_2.$$

Since

$$E(X_{Tj}) = \exp\left(\mu_T + \frac{\sigma_T^2}{2}\right), \ j = 1, \ldots, n_1 \text{ and } E(X_{Rj}) = \exp\left(\mu_R + \frac{\sigma_R^2}{2}\right), \ j = 1, \ldots, n_2,$$

the above test problem is equivalent to:

$$H_0: \frac{\exp\left(\mu_T + \frac{\sigma_T^2}{2}\right)}{\exp\left(\mu_R + \frac{\sigma_R^2}{2}\right)} \leq \theta_1 \text{ or } \frac{\exp\left(\mu_T + \frac{\sigma_T^2}{2}\right)}{\exp\left(\mu_R + \frac{\sigma_R^2}{2}\right)} \geq \theta_2$$

vs.

$$H_1: \theta_1 < \frac{\exp\left(\mu_T + \frac{\sigma_T^2}{2}\right)}{\exp\left(\mu_R + \frac{\sigma_R^2}{2}\right)} < \theta_2.$$

Assuming homogeneity of the variances, that is $\sigma_T^2 = \sigma_R^2 = \sigma^2$, the above expression reduces to:

$$H_0: \frac{\exp(\mu_T)}{\exp(\mu_R)} \leq \theta_1 \text{ or } \frac{\exp(\mu_T)}{\exp(\mu_R)} \geq \theta_2$$

vs.

$$H_1: \theta_1 < \frac{\exp(\mu_T)}{\exp(\mu_R)} < \theta_2$$

Taking logarithms, the corresponding test problem on the transformed scale results in:

$$H_0: \mu_T - \mu_R \leq \ln \theta_1 \text{ or } \mu_T - \mu_R \geq \ln \theta_2$$

vs.

$$H_1: \ln \theta_1 < \mu_T - \mu_R < \ln \theta_2,$$

which can be tested by two one-sided t-tests based on the transformed data. Hence, if the assumption of homogeneous variances holds, we obtain duality between the test problem based on the ratio of expected means on the original scale and the test problem based on the corresponding difference on the logarithmic scale. It is important to note that for unequal variances, i.e., $\sigma_T^2 \neq \sigma_R^2$, the corresponding duality only holds true for the ratio of medians on the original scale and the difference in means on the logarithmic scale:

$$H_0: \frac{M(X_T)}{M(X_R)} \leq \theta_1 \text{ or } \frac{M(X_T)}{M(X_R)} \geq \theta_2$$

vs.

$$H_1: \theta_1 < \frac{M(X_T)}{M(X_R)} < \theta_2.$$

Since $M(X_{Tj}) = \exp(\mu_T)$, $j = 1, \ldots, n_1$, and $M(X_{Rj}) = \exp(\mu_R)$, $j = 1, \ldots, n_2$, we have

$$H_0: \frac{\exp(\mu_T)}{\exp(\mu_R)} \leq \theta_1 \text{ or } \frac{\exp(\mu_T)}{\exp(\mu_R)} \geq \theta_2$$

vs.

$$H_1: \theta_1 < \frac{\exp(\mu_T)}{\exp(\mu_R)} < \theta_2,$$

which is equivalent to

$$H_0: \mu_T - \mu_R \leq \ln \theta_1 \text{ or } \mu_T - \mu_R \geq \ln \theta_2$$

vs.

$$H_1: \ln \theta_1 < \mu_T - \mu_R < \ln \theta_2.$$

In summary, assuming a normal distribution and expressing equivalence limits as fractions of the unknown reference mean requires statistical methods based on the ratio of population means. In the case of a lognormal distribution, this problem can be solved by a logarithmic transformation. However, the corresponding variances on the logarithmic scale must be equal in order to assure the duality between the test problems for the expected means on both the original and the logtransformed scale.

3.4   The *RT/TR* crossover design assuming an additive model

In the standard two-period, two-sequence crossover design, subjects are randomly allocated to two treatment sequences; in sequence 1, subjects receive the reference formulation (R) and test formulation (T) in periods 1 and 2, respectively, while in sequence 2, subjects receive the formulations in reverse order. Between period 1 and period 2 is a washout period, which has to be sufficiently long to ensure that the effect of the preceding formulation has been eliminated (see Table 3.5). This design will be referred to as the *RT/TR* design.

3.4.1   Additive model and effects

The following section solely deals with the additive model. This, for example, applies to logarithmically transformed pharmacokinetic characteristics such as AUC and C_{max}.

Let sequences and periods be indexed by i and k, $i, k = 1$, 2, respectively, and n_i subjects are randomized to sequence i. Let Y_{ijk} denote the outcome on the jth subject in the ith sequence during period k. The following additive model is considered:

$$Y_{ijk} = \mu_h + s_{ij} + \pi_k + \lambda_c + e_{ijk},$$

where μ_h is the effect of formulation h, where $h = R$ if $i = k$ and $h = T$ if $i \neq k$, π_k is the effect of the kth period, λ_c is the carryover effect of the corresponding formulation from period 1 to period 2, where $c = R$ if $i = 1$, $k = 2$, $c = T$ if $i = 2$, $k = 2$, and $\lambda_c = 0$ if $i = 1$, 2, $k = 1$, with the usual conditions for reparametrization $\pi_1 + \pi_2 = \lambda_R + \lambda_T = 0$.

The subject term s_{ij} is the random effect of the jth subject in sequence i and e_{ijk} is the random error term for subject j in period k and sequence i. It is assumed that s_{ij} are independent normally distributed with expected mean 0 and between-subject variance σ_B^2. The random errors e_{ijk} are also independent and normally distributed with expected mean 0 and within-subject variances σ_{WT}^2 and σ_{WR}^2 for the test and reference formulation, respectively. Furthermore, s_{ij} and e_{ijk} are assumed to be mutually independent. The intraindividual observations within a sequence are not independent and the corresponding covariance is $\sigma_{TR} = \sigma_B^2$. Under these assumptions the formulation variances are given by $\sigma_T^2 = \sigma_B^2 + \sigma_{WT}^2$ and $\sigma_R^2 = \sigma_B^2 + \sigma_{WR}^2$. Table 3.6 shows the layout of the random variables Y_{ijk}, $i, k = 1$, 2, $j = 1, \ldots, n_i$. The corresponding population means and variances are given in Table 3.7.

As given in the above additive model, the primary components of interest are the treatment, period and carryover effects. These effects are illustrated in the following

Table 3.5   The *RT/TR* design.

Sequence	Period 1	Washout	Period 2
1	R		T
2	T		R

Table 3.6 Layout for the *RT/TR* crossover design on the additive scale.

Sequence	Period 1	Period 2
1 (*RT*)	$Y_{1j1} = \mu_R + s_{1j} + \pi_1 + e_{1j1}$ $j = 1, \ldots, n_1$	$Y_{1j2} = \mu_T + s_{1j} + \pi_2$ $+ \lambda_R + e_{1j2}$ $j = 1, \ldots, n_1$
2 (*TR*)	$Y_{2j1} = \mu_T + s_{2j} + \pi_1 + e_{2j1}$ $j = 1, \ldots, n_2$	$Y_{2j2} = \mu_R + s_{2j} + \pi_2$ $+ \lambda_T + e_{2j2}$ $j = 1, \ldots, n_2$

Table 3.7 Expected means and variances for the *RT/TR* crossover design.

Sequence	Period 1	Period 2
1 (*RT*)	$E(Y_{1j1}) = \mu_R + \pi_1$ $Var(Y_{1j1}) = \sigma_R^2 = \sigma_B^2 + \sigma_{WR}^2$ $j = 1, \ldots, n_1$	$E(Y_{1j2}) = \mu_T + \pi_2 + \lambda_R$ $Var(Y_{1j2}) = \sigma_T^2 = \sigma_B^2 + \sigma_{WT}^2$ $j = 1, \ldots, n_1$
2 (*TR*)	$E(Y_{2j1}) = \mu_T + \pi_1$ $Var(Y_{2j1}) = \sigma_T^2 = \sigma_B^2 + \sigma_{WT}^2$ $j = 1, \ldots, n_2$	$E(Y_{2j2}) = \mu_R + \pi_2 + \lambda_T$ $Var(Y_{2j2}) = \sigma_R^2 = \sigma_B^2 + \sigma_{WR}^2$ $j = 1, \ldots, n_2$

sequence-by-period plots where the vertical axis represents the mean responses and the horizontal axis represents the periods.

Figures 3.8 (a) and (b) show examples where the difference in treatment effects is the same in both periods. However, in plot (b) the corresponding treatment difference in period 2 is on a higher level and hence, indicates a period difference.

Figures 3.8 (c) and (d) illustrate examples where the differences in treatment effects are not equal in both periods. In plot (c) the difference in period 2 is smaller than in period 1, and hence indicates a quantitative carryover difference. In plot (d) the treatment difference in period 2 is of the same absolute magnitude but differs in sign, which indicates a qualitative carryover difference. The latter will, for example, be observed in bioequivalence studies if the two sequences of subjects have different clearances and thereby different magnitudes of the resulting pharmacokinetic characteristics.

3.4.2   Parametric analysis based on *t*-tests

The additive model for the standard *RT/TR* design can be analyzed by a corresponding analysis of variance (ANOVA). However, Hills and Armitage (1979) reduced the above model to the two-sample situation and used simple *t*-tests for treatment, period and carryover effects. This technique will be presented in the following. Carryover effects are investigated first, because equality of these effects is necessary for an adequate assessment of treatment effects.

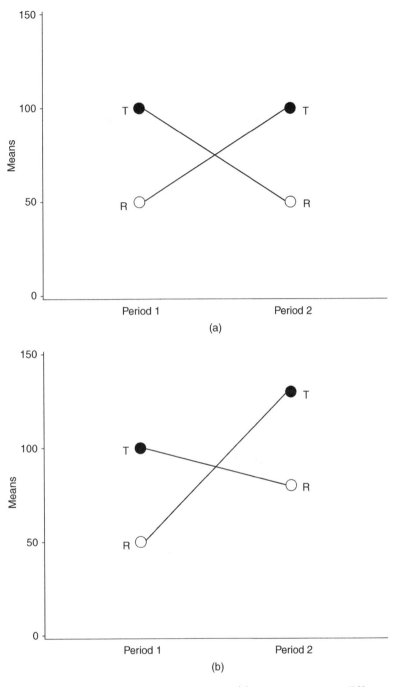

Figure 3.8 Sequence-by-period plots illustrating (a) only a treatment difference, (b) a treatment and a period difference, (c) treatment and quantitative carryover differences, and (d) treatment and qualitative carryover differences.

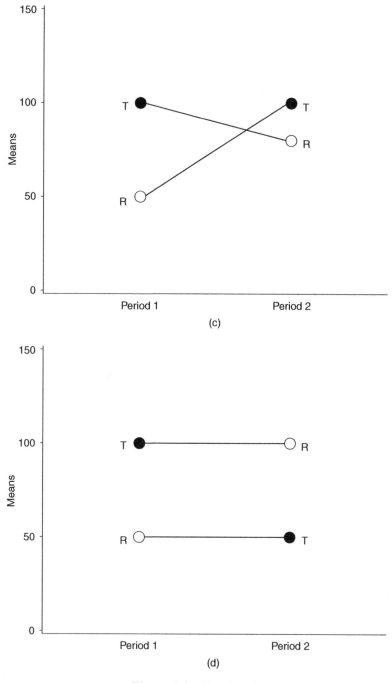

Figure 3.8 Continued.

3.4.2.1 Test for difference in carryover effects

For testing the difference in carryover effects, the intraindividual period sums Y_{ij}^S, $i = 1, 2, j = 1, \ldots, n_i$, of the observations for the first and second period are calculated as

$$Y_{1j}^S = Y_{1j1} + Y_{1j2}, \ j = 1, \ldots, n_1, \ \text{in sequence 1,}$$
$$Y_{2j}^S = Y_{2j1} + Y_{2j2}, \ j = 1, \ldots, n_2, \ \text{in sequence 2.}$$

The expected means and variances of these period sums are

$$E(Y_{1j}^S) = E(Y_{1j1}) + E(Y_{1j2}) = \mu_R + \pi_1 + \mu_T + \pi_2 + \lambda_R = \mu_T + \mu_R + \lambda_R,$$

because $\pi_1 + \pi_2 = 0$,

$$Var(Y_{1j}^S) = Var(Y_{1j1}) + Var(Y_{1j2}) + 2Cov(Y_{1j1}, Y_{1j2}) = \sigma_T^2 + \sigma_R^2 + 2\sigma_B^2, \ j = 1, \ldots, n_1,$$

and

$$E(Y_{2j}^S) = \mu_T + \mu_R + \lambda_T, \ Var(Y_{2j}^S) = \sigma_T^2 + \sigma_R^2 + 2\sigma_B^2, \ j = 1, \ldots, n_2.$$

Hence, calculating the period sums results in the following independent two-sample situation for normally distributed variables with identical variances:

$$Y_{1j}^S \sim N(\mu_T + \mu_R + \lambda_R, \sigma_*^2), \ j = 1, \ldots, n_1,$$
$$Y_{2j}^S \sim N(\mu_T + \mu_R + \lambda_T, \sigma_*^2), \ j = 1, \ldots, n_2,$$
$$\text{where } \sigma_*^2 = \sigma_T^2 + \sigma_R^2 + 2\sigma_B^2.$$

The corresponding means of the period sums for each sequence follow a normal distribution,

$$\overline{Y}_1^S \sim N\left(\mu_T + \mu_R + \lambda_R, \frac{\sigma_*^2}{n_1}\right)$$
$$\overline{Y}_2^S \sim N\left(\mu_T + \mu_R + \lambda_T, \frac{\sigma_*^2}{n_2}\right)$$

and hence, the difference in the means is normally distributed,

$$\overline{Y}_2^S - \overline{Y}_1^S \sim N\left(\lambda_T - \lambda_R, \sigma_*^2\left(\frac{1}{n_1} + \frac{1}{n_2}\right)\right).$$

Therefore, the difference in means, $\overline{Y}_2^S - \overline{Y}_1^S$, is an unbiased estimator of $\lambda = \lambda_T - \lambda_R$ and the corresponding two-sided $(1-\alpha)100\%$ confidence interval for the difference in carryover effects is

$$\left[\overline{Y}_2^S - \overline{Y}_1^S - t_{1-\alpha/2,n_1+n_2-2}\,\hat{\sigma}_*\sqrt{\frac{1}{n_1} + \frac{1}{n_2}}, \ \overline{Y}_2^S - \overline{Y}_1^S + t_{1-\alpha/2,n_1+n_2-2}\,\hat{\sigma}_*\sqrt{\frac{1}{n_1} + \frac{1}{n_2}}\right],$$

where

$$\hat{\sigma}_*^2 = \frac{1}{n_1 + n_2 - 2} \left(\sum_{j=1}^{n_1} \left(Y_{1j}^S - \overline{Y}_1^S \right)^2 + \sum_{j=1}^{n_2} \left(Y_{2j}^S - \overline{Y}_2^S \right)^2 \right).$$

The null hypothesis H_0 of no difference in carryover effects,

$$H_0: \lambda_T - \lambda_R = 0 \text{ vs. } H_1: \lambda_T - \lambda_R \neq 0,$$

can be rejected in favor of H_1 at significance level α, if

$$T_\lambda = \frac{\left| \overline{Y}_2^S - \overline{Y}_1^S \right|}{\hat{\sigma}_* \sqrt{\frac{1}{n_1} + \frac{1}{n_2}}} > t_{1-\alpha/2, n_1+n_2-2}.$$

It should be noted that the null hypothesis H_0 of no difference in carryover effects, i.e., $\lambda_T - \lambda_R = 0$, implies that $\lambda_T = \lambda_R = 0$. This follows directly from the constraint $\lambda_T + \lambda_R = 0$. Hence, the above null hypothesis of equality of carryover effects is equivalent to the null hypothesis of no carryover effects.

When assessing treatment effects, the fundamental assumption is the absence of carryover effects, which would again imply a reformulation of the test problem to ensure applicability of a direct test approach. For the sake of simplicity, it has been proposed to use a more liberal significance level for the above test, for example $\alpha = 0.10$; see also Jones and Kenward (2003) for a further discussion of this indirect approach. A direct approach for testing the absence of a relevant difference in carryover effects has been proposed by Wellek (2003). However, as discussed later in Chapter 4, carryover effects can be excluded in bioequivalence studies based on medical grounds since healthy volunteers are recruited and an adequate washout has to be chosen.

3.4.2.2   Test for difference in formulation effects

To test the difference in treatment effects, the intraindividual period differences Y_{ij}^P, $i = 1, 2, j = 1, \ldots, n_i$, of the observations between the first and second period are calculated as

$$Y_{1j}^P = Y_{1j1} - Y_{1j2}, \ j = 1, \ldots, n_1, \text{ in sequence 1,}$$

$$Y_{2j}^P = Y_{2j1} - Y_{2j2}, \ j = 1, \ldots, n_2, \text{ in sequence 2.}$$

The expected means and variances of these differences are

$$E(Y_{1j}^P) = E(Y_{1j1}) - E(Y_{1j2}) = \mu_R + \pi_1 - \mu_T - \pi_2 - \lambda_R$$

$$Var(Y_{1j}^P) = Var(Y_{1j1}) + Var(Y_{1j2}) - 2Cov(Y_{1j1}, Y_{1j2}) = \sigma_R^2 + \sigma_T^2 - 2\sigma_B^2, \ j = 1, \ldots, n_1,$$

and

$$E(Y_{2j}^P) = \mu_T + \pi_1 - \mu_R - \pi_2 - \lambda_T, \ Var(Y_{2j}^P) = \sigma_T^2 + \sigma_R^2 - 2\sigma_B^2, \ j = 1, \ldots, n_2.$$

Calculating the period differences results in the independent two-sample situation for normally distributed variables with identical variances:

$$Y_{1j}^P \sim N(\mu_R + \pi_1 - \mu_T - \pi_2 - \lambda_R, \sigma^2), \ j = 1, \ldots, n_1,$$
$$Y_{2j}^P \sim N(\mu_T + \pi_1 - \mu_R - \pi_2 - \lambda_T, \sigma^2), \ j = 1, \ldots, n_2,$$

where $\sigma^2 = \sigma_T^2 + \sigma_R^2 - 2\sigma_B^2$.

Due to the normality assumption, the distributions of the corresponding means of the period difference for each sequence are

$$\overline{Y}_1^P \sim N\left(\mu_R - \mu_T + \pi_1 - \pi_2 - \lambda_R, \frac{\sigma^2}{n_1}\right)$$

$$\overline{Y}_2^P \sim N\left(\mu_T - \mu_R + \pi_1 - \pi_2 - \lambda_T, \frac{\sigma^2}{n_2}\right)$$

and therefore,

$$\overline{Y}_2^P - \overline{Y}_1^P \sim N\left(2(\mu_T - \mu_R) - (\lambda_T - \lambda_R), \sigma^2\left(\frac{1}{n_1} + \frac{1}{n_2}\right)\right)$$

and if $\lambda_T - \lambda_R = 0$,

$$\overline{Y}_2^P - \overline{Y}_1^P \sim N\left(2(\mu_T - \mu_R), \sigma^2\left(\frac{1}{n_1} + \frac{1}{n_2}\right)\right).$$

Hence, the point estimator $\left(\overline{Y}_2^P - \overline{Y}_1^P\right)/2$ is an unbiased estimator of $\mu = \mu_T - \mu_R$ under the assumption of equal carryover effects, that is $\lambda_T = \lambda_R$, and the two-sided $(1-\alpha)100\,\%$ confidence interval for the difference in treatment effects is

$$\left[\frac{\overline{Y}_2^P - \overline{Y}_1^P}{2} - t_{1-\alpha/2, n_1+n_2-2}\frac{\hat{\sigma}}{2}\sqrt{\frac{1}{n_1} + \frac{1}{n_2}}, \frac{\overline{Y}_2^P - \overline{Y}_1^P}{2} + t_{1-\alpha/2, n_1+n_2-2}\frac{\hat{\sigma}}{2}\sqrt{\frac{1}{n_1} + \frac{1}{n_2}}\right],$$

where

$$\hat{\sigma}^2 = \frac{1}{n_1 + n_2 - 2}\left(\sum_{j=1}^{n_1}\left(Y_{1j}^P - \overline{Y}_1^P\right)^2 + \sum_{j=1}^{n_2}\left(Y_{2j}^P - \overline{Y}_2^P\right)^2\right).$$

Table 3.8 Sequence-by-period means for the *RT/TR* crossover design.

Sequence	Sample size	Period 1	Period 2
1 (*RT*)	n_1	$\overline{Y}_{1R1} = \frac{1}{n_1} \sum_{j=1}^{n_1} Y_{1j1}$	$\overline{Y}_{1T2} = \frac{1}{n_1} \sum_{j=1}^{n_1} Y_{1j2}$
2 (*TR*)	n_2	$\overline{Y}_{2T1} = \frac{1}{n_2} \sum_{j=1}^{n_2} Y_{2j1}$	$\overline{Y}_{2R2} = \frac{1}{n_2} \sum_{j=1}^{n_2} Y_{2j2}$

Under the assumption $\lambda_T = \lambda_R$, the null hypothesis H_0 of equality of treatment effects,

$$H_0 : \mu_T - \mu_R = 0 \text{ vs. } H_1 : \mu_T - \mu_R \neq 0$$

can be rejected at significance level α, if

$$T_\mu = \frac{\left| \dfrac{\overline{Y}_2^P - \overline{Y}_1^P}{2} \right|}{\dfrac{\hat{\sigma}}{2} \sqrt{\dfrac{1}{n_1} + \dfrac{1}{n_2}}} > t_{1-\alpha/2, n_1+n_2-2}.$$

The point estimator $\left(\overline{Y}_2^P - \overline{Y}_1^P \right) \Big/ 2$ can be expressed by the difference in the least squares means (LSMeans) for test and reference using the corresponding sequence-by-period means (see Table 3.8):

$$\frac{\overline{Y}_2^P - \overline{Y}_1^P}{2} = \overline{Y}_T - \overline{Y}_R$$

because

$$\overline{Y}_T = \frac{\overline{Y}_{1T2} + \overline{Y}_{2T1}}{2} = \frac{1}{2} \left(\frac{1}{n_1} \sum_{j=1}^{n_1} Y_{1j2} + \frac{1}{n_2} \sum_{j=1}^{n_2} Y_{2j1} \right)$$

$$\overline{Y}_R = \frac{\overline{Y}_{1R1} + \overline{Y}_{2R2}}{2} = \frac{1}{2} \left(\frac{1}{n_1} \sum_{j=1}^{n_1} Y_{1j1} + \frac{1}{n_2} \sum_{j=1}^{n_2} Y_{2j2} \right)$$

and

$$\frac{\overline{Y}_2^P - \overline{Y}_1^P}{2} = \frac{\overline{Y}_{2T1} - \overline{Y}_{2R2}}{2} - \frac{\overline{Y}_{1R1} - \overline{Y}_{1T2}}{2} = \frac{\overline{Y}_{1T2} + \overline{Y}_{2T1}}{2} - \frac{\overline{Y}_{1R1} + \overline{Y}_{2R2}}{2} = \overline{Y}_T - \overline{Y}_R.$$

Instead of using the LSMeans $\overline{Y}_T$ and $\overline{Y}_R$, the following simple means for test and reference may be applied:

$$\overline{Y}_T^* = \frac{1}{n_1 + n_2} \left(\sum_{j=1}^{n_1} Y_{1j2} + \sum_{j=1}^{n_2} Y_{2j1} \right)$$

$$\overline{Y}_R^* = \frac{1}{n_1 + n_2} \left(\sum_{j=1}^{n_1} Y_{1j1} + \sum_{j=1}^{n_2} Y_{2j2} \right)$$

and the expected means of these simple means, under the assumption of no difference in carryover effects, are

$$E(\overline{Y}_T^*) = \frac{1}{n_1 + n_2} \left(\sum_{j=1}^{n_1} E(Y_{1j2}) + \sum_{j=1}^{n_2} E(Y_{2j1}) \right)$$

$$= \frac{1}{n_1 + n_2} (n_1(\mu_T + \pi_2) + n_2(\mu_T + \pi_1))$$

and

$$E(\overline{Y}_R^*) = \frac{1}{n_1 + n_2} (n_1(\mu_R + \pi_1) + n_2(\mu_R + \pi_2)).$$

Thus, the expected mean of the difference $\overline{Y}_T^* - \overline{Y}_R^*$ is

$$E(\overline{Y}_T^* - \overline{Y}_R^*) = \frac{1}{n_1 + n_2} (n_1(\mu_T + \pi_2) + n_2(\mu_T + \pi_1) - n_1(\mu_R + \pi_1) - n_2(\mu_R + \pi_2))$$

$$= \frac{1}{n_1 + n_2} ((n_1 + n_2)(\mu_T - \mu_R) + \pi_1(n_2 - n_1) + \pi_2(n_1 - n_2))$$

$$= (\mu_T - \mu_R) + \frac{1}{n_1 + n_2} (\pi_1(n_2 - n_1) + \pi_2(n_1 - n_2)).$$

Hence, under the general assumption of equal carryover effects, and for balanced sample sizes, that is $n_1 = n_2$, or under the assumption of no period effects, that is $\pi_1 = \pi_2 = 0$, the difference in the simple means for test and reference is an unbiased estimator of the treatment difference. Obviously, for balanced sample sizes, the LSMeans for test and reference are equal to the corresponding simple means.

3.4.2.3 Test for difference in period effects

For testing the difference in period effects, the crossover differences Y_{ij}^C, $i = 1, 2, j = 1, \ldots, n_i$, of the observations between the first and second period are calculated as:

$$Y_{1j}^C = Y_{1j1} - Y_{1j2}, \; j = 1, \ldots, n_1, \text{ in sequence 1,}$$

$$Y_{2j}^C = Y_{2j2} - Y_{2j1}, \; j = 1, \ldots, n_2, \text{ in sequence 2.}$$

The expected means and variances of these differences are

$$E(Y_{1j}^C) = E(Y_{1j1}) - E(Y_{1j2}) = \mu_R + \pi_1 - \mu_T - \pi_2 - \lambda_R$$

$$Var(Y_{1j}^C) = Var(Y_{1j1}) + Var(Y_{1j2}) - 2Cov(Y_{1j1}, Y_{1j2}) = \sigma_R^2 + \sigma_T^2 - 2\sigma_B^2, \; j = 1, \ldots, n_1,$$

and

$$E(Y_{2j}^C) = \mu_R + \pi_2 + \lambda_T - \mu_T - \pi_1, \ Var(Y_{2j}^C) = \sigma_T^2 + \sigma_R^2 - 2\sigma_B^2, \ j = 1, \ldots, n_2.$$

Calculating the crossover differences results in the independent two-sample situation for normally distributed variables with identical variances:

$$Y_{1j}^C \sim N(\mu_R + \pi_1 - \mu_T - \pi_2 - \lambda_R, \sigma^2), \ j = 1, \ldots, n_1,$$
$$Y_{2j}^C \sim N(\mu_R + \pi_2 + \lambda_T - \mu_T - \pi_1, \sigma^2), \ j = 1, \ldots, n_2,$$
$$\text{where } \sigma^2 = \sigma_T^2 + \sigma_R^2 - 2\sigma_B^2.$$

The distributions of the means for the crossover differences are:

$$\overline{Y}_1^C \sim N\left(\mu_R - \mu_T + \pi_1 - \pi_2 - \lambda_R, \frac{\sigma^2}{n_1}\right)$$

$$\overline{Y}_2^C \sim N\left(\mu_R - \mu_T + \pi_2 - \pi_1 + \lambda_T, \frac{\sigma^2}{n_2}\right)$$

and, therefore

$$\overline{Y}_2^C - \overline{Y}_1^C \sim N\left(2(\pi_2 - \pi_1) + \lambda_T + \lambda_R, \sigma^2\left(\frac{1}{n_1} + \frac{1}{n_2}\right)\right)$$

$$\overline{Y}_2^C - \overline{Y}_1^C \sim N\left(2(\pi_2 - \pi_1), \sigma^2\left(\frac{1}{n_1} + \frac{1}{n_2}\right)\right),$$

because $\lambda_T + \lambda_R = 0$.

Hence, the point estimator $\left(\overline{Y}_2^C - \overline{Y}_1^C\right)\big/2$ is an unbiased estimator of $\pi = \pi_2 - \pi_1$, regardless of the presence of unequal carryover effects. The corresponding two-sided $(1 - \alpha)100\%$ confidence interval for the difference in period effects is

$$\left[\frac{\overline{Y}_2^C - \overline{Y}_1^C}{2} - t_{1-\alpha/2, n_1+n_2-2}\frac{\hat{\sigma}}{2}\sqrt{\frac{1}{n_1} + \frac{1}{n_2}}, \ \frac{\overline{Y}_2^C - \overline{Y}_1^C}{2} + t_{1-\alpha/2, n_1+n_2-2}\frac{\hat{\sigma}}{2}\sqrt{\frac{1}{n_1} + \frac{1}{n_2}}\right],$$

where

$$\hat{\sigma}^2 = \frac{1}{n_1 + n_2 - 2}\left(\sum_{j=1}^{n_1}\left(Y_{1j}^C - \overline{Y}_1^C\right)^2 + \sum_{j=1}^{n_2}\left(Y_{2j}^C - \overline{Y}_2^C\right)^2\right)$$

$$= \frac{1}{n_1 + n_2 - 2}\left(\sum_{j=1}^{n_1}\left(Y_{1j}^P - \overline{Y}_1^P\right)^2 + \sum_{j=1}^{n_2}\left(Y_{2j}^P - \overline{Y}_2^P\right)^2\right).$$

The null hypothesis H_0 of no difference in period effects,

$$H_0: \pi_1 - \pi_2 = 0 \ \text{vs.} \ H_1: \pi_1 - \pi_2 \neq 0$$

can be rejected at significance level α, if

$$T_\pi = \frac{\left| \dfrac{\overline{Y}_2^C - \overline{Y}_1^C}{2} \right|}{\dfrac{\hat{\sigma}}{2}\sqrt{\dfrac{1}{n_1} + \dfrac{1}{n_2}}} > t_{1-\alpha/2,\, n_1+n_2-2}.$$

The null hypothesis H_0 of no difference in period effects, i.e., $\pi_T - \pi_R = 0$, implies that $\pi_T = \pi_R = 0$, since $\pi_T + \pi_R = 0$.

3.4.3 Nonparametric analysis based on Wilcoxon rank sum tests

If the assumption of normality for the random variables is doubtful, the above t-tests to analyze the corresponding effects in the *RT/TR* design can be replaced by a nonparametric test procedure based on the Wilcoxon rank sum tests (Koch, 1972). As with the t-test for the parametric approach, the following nonparametric tests are based on period sums, period and crossover differences.

3.4.3.1 Test for difference in carryover effects

Let R_{2j}^S denote the rank of the period sum Y_{2j}^S, $j = 1, \ldots, n_2$, in the combined sample of size $n_1 + n_2$,

$$Y_{11}^S, \ldots, Y_{1n_1}^S, Y_{21}^S, \ldots, Y_{2n_2}^S$$

and let $R_2^S = \sum_{j=1}^{n_2} R_{2j}^S$ denote the sum of the ranks of the period sums for the second sequence in this joint ordering. The null hypothesis H_0 of no difference in carryover effects,

$$H_0 : \lambda_T - \lambda_R = 0 \text{ vs. } H_1 : \lambda_T - \lambda_R \neq 0$$

is rejected at significance level α, if

$$R_2^S \geq r_{1-\alpha/2,n_1,n_2} \text{ or } R_2^S \leq n_2(n_1 + n_2 + 1) - r_{1-\alpha/2,n_1,n_2},$$

where $r_{1-\alpha/2,n_1,n_2}$ denotes the $(1-\alpha/2)$ quantile of the Wilcoxon test statistic. The $(1-\alpha/2)$ quantiles are tabulated for different sample sizes in Hollander and Wolfe (1999).

The nonparametric point estimate and the corresponding two-sided $(1-\alpha)100\%$ confidence interval for $\lambda = \lambda_T - \lambda_R$ are calculated as follows. From the n_2 period sums, Y_{2j}^S, in the second sequence and the n_1 period sums, Y_{1j}^S, in the first sequence, $n_1 n_2$ pairwise differences, $D_k^S = Y_{2j*}^S - Y_{1j}^S$, $j* = 1, \ldots, n_2$, $j = 1, \ldots, n_1$, $k = 1, \ldots, n_1 n_2$, are calculated and ranked according to magnitude:

$$D_1^S \leq D_2^S \leq \cdots \leq D_{n_1 n_2}^S.$$

The nonparametric Hodges–Lehmann estimator (Hollander and Wolfe, 1999) of $\lambda = \lambda_T - \lambda_R$ is the median of the ranked differences D_k^S, $k = 1, \ldots, n_1 n_2$,

$$\hat{\lambda} = \begin{cases} D_{m+1}^S \text{ for } n_1 n_2 = 2m + 1 \\ \dfrac{D_m^S + D_{m+1}^S}{2} \text{ for } n_1 n_2 = 2m. \end{cases}$$

The nonparametric two-sided $(1 - \alpha)100\%$ confidence interval for $\lambda = \lambda_T - \lambda_R$ according to Moses (Hollander and Wolfe, 1999) is

$$[L_\lambda, U_\lambda],$$

where

$$L_\lambda = D_{C_{1-\alpha/2}}^S \text{ and } U_\lambda = D_{n_1 n_2 + 1 - C_{1-\alpha/2}}^S$$

and

$$C_{1-\alpha/2} = \frac{n_2(2n_1 + n_2 + 1)}{2} + 1 - r_{1-\alpha/2, n_1, n_2}.$$

3.4.3.2   Test for difference in formulation effects

The nonparametric test procedure for the treatment difference is based on the ranks R_{2j}^P of the period differences Y_{2j}^P, $j = 1, \ldots, n_2$, in the combined sample of size $n_1 + n_2$,

$$Y_{11}^P, \ldots, Y_{1n_1}^P, Y_{21}^P, \ldots, Y_{2n_2}^P$$

and $R_2^P = \sum_{j=1}^{n_2} R_{2j}^P$ denotes the sum of these ranks of the period differences. Under the assumption $\lambda_T = \lambda_R$, the null hypothesis of equality of treatment effects,

$$H_0 : \mu_T - \mu_R = 0 \text{ vs. } H_1 : \mu_T - \mu_R \neq 0$$

is rejected at significance level α, if

$$R_2^P \geq r_{1-\alpha/2, n_1, n_2} \text{ or } R_2^P \leq n_2(n_1 + n_2 + 1) - r_{1-\alpha/2, n_1, n_2}.$$

The nonparametric point estimate and the corresponding two-sided $(1 - \alpha)100\%$ confidence interval for the difference in treatment effects $\mu = \mu_T - \mu_R$ are calculated from the n_2 period differences, Y_{2j}^P, in the second sequence and the n_1 period differences, Y_{1j}^P, in the first sequence and the ranked $n_1 n_2$ pairwise differences $D_k^P = Y_{2j*}^P - Y_{1j}^P$, $j^* = 1, \ldots, n_2$, $j = 1, \ldots, n_1$, $k = 1, \ldots, n_1 n_2$,

$$D_1^P \leq D_2^P \leq \cdots \leq D_{n_1 n_2}^P.$$

The nonparametric Hodges–Lehmann estimator of $\mu = \mu_T - \mu_R$ is half the value of the median of the ranked differences D_k^P, $k = 1, \ldots, n_1 n_2$,

$$\hat{\mu} = \begin{cases} \dfrac{1}{2} D_{m+1}^P & \text{for } n_1 n_2 = 2m + 1 \\[2mm] \dfrac{1}{2} \left(\dfrac{D_m^P + D_{m+1}^P}{2} \right) & \text{for } n_1 n_2 = 2m \end{cases}$$

and the nonparametric two-sided $(1 - \alpha) 100\,\%$ confidence interval for $\mu = \mu_T - \mu_R$ is

$$\left[\frac{L_\mu}{2}, \frac{U_\mu}{2} \right],$$

where

$$L_\mu = D_{C_{1-\alpha/2}}^P \quad \text{and} \quad U_\mu = D_{n_1 n_2 + 1 - C_{1-\alpha/2}}^P$$

and

$$C_{1-\alpha/2} = \frac{n_2(2n_1 + n_2 + 1)}{2} + 1 - r_{1-\alpha/2, n_1, n_2}.$$

3.4.3.3 Test for difference in period effects

The nonparametric Wilcoxon rank sum test for the period effects is based on the ranks R_{2j}^C of the crossover differences Y_{2j}^C, $j = 1, \ldots, n_2$, in the combined sample of size $n_1 + n_2$,

$$Y_{11}^C, \ldots, Y_{1n_1}^C, Y_{21}^C, \ldots, Y_{2n_2}^C$$

and $R_2^C = \sum\limits_{j=1}^{n_2} R_{2j}^C$ denotes the sum of the ranks of these crossover differences. The null hypothesis H_0 of no difference in period effects,

$$H_0: \pi_1 - \pi_2 = 0 \quad \text{vs.} \quad H_1: \pi_1 - \pi_2 \neq 0$$

is rejected at significance level α, if

$$R_2^C \geq r_{1-\alpha/2, n_1, n_2} \quad \text{or} \quad R_2^C \leq n_2(n_1 + n_2 + 1) - r_{1-\alpha/2, n_1, n_2}.$$

The nonparametric point estimate and the corresponding two-sided $(1 - \alpha) 100\,\%$ confidence interval for $\pi = \pi_2 - \pi_1$ are calculated from the n_2 crossover differences Y_{2j}^C, the n_1 crossover differences Y_{1j}^C and the ranked $n_1 n_2$ pairwise differences $D_k^C = Y_{2j*}^C - Y_{1j}^C$, $j^* = 1, \ldots, n_2$, $j = 1, \ldots, n_1$, $k = 1, \ldots, n_1 n_2$,

$$D_1^C \leq D_2^C \leq \cdots \leq D_{n_1 n_2}^C.$$

The nonparametric Hodges–Lehmann estimator of $\pi = \pi_2 - \pi_1$ is half the value of the median of the ranked differences D_k^C, $k = 1, \ldots, n_1 n_2$,

$$\hat{\pi} = \begin{cases} \dfrac{1}{2} D_{m+1}^C & \text{for } n_1 n_2 = 2m + 1 \\ \dfrac{1}{2} \left(\dfrac{D_m^C + D_{m+1}^C}{2} \right) & \text{for } n_1 n_2 = 2m. \end{cases}$$

The nonparametric two-sided $(1 - \alpha) 100\%$ confidence interval for $\pi = \pi_2 - \pi_1$ according to Moses is

$$\left[\frac{L_\pi}{2}, \frac{U_\pi}{2} \right],$$

where

$$L_\pi = D_{C_{1-\alpha/2}}^C \text{ and } U_\pi = D_{n_1 n_2 + 1 - C_{1-\alpha/2}}^C$$

and

$$C_{1-\alpha/2} = \frac{n_2(2n_1 + n_2 + 1)}{2} + 1 - r_{1-\alpha/2, n_1, n_2}.$$

References

Berger, R.L. and Hsu, J.C. (1996) Bioequivalence trials, intersection union tests and equivalence confidence sets. *Statistical Science* **11**, 283–319.

Committee for Proprietary Medicinal Products (2001) *Note for guidance on the investigation of bioavailability and bioequivalence*. EMEA, London.

Fieller, E. (1954) Some problems in interval estimation. *Journal of the Royal Statistical Society B* **16**, 175–85.

Fisher, R.A. (1935) *The design of experiments*. Oliver and Boyd, London.

Food and Drug Administration (1992) *Guidance on statistical procedures for bioequivalence studies using a standard two-treatment crossover design*. Division of Bioequivalence, Rockville, MD.

Food and Drug Administration (2001) *Guidance for industry. Statistical approaches to establishing bioequivalence*. Center for Drug Evaluation and Research, Rockville, MD.

Hauschke, D., Kieser, M., Diletti, E. and Burke, M. (1999) Sample size determination for proving equivalence based on the ratio of two means for normally distributed data. *Statistics in Medicine* **18**, 93–105.

Hills, M. and Armitage, P. (1979) The two-period cross-over clinical trials. *British Journal of Clinical Pharmacology* **8**, 7–20.

Hollander, M. and Wolfe, D.A. (1999) *Nonparametric statistical methods* (2nd edition). Wiley & Sons, New York.

Jones, B. and Kenward, M.G. (2003) *Design and analysis of cross-over trials* (2nd edition). Chapman & Hall, Boca Raton.

Koch, G.G. (1972) The use of non-parametric methods in the statistical analysis of the two-period changeover design. *Biometrics* **28**, 577–84.

Schuirmann, D.J. (1987) A comparison of the two one-sided tests procedure and the power approach for assessing the equivalence of average bioavailability. *Journal of Pharmacokinetics and Biopharmaceutics* **15**, 657–80.

Wellek, S. (2003) *Testing statistical hypotheses of equivalence*. Chapman & Hall, Boca Raton.

4

Assessment of average bioequivalence in the *RT/TR* design

4.1 Introduction

In this chapter we discuss the underlying methodology for adequate statistical assessment of average bioequivalence as given in the following example. Hence, consideration is given to correct model specification, to adequate formulation of the underlying test problem, and to the determination of parametric and nonparametric point estimates and corresponding confidence intervals.

The example refers to a dose equivalence study (Steinijans *et al.*, 1989), comparing a pellet formulation at the same daily dose, but administered at different dosage strengths. The study had been stipulated by a regulatory authority in order to demonstrate that no relevant differences are to be expected *in vivo*, when switching from the available dose strengths of 200 and 300 mg to a new dose strength of 500 mg. In this randomized two-period, two-sequence crossover study with a one-week washout period, different capsule sizes of theophylline sustained release pellets were compared in 18 healthy male volunteers. Drug administration with 200 mg of tap water was 30 min after a standardized evening meal. Two capsules each of 200 and 300 mg theophylline served as reference, two capsules of 500 mg theophylline as test, all containing identical beads. In the acute part of the study, i.e., after the administration of the first dose, blood samples for the determination of theophylline in plasma were taken prior to and 1, 2, 3, 4, 5, 6, 8, 10, 12, 14, 16, 18, 20, 22, 24, 28, 36, 40, 44 and 48 hours after the evening administration. The linear trapezoidal rule was used to calculate the *AUC* up to 48 h, which was then extrapolated to infinity by means of the terminal monoexponential concentration-time curve.

Bioequivalence Studies in Drug Development: Methods and Applications   D. Hauschke, V. Steinijans and I. Pigeot
© 2007 John Wiley & Sons, Ltd

The subject numbers, treatment sequences, individual values of the characteristic $AUC = AUC(0 - \infty)$ and analysis of variance for the AUC under the assumption of a multiplicative model are given in Table 4.1; in addition, the within- and between-subject coefficients of variation and corresponding geometric means are derived. The analysis indicates a significant subject effect which reflects interindividual differences in clearance and hence in AUC. It also indicates no significant differences between formulations, sequences and periods. Additionally, the parametric and nonparametric point estimates and the corresponding 90 % confidence intervals are given for the ratio of expected means, $\exp(\mu_T)/\exp(\mu_R)$. The results reveal that with respect to the extent of absorption, equivalence can be concluded.

Figure 4.1 shows the sequence-by-period plot for the extent characteristic AUC. The results are given separately for each sequence in each period as geometric mean and the range corresponding to ± 1 standard deviation in the logarithmically transformed domain. The AUC values in the treatment sequence RT are higher than in the other

Table 4.1 Bioequivalence analysis for the primary extent characteristic $AUC(0 - \infty)$ $(\text{mg/L} \cdot \text{h})$ based on a multiplicative model, i.e., logarithmic transformation prior to data analysis. The subject numbers, treatment sequences and individual $AUCs$ are presented; Reference: $2 \cdot 200\,\text{mg} + 2 \cdot 300\,\text{mg}$ theophylline, Test: $2 \cdot 500\,\text{mg}$ theophylline. The analysis of variance, geometric means, as well as the parametric and nonparametric point estimates and 90 % confidence intervals are given for the ratio of expected means $\exp(\mu_T)/\exp(\mu_R)$.

Subject number	Sequence	Period 1	Period 2
1	*TR*	228.04	288.79
2	*RT*	339.03	329.76
3	*TR*	288.21	343.37
4	*RT*	242.64	258.19
5	*RT*	249.94	201.56
6	*TR*	217.97	225.77
7	*TR*	133.13	235.89
8	*RT*	184.32	249.64
9	*TR*	213.78	215.14
10	*TR*	248.98	245.48
11	*TR*	163.93	134.89
12	*RT*	209.30	231.98
13	*RT*	207.40	234.19
14	*TR*	245.92	223.39
15	*RT*	239.84	241.25
16	*RT*	211.24	255.60
17	*TR*	188.05	169.70
18	*RT*	230.36	256.55

Analysis of variance after logarithmic transformation of the individual *AUCs*.

Source of variation	Degrees of freedom	Sum of squares	Mean square	F-test	P-value
Between-subject					
Sequence	1	0.096373	0.096373	1.39	0.2561
Subject(sequence)	16	1.111719	0.069482	3.71	0.0063
Within-subject					
Formulation	1	0.000032	0.000032	0.00	0.9673
Period	1	0.044667	0.044667	2.38	0.1422
Residual	16	0.299892	0.018743		
Total	35	1.552683			

Between-subject $C\hat{V}_B = 16\%$, within-subject $C\hat{V}_W = 13.8\%$.

Geometric mean and 68 % range, i.e., $[\exp(\text{mean}(\ln AUC) - \text{sd}(\ln AUC)),$
$\exp(\text{mean}(\ln AUC) + \text{sd}(\ln AUC))]$.

	Period 1 Geometric mean	Period 2 Geometric mean	Both periods Geometric mean and 68 % range
Reference	231.64	224.11	227.84 [181.40, 286.18]
Test	209.26	249.02	228.28 [188.70, 276.16]

Point estimate and 90 % confidence interval for the ratio of expected means $\exp(\mu_T)/\exp(\mu_R)$.

Statistical method		Point estimate	Confidence limits lower	upper	Level of confidence
Parametric analysis	Two one-sided t-tests	1.00	0.925	1.085	0.90
Nonparametric analysis	Two one-sided Wilcoxon tests	1.03	0.942	1.097	0.9061

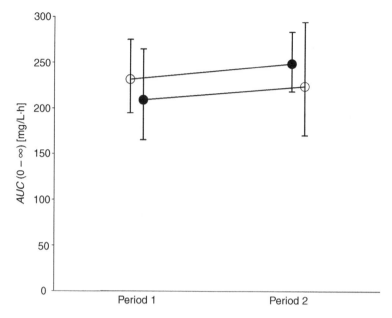

Figure 4.1 Sequence-by-period plot for the primary extent characteristic $AUC(0-\infty)$. The results are given separately for each sequence in each period as geometric mean and the range corresponding to ± 1 standard deviation in the logarithmically transformed domain, i.e., $[\exp(\text{mean}(\ln AUC) - \text{sd}(\ln AUC)), \exp(\text{mean}(\ln AUC) + \text{sd}(\ln AUC))]$, ($\circ$ = Reference, $\bullet$ = Test).

sequence, irrespective of the formulation. This may reflect a clearance difference between the subjects in the two sequences.

4.2 The *RT/TR* crossover design assuming a multiplicative model

The most commonly used design for the pharmacokinetic comparison of two formulations of the same drug substance is the two-period, two-sequence crossover design. By removing the between-subject variability from the residual variation, the crossover is considered to be the design of choice for bioequivalence studies. Hence, the FDA (1992, 2001) and the CPMP (2001) recommend the use of a crossover design, unless a parallel design is more appropriate for valid scientific reasons. One reason would be that the investigated substance has an unusually long half-live. For such a drug, the duration of a crossover would be unduly prolonged, bringing into question the assumption of intraindividual invariance of clearance, and increasing the risk of subjects dropping out of the study. However, the parallel group design is rarely used in practice because the number of subjects required to achieve the same power is usually much larger than for a crossover.

In the two-period, two-sequence crossover design, subjects, whether patients or healthy volunteers, are randomly allocated to two treatment sequences. In the first sequence, subjects receive the reference formulation (R) and test formulation (T) in periods 1 and 2, respectively. In the second sequence, subjects receive the formulations in reverse order, that is the test formulation and reference formulation in periods 1 and 2, respectively. Between the two periods is a washout period of about 5 to 6 half-lives, which has to be specified as sufficiently long as to ensure that all traces of the drug have been removed. This is usually confirmed by evidence of undetectable levels of the drug in a sample that has been drawn immediately prior to administration of the second formulation. This standard two-period, two-sequence crossover design will be referred to as *RT/TR* design.

4.2.1 Multiplicative model and effects

Let sequences and periods be indexed by i and k, $i, k = 1, 2$, respectively, and n_i subjects are randomized to sequence i. Let X_{ijk} denote the outcome of the underlying pharmacokinetic characteristic on the jth subject in the ith sequence during period k; then the following multiplicative model (Liu and Weng, 1992) is considered:

$$X_{ijk} = \exp(\mu_h + s_{ij} + \pi_k + \lambda_c + e_{ijk}),$$

where μ_h is the effect of formulation h, where $h = R$ if $i = k$ and $h = T$ if $i \neq k$; π_k is the effect of the kth period; λ_c is the carryover effect of the corresponding formulation from period 1 to period 2, where $c = R$ if $i = 1, k = 2$, $c = T$ if $i = 2, k = 2$, and $\lambda_c = 0$ if $i = 1, 2, k = 1$. The term s_{ij} denotes the random effect of the jth subject in sequence i and e_{ijk} is the random error term for subject j in period k and sequence i. Table 4.2 shows the layout of the random variables X_{ijk}, $i, k = 1, 2$ and $j = 1, \ldots, n_i$.

Taking logarithms of the pharmacokinetic outcomes transforms the multiplicative model on the original scale to the corresponding additive model on the logarithmic scale

$$Y_{ijk} = \ln X_{ijk} = \mu_h + s_{ij} + \pi_k + \lambda_c + e_{ijk},$$

Table 4.2 Layout for the *RT/TR* crossover design on the multiplicative scale.

Sequence	Period 1	Period 2
1 (*RT*)	$X_{1j1} = \exp(\mu_R + s_{1j} + \pi_1 + e_{1j1})$ $j = 1, \ldots, n_1$	$X_{1j2} = \exp(\mu_T + s_{1j} + \pi_2 + \lambda_R + e_{1j2})$ $j = 1, \ldots, n_1$
2 (*TR*)	$X_{2j1} = \exp(\mu_T + s_{2j} + \pi_1 + e_{2j1})$ $j = 1, \ldots, n_2$	$X_{2j2} = \exp(\mu_R + s_{2j} + \pi_2 + \lambda_T + e_{2j2})$ $j = 1, \ldots, n_2$

with the conditions for reparametrization $\pi_1 + \pi_2 = \lambda_R + \lambda_T = 0$. It is assumed that the subject effects s_{ij} are independent normally distributed with expected mean 0 and between-subject variance σ_B^2. The random errors e_{ijk} are independent and normally distributed with expected mean 0 and variances σ_{WT}^2 and σ_{WR}^2 for the test and reference treatment, respectively. Furthermore, the random terms s_{ij} and e_{ijk} are assumed to be mutually independent. Under these assumptions the formulation variances are given by $\sigma_T^2 = \sigma_B^2 + \sigma_{WT}^2$ and $\sigma_R^2 = \sigma_B^2 + \sigma_{WR}^2$. Note that the intraindividual observations within a sequence are not independent and the corresponding covariance is $\sigma_{TR} = \sigma_B^2$. Table 4.3 shows the layout of the random variables Y_{ijk}, $i, k = 1, 2$, $j = 1, \ldots, n_i$, and the corresponding expected means and variances are given in Table 4.4.

The between-subject variance σ_B^2 may result from physiological differences between the subjects, for example differences in clearance. In contrast to the parallel group design, the between-subject variance is removed from the residual term in crossover studies and, therefore, this parameter is only of minor interest in bioequivalence assessment.

The variances σ_{WT}^2 and σ_{WR}^2 cover within-subject variability, variability due to the random subject-by-formulation interaction and analytical error. Variation due to analytical error can be a problem if the plasma levels are close to the limit of quantification; this error can be examined by a repeated assay, but normally it is negligible in comparison to other sources of variation (Gaffney, 1992). The within-subject variability may be caused by changes in the external environment or changes in internal physiological parameters (e.g., due to circadian rhythms) or both (Alvares *et al.*, 1979). The random interaction

Table 4.3 Layout for the *RT/TR* crossover design on the additive scale, i.e., after logarithmic transformation.

Sequence	Period 1	Period 2
1 (*RT*)	$Y_{1j1} = \mu_R + s_{1j} + \pi_1 + e_{1j1}$ $j = 1, \ldots, n_1$	$Y_{1j2} = \mu_T + s_{1j} + \pi_2 + \lambda_R + e_{1j2}$ $j = 1, \ldots, n_1$
2 (*TR*)	$Y_{2j1} = \mu_T + s_{2j} + \pi_1 + e_{2j1}$ $j = 1, \ldots, n_2$	$Y_{2j2} = \mu_R + s_{2j} + \pi_2 + \lambda_T + e_{2j2}$ $j = 1, \ldots, n_2$

Table 4.4 Population means and variances for the *RT/TR* crossover design on the additive scale.

Sequence	Period 1	Period 2
1 (*RT*)	$E(Y_{1j1}) = \mu_R + \pi_1$ $Var(Y_{1j1}) = \sigma_R^2 = \sigma_B^2 + \sigma_{WR}^2$ $j = 1, \ldots, n_1$	$E(Y_{1j2}) = \mu_T + \pi_2 + \lambda_R$ $Var(Y_{1j2}) = \sigma_T^2 = \sigma_B^2 + \sigma_{WT}^2$ $j = 1, \ldots, n_1$
2 (*TR*)	$E(Y_{2j1}) = \mu_T + \pi_1$ $Var(Y_{2j1}) = \sigma_T^2 = \sigma_B^2 + \sigma_{WT}^2$ $j = 1, \ldots, n_2$	$E(Y_{2j2}) = \mu_R + \pi_2 + \lambda_T$ $Var(Y_{2j2}) = \sigma_R^2 = \sigma_B^2 + \sigma_{WR}^2$ $j = 1, \ldots, n_2$

component may be due to different variabilities of the two formulations or due to the existence of subgroups in the population. However, only replicated treatment designs permit the separate examination of the within-subject variability and the variability due to the random interaction (Gaffney, 1992; Ekbohm and Melander, 1989). In the standard two-period, two-sequence crossover design these variance components are confounded and it is not possible to separate them; consequently, they cannot be estimated separately. Thus, the variance component generally denoted as within-subject variability and estimated by the residual variance is composed of the true within-subject variability and the variability due to the subject-by-formulation interaction.

4.2.2 Test problem

Using the fact that if a random variable, Y, is normally distributed, i.e., $Y \sim N(\mu, \sigma^2)$, exponentiation, i.e., $X = \exp(Y)$, results in a lognormal distribution with expected mean $E(X) = \exp(\mu) \exp(\sigma^2/2)$ and median $M(X) = \exp(\mu)$. Expected means and medians of the random variables X_{ijk}, $i, k = 1, 2$, $j = 1, \ldots, n_i$, on the multiplicative scale can be calculated as in Table 4.5.

Let $\overline{X}_T$ and $\overline{X}_R$ denote the least squares means (LSMeans) on the multiplicative scale,

$$\overline{X}_T = \frac{1}{2}\left(\frac{1}{n_1}\sum_{j=1}^{n_1} X_{1j2} + \frac{1}{n_2}\sum_{j=1}^{n_2} X_{2j1}\right) \text{ and } \overline{X}_R = \frac{1}{2}\left(\frac{1}{n_1}\sum_{j=1}^{n_1} X_{1j1} + \frac{1}{n_2}\sum_{j=1}^{n_2} X_{2j2}\right).$$

The expected mean and median for the LSMean of test formulation on the multiplicative scale are:

$$E(\overline{X}_T) = E\left(\frac{1}{2}\left(\frac{1}{n_1}\sum_{j=1}^{n_1} X_{1j2} + \frac{1}{n_2}\sum_{j=1}^{n_2} X_{2j1}\right)\right)$$

$$= \frac{1}{2}\exp(\mu_T + \pi_2 + \lambda_R)\exp\left(\frac{\sigma_T^2}{2}\right) + \frac{1}{2}\exp(\mu_T + \pi_1)\exp\left(\frac{\sigma_T^2}{2}\right)$$

$$= \frac{1}{2}\exp(\mu_T)\exp\left(\frac{\sigma_T^2}{2}\right)\left(\exp(\pi_1) + \exp(\pi_2 + \lambda_R)\right)$$

Table 4.5 Layout of the population means and medians on the multiplicative scale.

Sequence	Period 1	Period 2
1 (RT)	$E(X_{1j1}) = \exp(\mu_R + \pi_1)\exp\left(\dfrac{\sigma_R^2}{2}\right)$ $M(X_{1j1}) = \exp(\mu_R + \pi_1)$ $j = 1, \ldots, n_1$	$E(X_{1j2}) = \exp(\mu_T + \pi_2 + \lambda_R)\exp\left(\dfrac{\sigma_T^2}{2}\right)$ $M(X_{1j2}) = \exp(\mu_T + \pi_2 + \lambda_R)$ $j = 1, \ldots, n_1$
2 (TR)	$E(X_{2j1}) = \exp(\mu_T + \pi_1)\exp\left(\dfrac{\sigma_T^2}{2}\right)$ $M(X_{2j1}) = \exp(\mu_T + \pi_1)$ $j = 1, \ldots, n_2$	$E(X_{2j2}) = \exp(\mu_R + \pi_2 + \lambda_T)\exp\left(\dfrac{\sigma_R^2}{2}\right)$ $M(X_{2j2}) = \exp(\mu_R + \pi_2 + \lambda_T)$ $j = 1, \ldots, n_2$

and

$$M(\overline{X}_T) = \frac{1}{2}\Big(\exp(\mu_T + \pi_2 + \lambda_R) + \exp(\mu_T + \pi_1) \Big)$$

$$= \frac{1}{2}\exp(\mu_T)\Big(\exp(\pi_1) + \exp(\pi_2 + \lambda_R) \Big).$$

In analogy, the expected mean and median for the mean of the reference can be derived as

$$E\left(\overline{X}_R\right) = \frac{1}{2}\exp\left(\mu_R\right)\exp\left(\frac{\sigma_R^2}{2}\right)\Big(\exp\left(\pi_1\right) + \exp\left(\pi_2 + \lambda_T\right)\Big),$$

$$M(\overline{X}_R) = \frac{1}{2}\exp(\mu_R)\Big(\exp(\pi_1) + \exp(\pi_2 + \lambda_T) \Big).$$

Calculating the ratios of the expected means and medians for the test and reference formulation results in

$$\frac{E(\overline{X}_T)}{E(\overline{X}_R)} = \frac{\dfrac{1}{2}\exp(\mu_T)\exp\left(\dfrac{\sigma_T^2}{2}\right)\Big(\exp(\pi_1) + \exp(\pi_2 + \lambda_R) \Big)}{\dfrac{1}{2}\exp(\mu_R)\exp\left(\dfrac{\sigma_R^2}{2}\right)\Big(\exp(\pi_1) + \exp(\pi_2 + \lambda_T) \Big)}$$

and

$$\frac{M(\overline{X}_T)}{M(\overline{X}_R)} = \frac{\dfrac{1}{2}\exp(\mu_T)\Big(\exp(\pi_1) + \exp(\pi_2 + \lambda_R) \Big)}{\dfrac{1}{2}\exp(\mu_R)\Big(\exp(\pi_1) + \exp(\pi_2 + \lambda_T) \Big)}.$$

Assuming that there is no difference in carryover effects, that is $\lambda_T - \lambda_R = 0$, which is equivalent to the assumption of no carryover effects $\lambda_T = \lambda_R = 0$ (see Section 3.4.2.1), a natural measure of average bioequivalence on the original scale (Mandallaz and Mau, 1981) is the following ratio of the medians which only depends on the formulation effects:

$$\frac{M(\overline{X}_T)}{M(\overline{X}_R)} = \frac{\dfrac{1}{2}\exp(\mu_T)(\exp(\pi_1) + \exp(\pi_2))}{\dfrac{1}{2}\exp(\mu_R)(\exp(\pi_1) + \exp(\pi_2))} = \frac{\exp(\mu_T)}{\exp(\mu_R)} = \exp(\mu_T - \mu_R).$$

Therefore, the parameter of interest in average bioequivalence testing is the ratio of medians

$$\frac{M(\overline{X}_T)}{M(\overline{X}_R)} = \frac{\exp(\mu_T)}{\exp(\mu_R)} = \exp(\mu_T - \mu_R).$$

In the traditional *RT/TR* crossover design it is assumed that the within-subject variances are independent of the formulation, $\sigma_{WT}^2 = \sigma_{WR}^2 = \sigma_W^2$, and that there are no carryover effects, resulting in the layout for the expected means and medians on the multiplicative scale as summarized in Table 4.6.

Under these assumptions, the ratio of expected means is equal to the ratio of medians

$$\frac{E(\overline{X}_T)}{E(\overline{X}_R)} = \frac{\frac{1}{2}\exp(\mu_T)\exp\left(\frac{\sigma_B^2 + \sigma_W^2}{2}\right)(\exp(\pi_1) + \exp(\pi_2))}{\frac{1}{2}\exp(\mu_R)\exp\left(\frac{\sigma_B^2 + \sigma_W^2}{2}\right)(\exp(\pi_1) + \exp(\pi_2))}$$

$$= \frac{\exp(\mu_T)}{\exp(\mu_R)} = \frac{M(\overline{X}_T)}{M(\overline{X}_R)}.$$

4.2.3 Estimation of the formulation difference

The difference of the least squares means for the test and reference formulation on the logarithmic scale can be calculated using the corresponding means of the period differences

$$\overline{Y}_T - \overline{Y}_R = \frac{\overline{Y}_2^P - \overline{Y}_1^P}{2},$$

where the intraindividual period differences Y_{ij}^P, $i = 1, 2$, $j = 1, \ldots, n_i$, of the observations between the first and second period are calculated as

$$Y_{1j}^P = Y_{1j1} - Y_{1j2}, j = 1, \ldots, n_1,$$
$$Y_{2j}^P = Y_{2j1} - Y_{2j2}, j = 1, \ldots, n_2.$$

Table 4.6 Layout of the expected means and medians on the multiplicative scale under the assumption of equal variances for test and reference formulation.

Period 1	Period 2
$E(X_{1j1}) = \exp(\mu_R + \pi_1)\exp\left(\frac{\sigma_B^2 + \sigma_W^2}{2}\right)$	$E(X_{1j2}) = \exp(\mu_T + \pi_2)\exp\left(\frac{\sigma_B^2 + \sigma_W^2}{2}\right)$
$M(X_{1j1}) = \exp(\mu_R + \pi_1)$	$M(X_{1j2}) = \exp(\mu_T + \pi_2)$
$j = 1, \ldots, n_1$	$j = 1, \ldots, n_1$
$E(X_{2j1}) = \exp(\mu_T + \pi_1)\exp\left(\frac{\sigma_B^2 + \sigma_W^2}{2}\right)$	$E(X_{2j2}) = \exp(\mu_R + \pi_2)\exp\left(\frac{\sigma_B^2 + \sigma_W^2}{2}\right)$
$M(X_{2j1}) = \exp(\mu_T + \pi_1)$	$M(X_{2j2}) = \exp(\mu_R + \pi_2)$
$j = 1, \ldots, n_2$	$j = 1, \ldots, n_2$

Table 4.7 Sequence-by-period means for the *RT/TR* crossover design.

Sequence	Sample size	Period 1	Period 2
1 (*RT*)	n_1	$\bar{Y}_{1R1} = \frac{1}{n_1} \sum_{j=1}^{n_1} Y_{1j1}$	$\bar{Y}_{1T2} = \frac{1}{n_1} \sum_{j=1}^{n_1} Y_{1j2}$
2 (*TR*)	n_2	$\bar{Y}_{2T1} = \frac{1}{n_2} \sum_{j=1}^{n_2} Y_{2j1}$	$\bar{Y}_{2R2} = \frac{1}{n_2} \sum_{j=1}^{n_2} Y_{2j2}$

Using the corresponding sequence-by-period means (Table 4.7), the difference can be formulated as

$$\frac{\bar{Y}_2^P - \bar{Y}_1^P}{2} = \frac{\bar{Y}_{2T1} + \bar{Y}_{1T2}}{2} - \frac{\bar{Y}_{1R1} + \bar{Y}_{2R2}}{2} = \bar{Y}_T - \bar{Y}_R,$$

because

$$\bar{Y}_1^P = \frac{1}{n_1} \sum_{j=1}^{n_1} Y_{1j1} - \frac{1}{n_1} \sum_{j=1}^{n_1} Y_{1j2} = \bar{Y}_{1R1} - \bar{Y}_{1T2}$$

$$\bar{Y}_2^P = \frac{1}{n_2} \sum_{j=1}^{n_2} Y_{2j1} - \frac{1}{n_2} \sum_{j=1}^{n_2} Y_{2j2} = \bar{Y}_{2T1} - \bar{Y}_{2R2}.$$

It was shown in Section 3.4.2.2 that

$$\bar{Y}_T - \bar{Y}_R = \frac{\bar{Y}_2^P - \bar{Y}_1^P}{2} \sim N\left(\mu_T - \mu_R + \frac{\lambda_T - \lambda_R}{2}, \frac{\sigma^2}{4}\left(\frac{1}{n_1} + \frac{1}{n_2}\right)\right),$$

where $\sigma^2 = \sigma_T^2 + \sigma_R^2 - 2\sigma_B^2$. Hence, under the assumption of equal carryover effects, that is $\lambda_T - \lambda_R = 0$, the difference of the LSMeans for test and reference formulations is an unbiased estimator of $\mu_T - \mu_R$, that is

$$E(\bar{Y}_T - \bar{Y}_R) = E\left(\frac{\bar{Y}_2^P - \bar{Y}_1^P}{2}\right) = \mu_T - \mu_R.$$

The corresponding estimator on the multiplicative scale after exponentiation of $\bar{Y}_T - \bar{Y}_R$ is

$$\exp(\bar{Y}_T - \bar{Y}_R)$$

$$= \exp\left(\frac{\bar{Y}_{1T2} + \bar{Y}_{2T1}}{2} - \frac{\bar{Y}_{1R1} + \bar{Y}_{2R2}}{2}\right)$$

$$= \exp\left(\frac{1}{2}\left(\left(\frac{1}{n_1}\sum_{j=1}^{n_1}\ln(X_{1j2}) + \frac{1}{n_2}\sum_{j=1}^{n_2}\ln(X_{2j1})\right) - \left(\frac{1}{n_1}\sum_{j=1}^{n_1}\ln(X_{1j1}) + \frac{1}{n_2}\sum_{j=1}^{n_2}\ln(X_{2j2})\right)\right)\right)$$

$$= \frac{\sqrt[2]{\sqrt[n_1]{\prod_{j=1}^{n_1} X_{1j2}}\ \sqrt[n_2]{\prod_{j=1}^{n_2} X_{2j1}}}}{\sqrt[2]{\sqrt[n_1]{\prod_{j=1}^{n_1} X_{1j1}}\ \sqrt[n_2]{\prod_{j=1}^{n_2} X_{2j2}}}}.$$

For a balanced design, that is $n_1 = n_2 = \dfrac{n}{2}$,

$$\exp\left(\overline{Y}_T - \overline{Y}_R\right) = \frac{\sqrt[n]{\prod_{j=1}^{n/2} X_{1j2}\ \prod_{j=1}^{n/2} X_{2j1}}}{\sqrt[n]{\prod_{j=1}^{n/2} X_{1j1}\ \prod_{j=1}^{n/2} X_{2j2}}} = \frac{\sqrt[n]{\prod_{j=1}^{n/2} X_{1j2}X_{2j1}}}{\sqrt[n]{\prod_{j=1}^{n/2} X_{1j1}X_{2j2}}}$$

which is the ratio of the geometric means for test and reference. However, it should be kept in mind that the ratio of these geometric means is not an unbiased estimate of $\exp(\mu_T - \mu_R)$, as

$$E(\exp(\overline{Y}_T - \overline{Y}_R)) = \exp(\mu_T - \mu_R)\exp\left(\frac{\sigma^2}{8}\left(\frac{1}{n_1} + \frac{1}{n_2}\right)\right) > \exp(\mu_T - \mu_R),$$

and $\exp\left((\sigma^2/8)\left(1/n_1 + 1/n_2\right)\right)$ is always greater than 1 for $\sigma^2 > 0$.

Hence, the ratio of geometric means always overestimates the parameter of interest, $\exp(\mu_T - \mu_R)$, and this amount may be substantial for large variances and small sample sizes (see Section 4.3.4).

Under the assumption of equal treatment variances, the variance of the estimator $\overline{Y}_T - \overline{Y}_R$ on the additive scale reduces to:

$$\sigma^2 = \sigma_T^2 + \sigma_R^2 - 2\sigma_B^2 = \sigma_B^2 + \sigma_W^2 + \sigma_B^2 + \sigma_W^2 - 2\sigma_B^2 = 2\sigma_W^2$$

and the distribution of the estimator $\overline{Y}_T - \overline{Y}_R$ is:

$$\overline{Y}_T - \overline{Y}_R \sim N\left(\mu_T - \mu_R, \frac{\sigma_W^2}{2}\left(\frac{1}{n_1} + \frac{1}{n_2}\right)\right).$$

4.3 Test procedures for bioequivalence assessment

4.3.1 Analysis of variance

In the traditional *RT/TR* crossover design it is assumed that the within-subject variances are independent of the formulations, $\sigma_{WT}^2 = \sigma_{WR}^2 = \sigma_W^2$, resulting in the analysis of variance table for the additive model given in Table 4.8.

The essential problem of the *RT/TR* crossover design concerns unbiased estimation of the formulation difference in the presence of different carryover effects, that is $\lambda_T \neq \lambda_R$. A failure to detect such an effect would lead to a biased estimate of the formulation difference. Therefore, Chow and Liu (2000) suggest performing a preliminary test for the presence of different carryover effects before comparing the formulations. The proposed strategy corresponds to the two-stage procedure of Grizzle (1965). If the result of the preliminary test is nonsignificant, e.g., *p*-value > 0.10, the conventional analysis for the crossover is performed assuming equal carryover effects. If the test is significant, the data from the second period are ignored and a two-sample *t*-test is performed using only the data from the first period. However, as Freeman (1989) has shown, the pretest is highly correlated with the analysis of formulation effects using only the data from the first period and, therefore, the actual significance level is higher than the nominal level even when there are no different carryover effects. Furthermore, the logic of the two-stage procedure is obviously false, because the failure to detect unequal carryover effects is not equivalent with the conclusion of equality in carryover effects (Senn, 1988).

Furthermore, carryover effects are confounded with sequence effects and treatment-by-period interaction. While different sequence effects per se would not bias the analysis, a difference in carryover effects and a treatment-by-period effect would lead to serious problems (Hauschke and Steinijans, 1997). In bioequivalence trials, carryover effects seldom occur if there is an adequate washout period between the periods. Furthermore, since healthy volunteers are recruited, their physical condition is unlikely to change from one period to another.

Therefore, in bioequivalence assessment, it is customary to include the factors formulation, subject, period and sequence in the multiplicative model

$$X_{ijk} = \exp(\mu_h + s_{ij} + \pi_k + v_i + e_{ijk}),$$

and the logarithmic transformation of the pharmacokinetic outcomes results in the corresponding additive model on the logarithmic scale

$$Y_{ijk} = \ln X_{ijk} = \mu_h + s_{ij} + \pi_k + v_i + e_{ijk}$$

where μ_h is the effect of formulation h, where $h = R$ if $i = k$ and $h = T$ if $i \neq k$; π_k is the effect of the kth period; v_i is the fixed sequence effect, $i, k = 1, 2$ and $j = 1, \ldots, n_i$; the usual reparametrization is applied to all fixed effects. It is assumed that the subject effects s_{ij} are independent normally distributed with expected mean 0 and between-subject variance σ_B^2, and e_{ijk} are independent and normally distributed with expected mean 0 and within-subject variances σ_W^2. The random terms s_{ij} and e_{ijk} are assumed to be

Table 4.8 Analysis of variance for the *RT/TR* crossover design including a carryover effect on the additive scale, i.e., after logarithmic transformation.

Source of variation	Degrees of freedom df	Sum of squares SS	Mean square $MS = SS/df$	Expected mean square	F-test
Between-subject					
Carryover	1	SS_{carry}	MS_{carry}	$r(\lambda_T - \lambda_R)^2 + 2\sigma_B^2 + \sigma_W^2$	$MS_{carry}/MS_{between}$
Residual	$n_1 + n_2 - 2$	$SS_{between}$	$MS_{between}$	$2\sigma_B^2 + \sigma_W^2$	$MS_{between}/MS_{within}$
Within-subject					
Formulation	1	SS_{form}	MS_{form}	$r((\mu_T - \mu_R) - (\lambda_T - \lambda_R)/2)^2 + \sigma_W^2$	MS_{form}/MS_{within}
Period	1	SS_{period}	MS_{period}	$r(\pi_2 - \pi_1)^2 + \sigma_W^2$	MS_{period}/MS_{within}
Residual	$n_1 + n_2 - 2$	SS_{within}	MS_{within}	σ_W^2	
Total	$2(n_1 + n_2) - 1$				

$r = \dfrac{2n_1 n_2}{n_1 + n_2}$

Table 4.9   Layout for the *RT/TR* crossover design on the additive scale in bioequivalence studies

Sequence	Period 1	Period 2
1 (*RT*)	$Y_{1j1} = \mu_R + s_{1j} + \pi_1 + v_1 + e_{1j1}$ $j = 1, \ldots, n_1$	$Y_{1j2} = \mu_T + s_{1j} + \pi_2 + v_1 + e_{1j2}$ $j = 1, \ldots, n_1$
2 (*TR*)	$Y_{2j1} = \mu_T + s_{2j} + \pi_1 + v_2 + e_{2j1}$ $j = 1, \ldots, n_2$	$Y_{2j2} = \mu_R + s_{2j} + \pi_2 + v_2 + e_{2j2}$ $j = 1, \ldots, n_2$

mutually independent. Table 4.9 shows the layout of the random variables Y_{ijk}, $i, k = 1, 2$, $j = 1, \ldots, n_i$.

The corresponding analysis of variance is given in Table 4.10. It should be noted that in practice, differences in formulations, sequences and periods are also termed as formulation, sequence and period effects, respectively. Obviously, the existence of a sequence effect has no influence on adequate assessment of the formulation effect.

The FDA guidance (1992) lists those conditions where the claim of bioequivalence is acceptable in the presence of a significant sequence effect. These conditions are those from which the possibility of a carryover effect or a treatment-by-period interaction can be eliminated:

'On the basis of these considerations, the Division of Bioequivalence has determined that an *in-vivo* standard two-treatment, two-period, two-sequence crossover bioequivalence study showing a statistically significant sequence effect may be acceptable provided

1. it is a single dose study

2. it includes only healthy, normal subjects

3. the drug is not an endogenous entity

4. more than adequate washout period has been allowed between the two phases of the study, and in the second phase, the predose biological matrix samples do not exhibit any detectable drug level in all subjects

5. the study meets all scientific and statistical criteria such as:

   - it is based upon an acceptable study protocol

   - it contains an acceptable validated assay methodology

   - appropriate statistical analyses of the data are performed

   - acceptable confidence intervals for the pharmacokinetic parameters are achieved.'

Table 4.10 Analysis of variance for the *RT/TR* crossover design including a sequence effect on the additive scale, i.e., after logarithmic transformation.

Source of variation	Degrees of freedom df	Sum of squares SS	Mean square $MS = SS/df$	Expected mean square	F-test
Between-subjects					
Sequence	1	SS_{seq}	MS_{seq}	$r(\nu_2 - \nu_1)^2 + 2\sigma_B^2 + \sigma_W^2$	$MS_{seq}/MS_{between}$
Subject(sequence)	$n_1 + n_2 - 2$	$SS_{between}$	$MS_{between}$	$2\sigma_B^2 + \sigma_W^2$	$MS_{between}/MS_{within}$
Within-subject					
Formulation	1	SS_{form}	MS_{form}	$r(\mu_T - \mu_R)^2 + \sigma_W^2$	MS_{form}/MS_{within}
Period	1	SS_{period}	MS_{period}	$r(\pi_2 - \pi_1)^2 + \sigma_W^2$	MS_{period}/MS_{within}
Residual	$n_1 + n_2 - 2$	SS_{within}	MS_{within}	σ_W^2	
Total	$2(n_1 + n_2) - 1$				

$r = \frac{2n_1 n_2}{n_1 + n_2}$

4.3.1.1   Example: Dose equivalence study

The Statistical Analysis System (SAS®, version 8.2, SAS Institute) is used to perform the analysis of variance for *AUC* in the dose equivalence study described in the introduction of this chapter. The following SAS® code, for the procedure 'proc glm', is used:

> *proc glm data=dose_equivalence;*
> > *class subject sequence period formulation;*
> > *model logAUC=sequence subject(sequence) period formulation;*
> > *random subject(sequence) / test;*
> > *run;*

and the corresponding output is provided in Table 4.11.

The results indicate no significant sequence effect (p-value = 0.2561) but a significant subject effect (p-value = 0.0063) which reflects interindividual differences in clearance and hence in *AUC*. Furthermore, the calculation reveals no significant period effect p-value = 0.1422) and no formulation effect (p-value = 0.9673). However, it should be noted that the test for formulation effect refers to the indirect test problem of equality of expected means versus difference in expected means,

$$H_0 : \exp(\mu_T) = \exp(\mu_R) \quad \text{vs.} \quad H_1 : \exp(\mu_T) \neq \exp(\mu_R)$$

and hence, this testing procedure cannot be used for equivalence assessment. The correct method will be presented in Section 4.3.2.

The estimate for the residual variance is $\hat{\sigma}_W^2 = MS_{within} = 0.018743$. For purposes of interpretation, it is more convenient to express the variability in terms of the coefficient of variation on the multiplicative scale (Hauschke *et al.*, 1994). It should be noted that due to the assumption of a lognormal distribution, the coefficient of variation is only a function of the corresponding variance. Under the assumption of equal treatment variances, the within-subject coefficient of variation CV_W is defined as

$$CV_W = \sqrt{\exp(\sigma_W^2) - 1}$$

and estimated by

$$C\hat{V}_W = \sqrt{\exp(MS_{within}) - 1}.$$

Whenever the square of coefficient of variation is small, $\ln(1 + CV_W^2) \approx CV_W^2$ holds; hence, in this case the square of coefficient of variation can be directly estimated via $C\hat{V}_W = \hat{\sigma}_W = \sqrt{MS_{within}}$. For example, the residual variance in the dose equivalence study is $\hat{\sigma}_W^2 = MS_{within} = 0.018743$ and corresponds to the within-subject coefficient of variation

$$C\hat{V}_W = \sqrt{\exp(MS_{within}) - 1}$$

$$= \sqrt{\exp(0.018743) - 1} = \sqrt{1.0189 - 1} = 0.138 \text{ or } 13.8 \text{ \%}.$$

Table 4.11   SAS® proc glm for the dose equivalence study.

```
data dose_equivalence;
  input subject sequence formulation $ period AUC;
  logAUC=log(AUC);
  datalines;
1     2  T  1  228.04
1     2  R  2  288.79
2     1  R  1  339.03
2     1  T  2  329.76
3     2  T  1  288.21
3     2  R  2  343.37
4     1  R  1  242.64
4     1  T  2  258.19
5     1  R  1  249.94
5     1  T  2  201.56
6     2  T  1  217.97
6     2  R  2  225.77
7     2  T  1  133.13
7     2  R  2  235.89
8     1  R  1  184.32
8     1  T  2  249.64
9     2  T  1  213.78
9     2  R  2  215.14
10    2  T  1  248.98
10    2  R  2  245.48
11    2  T  1  163.93
11    2  R  2  134.89
12    1  R  1  209.30
12    1  T  2  231.98
13    1  R  1  207.40
13    1  T  2  234.19
14    2  T  1  245.92
14    2  R  2  223.39
15    1  R  1  239.84
15    1  T  2  241.25
16    1  R  1  211.24
16    1  T  2  255.60
17    2  T  1  188.05
17    2  R  2  169.70
18    1  R  1  230.36
18    1  T  2  256.55
;
run;
```

Table 4.11   Continued.

```
proc glm data=dose_equivalence;
   class subject sequence period formulation;
   model logAUC=sequence subject(sequence) period formulation;
   random subject(sequence) / test;
   lsmeans formulation/pdiff cl alpha=0.1;
run;
quit;
```

The GLM Procedure

Class Level Information

Class	Levels	Values
subject	18	1 2 3 4 5 6 7 8 9 10 11 12 13 14 15 16 17 18
sequence	2	1 2
period	2	1 2
formulation	2	R T

Number of observations   36

The GLM Procedure

Dependent Variable: logAUC

Source	DF	Sum of Squares	Mean Square	F Value	Pr > F
Model	19	1.25279113	0.06593638	3.52	0.0071
Error	16	0.29989174	0.01874323		
Corrected Total	35	1.55268287			

R-Square	Coeff Var	Root MSE	logAUC Mean
0.806856	2.521469	0.136906	5.429611

Source	DF	Type I SS	Mean Square	F Value	Pr > F
sequence	1	0.09637288	0.09637288	5.14	0.0376
subject(sequence)	16	1.11171896	0.06948243	3.71	0.0063
period	1	0.04466680	0.04466680	2.38	0.1422
formulation	1	0.00003248	0.00003248	0.00	0.9673

Source	DF	Type III SS	Mean Square	F Value	Pr > F
sequence	1	0.09637288	0.09637288	5.14	0.0376
subject(sequence)	16	1.11171896	0.06948243	3.71	0.0063

```
period          1  0.04466680  0.04466680  2.38  0.1422
formulation  1  0.00003248  0.00003248  0.00  0.9673
```

The GLM Procedure

Source	Type III Expected Mean Square
sequence	Var(Error) + 2 Var(subject(sequence)) + Q(sequence)
subject (sequence)	Var(Error) + 2 Var(subject(sequence))
period	Var(Error) + Q(period)
formulation	Var(Error) + Q(formulation)

The GLM Procedure
Tests of Hypotheses for Mixed Model Analysis of Variance

Dependent Variable: logAUC

Source	DF	Type III SS	Mean Square	F Value	Pr > F
sequence	1	0.096373	0.096373	1.39	0.2561
Error	16	1.111719	0.069482		

Error: MS(subject(sequence))

Source	DF	Type III SS	Mean Square	F Value	Pr > F
subject(sequence)	16	1.111719	0.069482	3.71	0.0063
period	1	0.044667	0.044667	2.38	0.1422
formulation	1	0.000032479	0.000032479	0.00	0.9673
Error: MS(Error)	16	0.299892	0.018743		

Least Squares Means

formulation	logAUC LSMEAN	H0:LSMean1= LSMean2 Pr > |t|
R	5.42866089	0.9673
T	5.43056058	

formulation	logAUC LSMEAN	90% Confidence	Limits
R	5.428661	5.372323	5.484999
T	5.430561	5.374223	5.486899

Table 4.11   Continued.

Least Squares Means for Effect formulation			
		Difference	
		Between	90% Confidence Limits for
i	j	Means	LSMean(i)-LSMean(j)
1	2	-0.001900	-0.081574 0.077774

The approximation yields the following result:

$$C\hat{V}_W = \sqrt{MS_{within}} = \sqrt{0.018743} = 0.1369 \text{ or about } 13.7 \text{ \%}.$$

The between-subject variance σ_B^2 is also expressed by the between-subject coefficient of variation CV_B, defined as

$$CV_B = \sqrt{\exp(\sigma_B^2) - 1}$$

and estimated by

$$C\hat{V}_B = \sqrt{\exp\left(\frac{MS_{between} - MS_{within}}{2}\right) - 1}.$$

In the dose equivalence study the estimate of the between-subject coefficient of variation is

$$C\hat{V}_B = \sqrt{\exp\left(\frac{MS_{between} - MS_{within}}{2}\right) - 1}$$

$$= \sqrt{\exp\left(\frac{0.069482 - 0.018743}{2}\right) - 1} = 0.16 \text{ or } 16 \text{ \%}.$$

The power in a bioequivalence study, and hence the sample size, depends only on the within-subject coefficient of variation (see Chapter 5). Nevertheless, the calculation of the between-subject coefficient of variation allows a clinical interpretation, e.g., large values of CV_B may have implications with regard to individualized dosing (Hauschke *et al.*, 1994).

4.3.2   Two one-sided *t*-tests and $(1 - 2\alpha)100\ \%$ confidence interval

Let $\exp(\mu_T)/\exp(\mu_R) = \exp(\mu_T - \mu_R)$ be the ratio of the expected median values of the test and the reference formulation on the original scale. As shown in Section 4.2.2, under the assumption of equal formulation variances and no carryover effects, the ratio of medians is equal to the ratio of means on the original scale. If the equivalence range is denoted by (θ_1, θ_2), where $0 < \theta_1 < 1 < \theta_2$, then the following test problem for equivalence is considered:

$$H_0 : \exp(\mu_T - \mu_R) \leq \theta_1 \ \text{ or } \ \exp(\mu_T - \mu_R) \geq \theta_2$$

vs.

$$H_1 : \theta_1 < \exp(\mu_T - \mu_R) < \theta_2.$$

After logarithmic transformation, the above test problem becomes

$$H_0 : \mu_T - \mu_R \leq \ln \theta_1 \ \text{ or } \ \mu_T - \mu_R \geq \ln \theta_2$$

vs.

$$H_1 : \ln \theta_1 < \mu_T - \mu_R < \ln \theta_2.$$

Testing this two-sided equivalence problem is equivalent to simultaneous testing of the following two one-sided hypotheses (two one-sided testing or TOST, Schuirmann, 1987):

$$H_{01} : \mu_T - \mu_R \leq \ln \theta_1 \quad \text{vs.} \quad H_{11} : \mu_T - \mu_R > \ln \theta_1$$

and

$$H_{02} : \mu_T - \mu_R \geq \ln \theta_2 \quad \text{vs.} \quad H_{12} : \mu_T - \mu_R < \ln \theta_2.$$

Equivalence can be concluded at significance level α, if both null hypotheses H_{01} and H_{02} are rejected at level α, that is

$$T_{\ln \theta_1} = \frac{\overline{Y}_T - \overline{Y}_R - \ln \theta_1}{\hat{\sigma}_W \sqrt{\frac{1}{2}\left(\frac{1}{n_1} + \frac{1}{n_2}\right)}} > t_{1-\alpha, n_1+n_2-2}$$

and

$$T_{\ln \theta_2} = \frac{\overline{Y}_T - \overline{Y}_R - \ln \theta_2}{\hat{\sigma}_W \sqrt{\frac{1}{2}\left(\frac{1}{n_1} + \frac{1}{n_2}\right)}} < -t_{1-\alpha, n_1+n_2-2},$$

where $t_{1-\alpha, n_1+n_2-2}$ is the $(1 - \alpha)$ quantile of the central *t*-distribution with $n_1 + n_2 - 2$ degrees of freedom, $\overline{Y}_T$ and $\overline{Y}_R$ are the least squares means of the test and reference treatment and $\hat{\sigma}_W^2$ is the mean square, MS_{within}, from the ANOVA after logarithmic transformation.

Rejection of H_{01} by $T_{\ln\theta_1}$ at level α implies that

$$\frac{\overline{Y}_T - \overline{Y}_R - \ln\theta_1}{\hat{\sigma}_W\sqrt{\frac{1}{2}\left(\frac{1}{n_1}+\frac{1}{n_2}\right)}} > t_{1-\alpha,n_1+n_2-2}$$

$$\Leftrightarrow \quad \overline{Y}_T - \overline{Y}_R - \ln\theta_1 > t_{1-\alpha,n_1+n_2-2}\,\hat{\sigma}_W\sqrt{\frac{1}{2}\left(\frac{1}{n_1}+\frac{1}{n_2}\right)}$$

$$\Leftrightarrow \quad \overline{Y}_T - \overline{Y}_R - t_{1-\alpha,n_1+n_2-2}\,\hat{\sigma}_W\sqrt{\frac{1}{2}\left(\frac{1}{n_1}+\frac{1}{n_2}\right)} > \ln\theta_1.$$

In analogy, rejection of H_{02} by $T_{\ln\theta_2}$ at level α implies that

$$\frac{\overline{Y}_T - \overline{Y}_R - \ln\theta_2}{\hat{\sigma}_W\sqrt{\frac{1}{2}\left(\frac{1}{n_1}+\frac{1}{n_2}\right)}} < -t_{1-\alpha,n_1+n_2-2}$$

$$\Leftrightarrow \quad \overline{Y}_T - \overline{Y}_R - \ln\theta_2 < -t_{1-\alpha,n_1+n_2-2}\,\hat{\sigma}_W\sqrt{\frac{1}{2}\left(\frac{1}{n_1}+\frac{1}{n_2}\right)}$$

$$\Leftrightarrow \quad \overline{Y}_T - \overline{Y}_R + t_{1-\alpha,n_1+n_2-2}\,\hat{\sigma}_W\sqrt{\frac{1}{2}\left(\frac{1}{n_1}+\frac{1}{n_2}\right)} < \ln\theta_2.$$

Thus, rejection of H_{01} and H_{02} at level α is equivalent to

$$\left[\overline{Y}_T - \overline{Y}_R - t_{1-\alpha,n_1+n_2-2}\,\hat{\sigma}_W\sqrt{\frac{1}{2}\left(\frac{1}{n_1}+\frac{1}{n_2}\right)},\ \overline{Y}_T - \overline{Y}_R + t_{1-\alpha,n_1+n_2-2}\,\hat{\sigma}_W\sqrt{\frac{1}{2}\left(\frac{1}{n_1}+\frac{1}{n_2}\right)}\right]$$

$$\subset (\ln\theta_1, \ln\theta_2).$$

Exponential transformation of the $(1-2\alpha)100\%$ confidence limits in the logarithmically transformed domain yields $(1-2\alpha)100\%$ confidence limits for the ratio of expected means $\exp(\mu_T - \mu_R)$ and the equivalent relationship:

$$\left[\exp\left(\overline{Y}_T - \overline{Y}_R - t_{1-\alpha,n_1+n_2-2}\,\hat{\sigma}_W\sqrt{\frac{1}{2}\left(\frac{1}{n_1}+\frac{1}{n_2}\right)}\right),\ \exp\left(\overline{Y}_T - \overline{Y}_R + t_{1-\alpha,n_1+n_2-2}\,\hat{\sigma}_W\sqrt{\frac{1}{2}\left(\frac{1}{n_1}+\frac{1}{n_2}\right)}\right)\right]$$

$$\subset (\theta_1, \theta_2).$$

Hence, the following common rule is applied in practice. Equivalence is concluded for the underlying pharmacokinetic characteristic at level α, if the $(1-2\alpha)100\%$ confidence interval for $\exp(\mu_T - \mu_R)$ is included in the bioequivalence range.

4.3.2.1 Example: Dose equivalence study

The parametric analysis will be illustrated using the data from the dose equivalence study (see Section 4.1). The formulation-by-period means, variances and the corresponding 68 % ranges (mean ± standard deviation) are defined by:

$$\bar{Y}_{1T2} = \frac{1}{n_1} \sum_{j=1}^{n_1} Y_{1j2}, \bar{Y}_{2T1} = \frac{1}{n_2} \sum_{j=1}^{n_2} Y_{2j1}$$

$$\hat{\sigma}_{1T2} = \frac{1}{n_1 - 1} \sum_{j=1}^{n_1} (Y_{1j2} - \bar{Y}_{1T2})^2, \ \hat{\sigma}_{2T1} = \frac{1}{n_2 - 1} \sum_{j=1}^{n_2} (Y_{2j1} - \bar{Y}_{2T1})^2$$

$$[\bar{Y}_{1T2} - \hat{\sigma}_{1T2}, \bar{Y}_{1T2} + \hat{\sigma}_{1T2}], [\bar{Y}_{2T1} - \hat{\sigma}_{2T1}, \bar{Y}_{2T1} + \hat{\sigma}_{2T1}]$$

for the test formulation and

$$\bar{Y}_{1R1} = \frac{1}{n_1} \sum_{j=1}^{n_1} Y_{1j1}, \bar{Y}_{2R2} = \frac{1}{n_2} \sum_{j=1}^{n_2} Y_{2j2}$$

$$\hat{\sigma}_{1R1} = \frac{1}{n_1 - 1} \sum_{j=1}^{n_1} (Y_{1j1} - \bar{Y}_{1R1})^2, \ \hat{\sigma}_{2R2} = \frac{1}{n_2 - 1} \sum_{j=1}^{n_2} (Y_{2j2} - \bar{Y}_{2R2})^2$$

$$[\bar{Y}_{1R1} - \hat{\sigma}_{1R1}, \bar{Y}_{1R1} + \hat{\sigma}_{1R1}], [\bar{Y}_{2R2} - \hat{\sigma}_{2R2}, \bar{Y}_{2R2} + \hat{\sigma}_{2R2}]$$

for the reference formulation. Empirical results for the dose equivalence study are given in Table 4.12. Exponential transformation of these results yields the corresponding sequence-by-period geometric means and 68 % ranges on the multiplicative scale. Table 4.13 shows the values for the dose equivalence study and these values are used to construct the sequence-by-period plot (Figure 4.1).

Table 4.12 Formulation-by-period means, standard deviations and corresponding 68 % ranges for the dose equivalence study on the additive scale, i.e., after logarithmic transformation.

Treatment	Period 1	Period 2
Test	$\bar{Y}_{2T1} = 5.3436$ $\hat{\sigma}_{2T1} = 0.23553$ $[\bar{Y}_{2T1} - \hat{\sigma}_{2T1}, \bar{Y}_{2T1} + \hat{\sigma}_{2T1}] =$ $[5.1081, 5.5791]$	$\bar{Y}_{1T2} = 5.5175$ $\hat{\sigma}_{1T2} = 0.13051$ $[\bar{Y}_{1T2} - \hat{\sigma}_{1T2}, \bar{Y}_{1T2} + \hat{\sigma}_{1T2}] =$ $[5.3870, 5.6480]$
Reference	$\bar{Y}_{1R1} = 5.4452$ $\hat{\sigma}_{1R1} = 0.17229$ $[\bar{Y}_{1R1} - \hat{\sigma}_{1R1}, \bar{Y}_{1R1} + \hat{\sigma}_{1R1}] =$ $[5.2729, 5.6175]$	$\bar{Y}_{2R2} = 5.4121$ $\hat{\sigma}_{2R2} = 0.27251$ $[\bar{Y}_{2R2} - \hat{\sigma}_{2R2}, \bar{Y}_{2R2} + \hat{\sigma}_{2R2}] =$ $[5.1396, 5.6847]$

Table 4.13 Formulation-by-period geometric means and corresponding 68 % ranges for the dose equivalence study on the multiplicative scale.

Treatment	Period 1	Period 2
Test	$\exp(\bar{Y}_{2T1}) = 209.2640$ $[\exp(\bar{Y}_{2T1} - \hat{\sigma}_{2T1}),$ $\exp(\bar{Y}_{2T1} + \hat{\sigma}_{2T1})]$ $= [165.3502, 264.8403]$	$\exp(\bar{Y}_{1T2}) = 249.0179$ $[\exp(\bar{Y}_{1T2} - \hat{\sigma}_{1T2}),$ $\exp(\bar{Y}_{1T2} + \hat{\sigma}_{1T2})]$ $= [218.5506, 283.7325]$
Reference	$\exp(\bar{Y}_{1R1}) = 231.6382$ $[\exp(\bar{Y}_{1R1} - \hat{\sigma}_{1R1}),$ $\exp(\bar{Y}_{1R1} + \hat{\sigma}_{1R1})]$ $= [194.9772, 275.1925]$	$\exp(\bar{Y}_{2R2}) = 224.1118$ $[\exp(\bar{Y}_{2R2} - \hat{\sigma}_{2R2}),$ $\exp(\bar{Y}_{2R2} + \hat{\sigma}_{2R2})]$ $= [170.6542, 294.3150]$

Calculation of the geometric means for both periods for test is done as follows:

$$\exp(\bar{Y}_T) = \exp\left(\frac{\bar{Y}_{1T2} + \bar{Y}_{2T1}}{2}\right) = \exp(5.4306) = 228.2772 \approx 228.28$$

and the geometric 68 % range is

$$[\exp(\bar{Y}_T - \hat{\sigma}_T), \exp(\bar{Y}_T + \hat{\sigma}_T)],$$

where

$$\hat{\sigma}_T^2 = \frac{1}{n_1 + n_2 - 2}\left((n_1 - 1)\hat{\sigma}_{1T2}^2 + (n_2 - 1)\hat{\sigma}_{2T1}^2\right)$$

$$= \frac{1}{16}(8 \times 0.0555 + 8 \times 0.0170) = 0.0363$$

and

$$\left[\exp(\bar{Y}_T - \hat{\sigma}_T), \exp(\bar{Y}_T + \hat{\sigma}_T)\right] = [188.70, 276.16].$$

In analogy, the calculation of the geometric mean and 68 % range for reference across both periods is

$$\exp(\bar{Y}_R) = \exp\left(\frac{\bar{Y}_{1R1} + \bar{Y}_{2R2}}{2}\right) = \exp(5.4287) = 227.8439 \approx 227.84$$

and

$$\left[\exp(\bar{Y}_R - \hat{\sigma}_R), \exp(\bar{Y}_R + \hat{\sigma}_R)\right] = [181.40, 286.18],$$

where

$$\hat{\sigma}_R^2 = \frac{1}{n_1 + n_2 - 2}\left((n_1 - 1)\hat{\sigma}_{1R1}^2 + (n_2 - 1)\hat{\sigma}_{2R2}^2\right)$$

$$= \frac{1}{16}(8 \times 0.0297 + 8 \times 0.0743) = 0.0520.$$

The point estimate of the parameter of interest, $\exp(\mu_T)/\exp(\mu_R) = \exp(\mu_T - \mu_R)$, is given as:

$$\exp(\bar{Y}_T - \bar{Y}_R) = \exp(5.4306 - 5.4287) = 1.0019 \approx 1.00,$$

which is equivalent to calculating the ratio of geometric means for test and reference on the multiplicative scale:

$$\exp(\bar{Y}_T - \bar{Y}_R)\frac{\sqrt[n]{\prod\limits_{j=1}^{n/2} X_{1j2}\prod\limits_{j=1}^{n/2} X_{2j1}}}{\sqrt[n]{\prod\limits_{j=1}^{n/2} X_{1j1}\prod\limits_{j=1}^{n/2} X_{2j2}}} = \frac{228.2772}{227.8439} = 1.0019 \approx 1.00.$$

Calculation of the $(1 - 2\alpha)100\%$ confidence interval,

$$\left[\bar{Y}_T - \bar{Y}_R - t_{1-\alpha, n_1+n_2-2}\hat{\sigma}_W\sqrt{\frac{1}{2}\left(\frac{1}{n_1} + \frac{1}{n_2}\right)}, \bar{Y}_T - \bar{Y}_R + t_{1-\alpha, n_1+n_2-2}\hat{\sigma}_W\sqrt{\frac{1}{2}\left(\frac{1}{n_1} + \frac{1}{n_2}\right)}\right]$$

requires specification of the significance level. According to regulatory requirements for bioequivalence, this value is set to $\alpha = 0.05$ and hence, the statistical assessment is based on the two-sided 90 % confidence interval. The $(1 - \alpha) = 0.95$ quantile, $t_{0.95, n_1+n_2-2} = t_{0.95, 16}$ of the central t-distribution with 16 degrees of freedom, is $t_{0.95, 16} = 1.7459$.

Table 4.11 provides the estimate $\hat{\sigma}_W = \sqrt{MSE_{within}} = \sqrt{0.01874323} = 0.1369$ and the 90 % confidence interval for $\mu_T - \mu_R$ is

$$\left[\bar{Y}_T - \bar{Y}_R - t_{1-\alpha, n_1+n_2-2}\hat{\sigma}_W\sqrt{\frac{1}{2}\left(\frac{1}{n_1} + \frac{1}{n_2}\right)}, \bar{Y}_T - \bar{Y}_R + t_{1-\alpha, n_1+n_2-2}\hat{\sigma}_W\sqrt{\frac{1}{2}\left(\frac{1}{n_1} + \frac{1}{n_2}\right)}\right]$$

$$= \left[5.4306 - 5.4287 - 1.7459 \times 0.1369\sqrt{\frac{1}{9}}, 5.4306 - 5.4287 + 1.7459 \times 0.1369\sqrt{\frac{1}{9}}\right]$$

$$= [-0.0778, 0.08158]$$

and hence, the 90 % confidence interval for $\exp(\mu_T - \mu_R)$ is

$$[\exp(-0.0778), \exp(0.08158)] = [0.925, 1.085].$$

It should be noted that the 90 % confidence interval for $\mu_R - \mu_T$ is provided by SAS®
using the additional statement

lsmeans formulation/pdiff cl alpha = 0.1;

reversing the signs and an exponential transformation of these results yields the above
90 % confidence interval.

The 90 % confidence interval for $\exp(\mu_T - \mu_R)$ is included in the equivalence range
of (0.80, 1.25) and therefore, equivalence with respect to the extent of absorption can be
concluded.

4.3.3 Two one-sided Wilcoxon rank sum tests and $(1 - 2\alpha)100$ % confidence interval

The nonparametric procedure according to Hauschke *et al.* (1990) is an alternative to the
parametric analysis proposed by Schuirmann (1987) and can be applied in conjunction to
increase robustness.

For equal formulation variances, equal carryover effects and a symmetrical distribution
on the additive scale for the underlying pharmacokinetic characteristic, the ratio of the
expected mean values of the test and the reference formulation on the multiplicative scale
is equal to the ratio of medians and hence the parameter of interest is

$$\frac{\exp(\mu_T)}{\exp(\mu_R)} = \exp(\mu_T - \mu_R) = \frac{E(X_T)}{E(X_R)} = \frac{M(X_T)}{M(X_R)}.$$

The test problem for equivalence can be written as

$$H_0 : \exp(\mu_T - \mu_R) \leq \theta_1 \text{ or } \exp(\mu_T - \mu_R) \geq \theta_2$$

vs.

$$H_1 : \theta_1 < \exp(\mu_T - \mu_R) < \theta_2.$$

This is equivalent to simultaneous testing of the following two one-sided hypotheses:

$$H_{01} : \mu_T - \mu_R \leq \ln \theta_1 \text{ vs. } H_{11} : \mu_T - \mu_R > \ln \theta_1$$

and

$$H_{02} : \mu_T - \mu_R \geq \ln \theta_2 \text{ vs. } H_{12} : \mu_T - \mu_R < \ln \theta_2.$$

As with the parametric method, the null hypothesis H_0 can be rejected at level α if
both one-sided null hypotheses H_{01} and H_{02} are rejected, each at level α, by the respective
Wilcoxon rank sum test (Hauschke *et al.*, 1990). The nonparametric test procedure is

also based on the intraindividual period differences $Y_{ij}^P, i = 1, 2, \quad j = 1, \ldots, n_i$, of the observations between the first and second period

$$Y_{1j}^P = Y_{1j1} - Y_{1j2}, \ j = 1, \ldots, n_1, \ \text{in sequence 1,}$$

$$Y_{2j}^P = Y_{2j1} - Y_{2j2}, \ j = 1, \ldots, n_2, \ \text{in sequence 2.}$$

Let $R_{2j}^P(2\ln\theta_1)$ denote the rank of the modified period difference $Y_{2j}^P - 2\ln\theta_1$, $j = 1, \ldots, n_2$, in the combined sample of size $n_1 + n_2$,

$$Y_{11}^P, \ldots, Y_{1n_1}^P, Y_{21}^P - 2\ln\theta_1, \ldots, Y_{2n_2}^P - 2\ln\theta_1$$

and $R_{2j}^P(2\ln\theta_2)$ denote the rank of $Y_{2j}^P - 2\ln\theta_2, j = 1, \ldots, n_2$, in the combined sample of size $n_1 + n_2$,

$$Y_{11}^P, \ldots, Y_{1n_1}^P, Y_{21}^P - 2\ln\theta_2, \ldots, Y_{2n_2}^P - 2\ln\theta_2,$$

where $R_2^P(2\ln\theta_1) = \sum_{j=1}^{n_2} R_{2j}^P(2\ln\theta_1)$ and $R_2^P(2\ln\theta_2) = \sum_{j=1}^{n_2} R_{2j}^P(2\ln\theta_2)$ denote the sums of the ranks, respectively. The null hypotheses H_{01} and H_{02} are rejected at significance level α, if

$$R_2^P(2\ln\theta_1) \geq r_{1-\alpha,n_1,n_2}$$

and

$$R_2^P(2\ln\theta_2) \leq n_2(n_1 + n_2 + 1) - r_{1-\alpha,n_1,n_2},$$

where $r_{1-\alpha,n_1,n_2}$ denotes the $(1 - \alpha)$ quantile of the Wilcoxon test statistic. The $(1 - \alpha)$ quantiles are tabulated for different sample sizes in Hollander and Wolfe (1999). In analogy to the parametric method, the following relationship between the two one-sided Wilcoxon tests and the associated nonparametric confidence interval holds true (Hauschke et al., 1990). Rejecting H_{01} and H_{02} by Wilcoxon rank sum tests at level α is equivalent to the inclusion of the corresponding nonparametric $(1 - 2\alpha)100\%$ confidence interval for $\mu = \mu_T - \mu_R$ in the range $(\ln\theta_1, \ln\theta_2)$.

The nonparametric $(1 - 2\alpha)100\%$ confidence interval for $\mu = \mu_T - \mu_R$ according to Moses, is calculated from the n_2 period differences Y_{2j}^P in the second sequence and the n_1 period differences Y_{1j}^P in the first sequence and the ranked $n_1 n_2$ pairwise differences $D_k^P = Y_{2j*}^P - Y_{1j}^P, j^* = 1, \ldots, n_2, j = 1, \ldots, n_1, k = 1, \ldots, n_1 n_2$,

$$D_1^P \leq D_2^P \leq \cdots \leq D_{n_1 n_2}^P.$$

The nonparametric Hodges–Lehmann estimator of $\mu = \mu_T - \mu_R$ is half the value of the median of the ranked differences D_k^P, $k = 1, \ldots, n_1 n_2$,

$$
\hat{\mu} = \begin{cases} \dfrac{1}{2} D_{m+1}^P & \text{for } n_1 n_2 = 2m + 1 \\[2ex] \dfrac{1}{2} \left(\dfrac{D_m^P + D_{m+1}^P}{2} \right) & \text{for } n_1 n_2 = 2m. \end{cases}
$$

The nonparametric two-sided $(1 - 2\alpha)100\%$ confidence interval for $\mu = \mu_T - \mu_R$ is given as

$$
\left[\frac{L_\mu}{2}, \frac{U_\mu}{2} \right]
$$

where

$$
L_\mu = D_{C_\alpha}^P \text{ and } U_\mu = D_{n_1 n_2 + 1 - C_\alpha}^P
$$

and

$$
C_\alpha = \frac{n_2(2n_1 + n_2 + 1)}{2} + 1 - r_{1-\alpha, n_1, n_2}.
$$

Exponential transformation of the $(1 - 2\alpha)100\%$ confidence limits in the logarithmically transformed domain yields $(1 - 2\alpha)100\%$ confidence limits for $\exp(\mu_T - \mu_R)$, the ratio of the expected means or medians of test and reference.

4.3.3.1   Example: Dose equivalence study

Calculation of the nonparametric point estimate and corresponding 90 % confidence interval will be illustrated using the data from the dose equivalence study. The $n_1 n_2 = 9 \times 9 = 81$ ordered differences D_k^P, $k = 1, \ldots, 81$, are listed In Table 4.14.

Table 4.14   Ordered pairwise differences for the dose equivalence study on the additive scale, i.e., after logarithmic transformation.

−0.7872,	−0.5998,	−0.5662,	−0.5099,	−0.4692,	−0.4644,	−0.4513,	−0.4506,	−0.3903,
−0.3814,	−0.2687,	−0.2639,	−0.2503,	−0.2303,	−0.2215,	−0.2028,	−0.2010,	−0.1741,
−0.1693,	−0.1333,	−0.1285,	<u>−0.1190</u>,	−0.1147,	−0.1130,	−0.1125,	−0.0722,	−0.0674,
−0.0629,	−0.0536,	−0.0456,	−0.0341,	−0.0293,	−0.0202,	−0.0136,	−0.0005,	0.0155,
0.0200,	0.0270,	0.0558,	0.0672,	<u>0.0677</u>,	0.0684,	0.0725,	0.0750,	0.0763,
0.0863,	0.0965,	0.1013,	0.1019,	0.1085,	0.1151,	0.1170,	0.1218,	0.1282,
0.1356,	0.1555,	0.1582,	0.1648,	0.1673,	<u>0.1843</u>,	0.1990,	0.2008,	0.2038,
0.2048,	0.2056,	0.2104,	0.2176,	0.2242,	0.2571,	0.2682,	0.2867,	0.2933,
0.2970,	0.2979,	0.3027,	0.3165,	0.3175,	0.3856,	0.3994,	0.4060,	0.4983

The nonparametric Hodges–Lehmann estimate $\hat{\mu}$, of $\mu = \mu_T - \mu_R$, is half the value of the median of the $9 \times 9 = 2 \times 40 + 1$ differences

$$\hat{\mu} = \frac{1}{2}D_{41}^P = \frac{0.0677}{2}$$

and the nonparametric estimate of $\exp(\mu_T - \mu_R)$ is $\exp(\hat{\mu}) = \exp(0.0677/2) = 1.034$.

The indices $(l, u) = (C_\alpha, n_1 n_2 + 1 - C_\alpha)$, corresponding to those of the ranked differences $D_k = Y_{2j*}^P - Y_{1j}^P$, $j^* = 1, \ldots, n_2, j = 1, \ldots, n_1, k = 1, \ldots, n_1 n_2$, that form the 90 % confidence limits are presented in Table 4.15 for total sample sizes of $n = n_1 + n_2 = 12$ to 36. Note that due to the discrete distribution of the Wilcoxon test, it is not possible to achieve the confidence level exactly. Therefore, the exact level of confidence is also given in Table 4.15.

For $n_1 = n_2 = 9$, the indices (l, u) are obtained as $(22, 60)$ and therefore,

$$L_\mu = D_{C_{0.05}} = D_l^P = D_{22}^P = -0.1190 \text{ and } U_\mu = D_{82-C_{0.05}}^P = D_u^P = D_{60}^P = 0.1843.$$

Thus, the nonparametric two-sided 90 % confidence interval for $\mu_T - \mu_R$ is

$$\left[\left(\frac{L_\mu}{2} \right), \left(\frac{U_\mu}{2} \right) \right] = \left[\left(\frac{-0.1190}{2} \right), \left(\frac{0.1843}{2} \right) \right].$$

Exponential transformation of these confidence limits yields the 90 % confidence interval for $\exp(\mu_T - \mu_R)$:

$$\left[\exp\left(\frac{L_\mu}{2} \right), \exp\left(\frac{U_\mu}{2} \right) \right]$$

$$= \left[\exp\left(\frac{-0.1190}{2} \right), \exp\left(\frac{0.1843}{2} \right) \right] = [0.942, 1.097]$$

and the exact confidence level of this interval is 0.9061.

4.3.3.2 Analysis of time to maximum concentration

Where there is no pharmacokinetic or other justification for a transformation of the pharmacokinetic characteristics, e.g., t_{max}, the characteristics are analyzed by an ANOVA assuming an additive model for the original observations with the usual assumptions for the fixed and random effects (see Section 4.3.1)

$$X_{ijk} = \mu_h + s_{ij} + \pi_k + v_i + e_{ijk}.$$

Table 4.15 Indices (l, u) for the construction of the nonparametric 90 % confidence intervals. Listed below each pair of indices is the exact confidence coefficient.

n_2	$n_1=6$	7	8	9	10	11	12	13	14	15	16	17	18
6	8, 29 0.9069	9, 34 0.9266	11, 38 0.9187	13, 42 0.9121	15, 46 0.9066	17, 50 0.9017	18, 55 0.9169	20, 59 0.9126	22, 63 0.9087	24, 67 0.9052	26, 71 0.9020	27, 76 0.9135	29, 80 0.9105
7	9, 34 0.9266	12, 38 0.9027	14, 43 0.9061	16, 48 0.9093	18, 53 0.9122	20, 58 0.9147	22, 63 0.9169	25, 67 0.9032	27, 72 0.9062	29, 77 0.9089	31, 82 0.9113	34, 86 0.9005	36, 91 0.9033
8	11, 38 0.9187	14, 43 0.9061	16, 49 0.9170	19, 54 0.9073	21, 60 0.9169	24, 65 0.9092	27, 70 0.9021	29, 76 0.9110	32, 81 0.9050	34, 87 0.9127	37, 92 0.9074	40, 97 0.9025	42, 103 0.9095
9	13, 42 0.9121	16, 48 0.9093	19, 54 0.9073	22, 60 0.9061	25, 66 0.9053	28, 72 0.9048	31, 78 0.9045	34, 84 0.9044	37, 90 0.9044	40, 96 0.9045	43, 102 0.9046	46, 108 0.9048	49, 114 0.9049
10	15, 46 0.9066	18, 53 0.9122	21, 60 0.9169	25, 66 0.9053	28, 73 0.9108	32, 79 0.9014	35, 86 0.9069	38, 93 0.9117	42, 99 0.9044	45, 106 0.9090	49, 112 0.9026	52, 119 0.9071	56, 125 0.9013
11	17, 50 0.9017	20, 58 0.9147	24, 65 0.9092	28, 72 0.9048	32, 79 0.9014	35, 87 0.9121	39, 94 0.9092	43, 101 0.9067	47, 108 0.9046	51, 115 0.9027	55, 122 0.9011	58, 130 0.9094	62, 137 0.9078
12	18, 55 0.9169	22, 63 0.9169	27, 70 0.9021	31, 78 0.9045	35, 86 0.9069	39, 94 0.9092	43, 102 0.9113	48, 109 0.9024	52, 117 0.9050	56, 125 0.9074	61, 132 0.9001	65, 140 0.9027	69, 148 0.9051
13	20, 59 0.9126	25, 67 0.9032	29, 76 0.9110	34, 84 0.9044	38, 93 0.9117	43, 101 0.9067	48, 109 0.9024	52, 118 0.9092	57, 126 0.9055	62, 134 0.9023	66, 143 0.9084	71, 151 0.9055	76, 159 0.9029
14	22, 63 0.9087	27, 72 0.9062	32, 81 0.9050	37, 90 0.9044	42, 99 0.9044	47, 108 0.9046	52, 117 0.9050	57, 126 0.9055	62, 135 0.9061	67, 144 0.9068	72, 153 0.9075	78, 161 0.9000	83, 170 0.9011
15	24, 67 0.9052	29, 77 0.9089	34, 87 0.9127	40, 96 0.9045	45, 106 0.9090	51, 115 0.9027	56, 125 0.9074	62, 134 0.9023	67, 144 0.9068	73, 153 0.9025	78, 163 0.9067	84, 172 0.9030	89, 182 0.9070
16	26, 71 0.9020	31, 82 0.9113	37, 92 0.9074	43, 102 0.9046	49, 112 0.9026	55, 122 0.9011	61, 132 0.9001	66, 143 0.9084	72, 153 0.9075	78, 163 0.9067	84, 173 0.9062	90, 183 0.9058	96, 193 0.9054
17	27, 76 0.9135	34, 86 0.9005	40, 97 0.9025	46, 108 0.9048	52, 119 0.9071	58, 130 0.9094	65, 140 0.9027	71, 151 0.9055	78, 161 0.9000	84, 172 0.9030	90, 183 0.9058	97, 193 0.9013	103, 204 0.9041
18	29, 80 0.9105	36, 91 0.9033	42, 103 0.9095	49, 114 0.9049	56, 125 0.9013	62, 137 0.9078	69, 148 0.9051	76, 159 0.9029	83, 170 0.9011	89, 182 0.9070	96, 193 0.9054	103, 204 0.9041	110, 215 0.9029

The following SAS® code can be used for calculating the ANOVA and the 90 %confidence interval:

proc glm data=dataset;
        class subject sequence period formulation;
        model characteristic=sequence subject(sequence) period formulation;
        random subject(sequence) / test;
        lsmeans formulation / pdiff cl alpha=0.1;
        run;

However, for the rate characteristic time to maximum concentration, t_{max}, the CPMP guideline (2001) strongly recommends the application of nonparametric techniques to the untransformed data. The parameter of interest is the difference of expected medians for test and reference

$$M(X_T) - M(X_R) = \mu_T - \mu_R.$$

The test problem for equivalence is again:

$$H_0 : \mu_T - \mu_R \leq \delta_1 \text{ or } \mu_T - \mu_R \geq \delta_2$$

vs.

$$H_1 : \delta_1 < \mu_T - \mu_R < \delta_2,$$

which is equivalent to simultaneous testing of the following two one-sided hypotheses:

$$H_{01} : \mu_T - \mu_R \leq \delta_1 \text{ vs. } H_{11} : \mu_T - \mu_R > \delta_1$$

and

$$H_{02} : \mu_T - \mu_R \geq \delta_2 \text{ vs. } H_{12} : \mu_T - \mu_R < \delta_2.$$

The equivalence range (δ_1, δ_2) is expressed in absolute values, for example in hours, and must be clinically determined (CPMP, 2001). As with the multiplicative model, the null hypothesis H_0 can be rejected at level α if both one-sided null hypotheses H_{01} and H_{02} are rejected, each at level α, by the respective Wilcoxon test. The nonparametric test procedure in the additive model is based on the period differences of the untransformed data,

$$X_{1j}^P = X_{1j1} - X_{1j2}, j = 1, \ldots, n_1,$$
$$X_{2j}^P = X_{2j1} - X_{2j2}, j = 1, \ldots, n_2.$$

Let $R_{2j}^P(2\delta_1)$ denote the rank of $X_{2j}^P - 2\delta_1$, $j = 1, \ldots, n_2$, in the combined sample of size $n_1 + n_2$,

$$X_{11}^P, \ldots, X_{1n_1}^P, X_{21}^P - 2\delta_1, \ldots, X_{2n_2}^P - 2\delta_1$$

and $R^P_{2j}(2\delta_2)$ is the rank of $X^P_{2j} - 2\delta_2$, $j = 1, \ldots, n_2$, in the combined sample of size $n_1 + n_2$,

$$X^P_{11}, \ldots, X^P_{1n_1}, X^P_{21} - 2\delta_2, \ldots, X^P_{2n_2} - 2\delta_2.$$

$R^P_2(2\delta_1) = \sum_{j=1}^{n_2} R^P_{2j}(2\delta_1)$ and $R^P_2(2\delta_2) = \sum_{j=1}^{n_2} R^P_{2j}(2\delta_2)$ denote the sums of the ranks, respectively. The null hypotheses H_{01} and H_{02} are rejected, if

$$R^P_2(2\delta_1) \geq r_{1-\alpha, n_1, n_2}$$

and

$$R^P_2(2\delta_2) \leq n_2(n_1 + n_2 + 1) - r_{1-\alpha, n_1, n_2},$$

where $r_{1-\alpha, n_1, n_2}$ denotes the $(1 - \alpha)$ quantile of the usual Wilcoxon test statistic. In analogy to the method based on the multiplicative model, the following relationship between the two one-sided tests and the confidence interval holds true: Rejecting H_{01} and H_{02} by Wilcoxon tests at level α is equivalent to the inclusion of the corresponding nonparametric $(1 - 2\alpha)100\%$ confidence interval for $\mu = \mu_T - \mu_R$ in the range (δ_1, δ_2). The nonparametric $(1 - 2\alpha)100\%$ confidence interval according to Moses for $\mu = \mu_T - \mu_R$, is calculated from the n_2 period differences X^P_{2j} in the second sequence and the n_1 period differences X^P_{1j} in the first sequence and the ranked $n_1 n_2$ pairwise differences $G^P_k = X^P_{2j*} - X^P_{1j}$, $j^* = 1, \ldots, n_2$, $j = 1, \ldots, n_1$, $k = 1, \ldots, n_1 n_2$,

$$G^P_1 \leq G^P_2 \leq \cdots \leq G^P_{n_1 n_2}.$$

The nonparametric Hodges–Lehmann estimator of $\mu = \mu_T - \mu_R$ is half the value of the median of the ranked differences G^P_k, $k = 1, \ldots, n_1 n_2$,

$$\hat{\mu} = \begin{cases} \dfrac{1}{2} G^P_{m+1} & \text{for } n_1 n_2 = 2m + 1 \\[2mm] \dfrac{1}{2} \left(\dfrac{G^P_m + G^P_{m+1}}{2} \right) & \text{for } n_1 n_2 = 2m \end{cases}$$

and the nonparametric two-sided $(1 - 2\alpha)100\%$ confidence interval is given as

$$\left[\frac{L_\mu}{2}, \frac{U_\mu}{2} \right]$$

where

$$L_\mu = G^P_{C_\alpha} \quad \text{and} \quad U_\mu = G^P_{n_1 n_2 + 1 - C_\alpha}$$

and

$$C_\alpha = \frac{n_2(2n_1 + n_2 + 1)}{2} + 1 - r_{1-\alpha, n_1, n_2}.$$

Again, Table 4.15 can be used for the calculation of the 90 % confidence limits for total sample sizes of $n = n_1 + n_2 = 12$ to 36.

4.3.4 Bioequivalence ranges

According to the CPMP (2001) guideline, bioequivalence can be concluded if the 90 % confidence interval lies within the acceptance range of (0.80, 1.25) for the relative bioavailability measure AUC. This is also the case for the rate characteristic C_{max} but in certain cases a wider interval of (0.75, 1.333) for C_{max} may be acceptable if it is based on sound medical grounds. The characteristic t_{max} should be analyzed based on untransformed data and the nonparametric 90 % confidence interval should lie within a clinically determined acceptance range. The bioequivalence standards required by the FDA (1992, 2001) are that the 90 % confidence interval for AUC and C_{max} must be within the equivalence range (0.80, 1.25).

In Canada (Health Canada, 1996), only the 90 % confidence interval for AUC is required to be within the interval (0.80, 1.25). With regard to C_{max}, the Canadian guideline requires merely that the point estimate and not the entire 90 % confidence interval has to be within the acceptance range of (0.80, 1.25). Hence, from a statistical point of view, the criterion for C_{max} is solely based on the ratio of geometric means for test and reference formulation. However, as shown in Section 4.2.3, this estimator is biased and in the following the extent of bias is investigated for small sample sizes and highly variable drugs.

Assuming a balanced design, that is $n_1 = n_2 = \frac{n}{2}$,

$$E\left(\exp(\overline{Y}_T - \overline{Y}_R)\right) = \exp(\mu_T - \mu_R)\exp\left(\frac{\sigma_W^2}{n}\right) > \exp(\mu_T - \mu_R),$$

because the term $\exp\left(\frac{\sigma_W^2}{n}\right)$ is always greater than 1 for $\sigma_W^2 > 0$. Using the relation $\sigma_W^2 = \ln(1 + CV_W^2)$, the above expression can be reformulated as

$$\exp(\mu_T - \mu_R)\exp\left(\frac{\sigma_W^2}{n}\right) = \exp(\mu_T - \mu_R)\exp\left(\frac{\ln(1 + CV_W^2)}{n}\right).$$

In Table 4.16, the term $\exp\left(\frac{\ln(1 + CV_W^2)}{n}\right)$ is calculated for various coefficients of variation $CV_W = 0.30, \ldots, 0.80$ and total sample sizes $n = 12, 16$.

For example, for $n = 12$ and $CV_W = 0.6$,

$$\exp\left(\frac{\ln(1 + CV_W^2)}{n}\right) = \exp\left(\frac{\ln(1 + 0.6^2)}{12}\right) = 1.026,$$

which implies an overestimation of about 2.6 %. Hence, the bias-corrected value of an empirical ratio of geometric means of 0.82 is 0.82/1.026 = 0.799. Thus, it becomes obvious that an erroneous decision in favor of equivalence would have been made based on the uncorrected geometric mean. However, an empirical value of 1.28 would have led to the decision of inequivalence while the bias-corrected value of 1.247 would have implied equivalence.

Table 4.16 Overestimation of the geometric means for different total sample sizes and coefficients of variation.

$CV_W(\%)$	Total sample size n	$\exp\left(\dfrac{\ln(1+CV_W^2)}{n}\right)$
30	12	1.007
	16	1.005
40	12	1.012
	16	1.009
50	12	1.019
	16	1.014
60	12	1.026
	16	1.019
70	12	1.034
	16	1.025
80	12	1.042
	16	1.031

Furthermore, from a statistical point of view the presentation of a point estimate should always be accompanied by a corresponding confidence interval. For example, for $n = 12$, $CV_W = 0.6$, and the above empirical ratios of geometric means of 0.82 and 1.28, respectively, the 90 % confidence intervals for $\exp(\mu_T - \mu_R)$ are

$$\left[\exp\left(\ln(0.82) - 1.65 \times \sqrt{\frac{\ln(1+0.6^2)}{6}}\right), \exp\left(\ln(0.82) + 1.65 \times \sqrt{\frac{\ln(1+0.6^2)}{6}}\right)\right]$$

$$= [0.56, 1.19]$$

and

$$\left[\exp\left(\ln(1.28) - 1.65 \times \sqrt{\frac{\ln(1+0.6^2)}{6}}\right), \exp\left(\ln(1.28) + 1.65 \times \sqrt{\frac{\ln(1+0.6^2)}{6}}\right)\right]$$

$$= [0.88, 1.86],$$

where 1.65 is the 95 % quantile from the standard normal distribution.

When assessing the point estimates together with the 90 % confidence intervals, a positive claim of equivalence for the rate of absorption might be difficult to reach not only from a statistical, but also from a regulatory, point of view.

In summary, for small sample sizes, highly variable drugs, and ratios of geometric means not far away from the acceptance limits 0.8 or 1.25, this procedure might lead to wrong decisions. Furthermore, it is not sufficient to focus solely on point estimates, ignoring the variability of the corresponding estimator. Hence, the Canadian requirement for the assessment of the rate characteristic C_{max} should be reconsidered by the regulatory authority.

4.4 Conclusions

The statistical analysis of two-period crossover bioequivalence studies has been consolidated through the work of Schuirmann (1987) and Hauschke *et al.* (1990). The decision in favor of bioequivalence is based on the inclusion of the classical 90 % confidence interval for the ratio of expected means in the respective bioequivalence range, assuming a multiplicative model. This decision is equivalent to the rejection of two one-sided hypotheses by means of two one-sided tests.

According to regulatory requirements, the primary analysis for pharmacokinetic characteristics following a multiplicative model, e.g., AUC and C_{max}, is the parametric analysis. However, the corresponding nonparametric analysis should be performed in conjunction, in order to demonstrate the robustness of the results. In the case of untransformed data such as t_{max}, the nonparametric procedure is recommended for the analysis.

References

Alvares, A.P., Kappas, A., Eiseman, J.L., Anderson, K.E., Patnaik, C.B., Pantuck, E.J., Hsiao, K.C., Garland, W.A. and Conney, A.H. (1979) Intraindividual variation in drug absorption. *Clinical Pharmacology and Therapeutics* **26**, 407–19.

Chow, S-C. and Liu, J-P. (2000) *Design and analysis of bioavailability and bioequivalence studies* (2nd edition). Marcel Dekker, New York.

Committee for Proprietary Medicinal Products (2001) *Note for guidance on the investigation of bioavailability and bioequivalence*. EMEA, London.

Ekbohm, G. and Melander, H. (1989) The subject-by-formulation interaction as a criterion of interchangeability of drugs. *Biometrics* **45**, 1249–54.

Food and Drug Administration (1992) *Guidance on statistical procedures for bioequivalence studies using a standard two-treatment crossover design*. Division of Bioequivalence, Rockville, MD.

Food and Drug Administration (2001) *Guidance for industry. Statistical approaches to establishing bioequivalence*. Center for Drug Evaluation and Research, Rockville, MD.

Freeman, P.R. (1989) The performance of the two-stage analysis of two-treatment, two-period crossover trials. *Statistics in Medicine* **8**, 1421–32.

Gaffney, M. (1992) Variance components in comparative bioavailability studies. *Journal of Pharmaceutical Science* **81**, 315–17.

Grizzle, J.E. (1965) The two-period change-over and its use in clinical trials. *Biometrics* **21**, 467–80.

Hauschke, D. and Steinijans, V.W. (1997) Crossover trials in bioequivalence assessment. In: Vollmar, J. and Hothorn, L. (eds) *Biometrics in the Pharmaceutical Industry*, 27–40, Gustav Fischer, Stuttgart.

Hauschke, D., Steinijans, V.W. and Diletti, E. (1990) A distribution-free procedure for the statistical analysis of bioequivalence studies. *International Journal of Clinical Pharmacology, Therapy and Toxicology* **28**, 72–8.

Hauschke, D., Steinijans, V.W., Diletti, E., Schall, R., Luus, H.G., Elze, M. and Blume, H. (1994) Presentation of the intrasubject coefficient of variation for sample size planning in bioequivalence studies. *International Journal of Clinical Pharmacology, Therapy and Toxicology* **32**, 376–8.

Health Canada (1996) *Guidance for industry. Conduct and analysis of bioavailability and bioequivalence studies. Part B: oral modified release formulations.* Ottawa.

Hollander, M. and Wolfe, D.A. (1999) *Nonparametric statistical methods* (2nd edition). Wiley & Sons, New York.

Liu, J-P. and Weng, C-S. (1992) Estimation of direct formulation effect under the log-normal distribution in bioavailability/bioequivalence studies. *Statistics in Medicine* **11**, 881–96.

Mandallaz, D. and Mau, J. (1981) Comparison of different methods for decision-making in bioequivalence assessment. *Biometrics* **37**, 213–22.

SAS Institute Inc., SAS Campus Drive, Cary, North Carolina 27513, USA.

Schuirmann, D.J. (1987) A comparison of the two one-sided tests procedure and the power approach for assessing the equivalence of average bioavailability. *Journal of Pharmacokinetics and Biopharmaceutics* **15**, 657–80.

Senn, S. (1988) Cross-over trials, carry-over effects and the art of self-delusion. *Statistics in Medicine* **7**, 1099–1101.

Steinijans, V.W., Sauter, R., Jonkman, J.H., Schulz, H., Stricker, H. and Blume, H. (1989) Bioequivalence studies: single vs multiple dose. *International Journal of Clinical Pharmacology, Therapy and Toxicology* **27**, 261–6.

5

Power and sample size determination for testing average bioequivalence in the *RT/TR* design

5.1 Introduction

The note for guidance on the investigation of bioavailability and bioequivalence (CPMP, 2001) requires that the number of subjects in the underlying crossover design be determined by the variability of the primary pharmacokinetic characteristic, the significance level, the power, and by the expected deviation from the reference. Furthermore, it is recommended that generally the minimum total sample size should be not less than 12 subjects.

Based on the earlier work of Owen (1965), Phillips (1990) addressed the issue of sample size determination under a standard *RT/TR* crossover design for the additive model assuming normality for the untransformed pharmacokinetic characteristic. Liu and Chow (1992) provided corresponding approximate formulas for sample size calculation.

However, international harmonization of guidelines for bioequivalence assessment (CPMP, 1991, 2001; FDA, 1992, 2001) has led to the acceptance of a multiplicative model for all concentration-related pharmacokinetic characteristics, which suggests a lognormal distribution in the case of a parametric analysis (see Chapter 4). Therefore, Diletti *et al.* (1991, 1992) derived sample sizes for the more relevant multiplicative model for various deviations from the reference and various within-subject coefficients of variation. The methodology is illustrated in this chapter for the balanced *RT/TR* crossover design, and sample sizes necessary to attain a power of at least 0.80 and 0.90 are presented under

Bioequivalence Studies in Drug Development: Methods and Applications   D. Hauschke, V. Steinijans and I. Pigeot
© 2007 John Wiley & Sons, Ltd

different assumptions. Additionally, the appropriateness of the corresponding approximate formulas according to Hauschke *et al.* (1992) is discussed.

Although the experienced biostatistician is able to perform power and sample size determination without off-the-shelf programs, software routines facilitate application of the techniques by less experienced researchers. nQuery Advisor® (Elashoff, 2005) is a statistical software package, which provides the user with the most commonly used procedures for power and sample size calculation. The application of this program is illustrated at the end of this chapter for sample size determination in bioequivalence studies. The applied algorithm corresponds to the exact method provided by Diletti *et al.* (1991).

5.2 Challenging the classical approach

Although the assumption of a lognormal distribution is widely accepted by regulatory authorities for all concentration-related characteristics (CPMP, 2001; FDA, 1992, 2001), Chow and Liu (2000), and recently Patterson and Jones (2006), reproduced the results of Phillips (1990) for the additive model under the normality assumption for the untransformed pharmacokinetic characteristics

$$X_{ijk} = \mu_h + s_{ij} + \pi_k + e_{ijk},$$

where i denotes the sequence, $i = 1, 2, j$ denotes the subjects within sequence i, $j = 1, \ldots, n_i$, π_k is the effect of the kth period, $k = 1, 2$, with the side condition $\pi_1 + \pi_2 = 0$, and μ_h is the effect of formulation, with $h = R$ if $i = k$ and $h = T$ if $i \neq k$. Sequence effects are not included in the model because these effects have no influence on the investigation of the formulation effect (see Section 4.3.1) and, therefore, they are not relevant for power and sample size determination (Hauschke and Steinijans, 1997). It is assumed that s_{ij} and e_{ijk} are independent normally distributed with expected means 0 and variances σ_B^2 and σ_W^2, respectively. Furthermore, s_{ij} and e_{ijk} are assumed to be mutually independent.

The test problem for equivalence,

$$H_0: \ \mu_T - \mu_R \leq \delta_1 \text{ or } \mu_T - \mu_R \geq \delta_2$$

vs.

$$H_1: \delta_1 < \mu_T - \mu_R < \delta_2,$$

$\delta_1 < 0 < \delta_2$, is split into two one-sided test problems:

$$H_{01}: \mu_T - \mu_R \leq f_1\mu_R \quad \text{vs.} \quad H_{11}: \mu_T - \mu_R > f_1\mu_R$$

and

$$H_{02}: \mu_T - \mu_R \geq f_2\mu_R \quad \text{vs.} \quad H_{12}: \mu_T - \mu_R < f_2\mu_R,$$

where the equivalence range is described as $(\delta_1, \delta_2) = (f_1\mu_R, f_2\mu_R)$, $\mu_R \neq 0$.

The null hypothesis H_0 is rejected at a significance level α, if both null hypotheses H_{01} and H_{02} are rejected at level α, that is

$$T_{f_1\mu_R} = \frac{\overline{X}_T - \overline{X}_R - f_1\mu_R}{\hat{\sigma}_W \sqrt{\frac{1}{2}\left(\frac{1}{n_1} + \frac{1}{n_2}\right)}} > t_{1-\alpha,n_1+n_2-2}$$

and

$$T_{f_2\mu_R} = \frac{\overline{X}_T - \overline{X}_R - f_2\mu_R}{\hat{\sigma}_W \sqrt{\frac{1}{2}\left(\frac{1}{n_1} + \frac{1}{n_2}\right)}} < -t_{1-\alpha,n_1+n_2-2}.$$

For power and sample size determination, a balanced *RT/TR* crossover design is assumed, i.e., $n_1 = n_2 = n/2$, resulting in

$$T_{f_1\mu_R} = \frac{\overline{X}_T - \overline{X}_R - f_1\mu_R}{\hat{\sigma}_W \sqrt{\frac{2}{n}}} > t_{1-\alpha,n-2}$$

and

$$T_{f_2\mu_R} = \frac{\overline{X}_T - \overline{X}_R - f_2\mu_R}{\hat{\sigma}_W \sqrt{\frac{2}{n}}} < -t_{1-\alpha,n-2}.$$

The power of the test procedure is the probability that the null hypothesis H_0, in this case inequivalence, is rejected if the alternative hypothesis H_1, in this case equivalence, is true. In other words, the probability of correctly accepting equivalence is called the power of the test procedure,

$$P(T_{f_1\mu_R} > t_{1-\alpha,n-2} \quad \text{and} \quad T_{f_2\mu_R} < -t_{1-\alpha,n-2} | f_1\mu_R < \mu_T - \mu_R < f_2\mu_R , \sigma_W).$$

The power calculation is based on the following relations:

$$Var(\overline{X}_T - \overline{X}_R - f_1\mu_R) = Var(\overline{X}_T - \overline{X}_R - f_2\mu_R) = Var(\overline{X}_T - \overline{X}_R)$$
$$Cov(\overline{X}_T - \overline{X}_R - f_1\mu_R, \overline{X}_T - \overline{X}_R - f_2\mu_R)$$
$$= Cov(\overline{X}_T - \overline{X}_R, \overline{X}_T - \overline{X}_R) = Var(\overline{X}_T - \overline{X}_R)$$

and hence,

$$Corr(\overline{X}_T - \overline{X}_R - f_1\mu_R, \overline{X}_T - \overline{X}_R - f_2\mu_R)$$

$$= \frac{Cov(\overline{X}_T - \overline{X}_R - f_1\mu_R, \overline{X}_T - \overline{X}_R - f_2\mu_R)}{\sqrt{Var(\overline{X}_T - \overline{X}_R - f_1\mu_R)Var(\overline{X}_T - \overline{X}_R - f_2\mu_R)}}$$

$$= \frac{Var(\overline{X}_T - \overline{X}_R)}{Var(\overline{X}_T - \overline{X}_R)} = 1.$$

The variable $(n-2)\hat{\sigma}_W^2/\sigma_W^2$ is χ^2-distributed with $n-2$ degrees of freedom and independent of $\overline{X}_T - \overline{X}_R - f_1\mu_R$ and $\overline{X}_T - \overline{X}_R - f_2\mu_R$, respectively. Therefore, the random vector $(T_{f_1\mu_R}, T_{f_2\mu_R})$ has a bivariate noncentral t-distribution with $n-2$ degrees of freedom, $Corr(T_{f_1\mu_R}, T_{f_2\mu_R}) = 1$, and noncentrality parameters

$$\Delta_1 = \frac{\mu_T - \mu_R - f_1\mu_R}{\sigma_W\sqrt{\dfrac{2}{n}}} = \frac{\dfrac{\mu_T - \mu_R}{\mu_R} - f_1}{\sigma_W\sqrt{\dfrac{2}{n}}} = \frac{\dfrac{\mu_T - \mu_R}{\mu_R} - f_1}{CV_R\sqrt{\dfrac{2}{n}}}$$

and

$$\Delta_2 = \frac{\mu_T - \mu_R - f_2\mu_R}{\sigma_W\sqrt{\dfrac{2}{n}}} = \frac{\dfrac{\mu_T - \mu_R}{\mu_R} - f_2}{CV_R\sqrt{\dfrac{2}{n}}}.$$

The above expression for the power can be calculated by the difference of two definite integrals which depend on Δ_1 and Δ_2 (see Appendix at end of chapter). Owen (1965) has provided the exact form of these integrals and an algorithm for their calculation.

For power and corresponding sample size determination, Chow and Liu (2000) assumed an equivalence range of $(f_1\mu_R, f_2\mu_R) = (-0.20\mu_R, 0.20\mu_R)$ which corresponds to the former $\pm 20\%$ criteria. In Figure 5.1 the power curves are shown for a significance level $\alpha = 0.05$, total sample sizes of $n = 12, 18, 24, 36, 48$, a coefficient of variation of $CV_R = \sigma_W/\mu_R = 20\%$, and values from the corresponding alternative $-0.20 < (\mu_T - \mu_R)/\mu_R < 0.20$.

Obviously, the equivalence limits are unknown because the population mean of the reference, μ_R, is unknown. Hence, Chow and Liu (2000) proposed a testing procedure that cannot be calculated in practice since both test statistics, $T_{f_1\mu_R}$ and $T_{f_2\mu_R}$, are based on μ_R. Chow and Liu (2000) circumvented this issue by suggesting replacement of the unknown population mean μ_R by the empirical mean $\overline{X}_R$, resulting in the equivalence range of $(f_1\overline{X}_R, f_2\overline{X}_R)$ and the null hypothesis H_0 is rejected at a significance level α, if

$$T_{f_1\overline{X}_R} = \frac{\overline{X}_T - \overline{X}_R - f_1\overline{X}_R}{\hat{\sigma}_W\sqrt{\dfrac{1}{2}\left(\dfrac{1}{n_1} + \dfrac{1}{n_2}\right)}} > t_{1-\alpha, n_1+n_2-2}$$

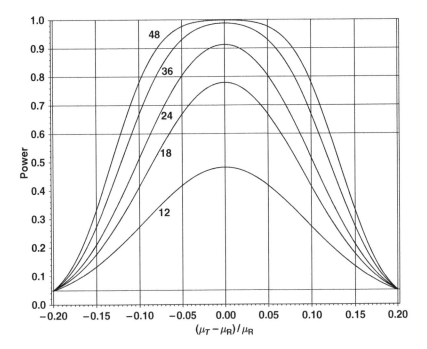

Figure 5.1 Probability of correctly concluding equivalence (power) in the case of an additive model as a function of values from $(\mu_T - \mu_R)/\mu_R = f$, $f_1 = -0.20 < f < 0.20 = f_2$. The power curves refer to a significance level of $\alpha = 0.05$, total sample sizes of $n = 12,\ 18,\ 24,\ 36,\ 48$, and a coefficient of variation of $CV_R = \sigma_W/\mu_R = 20\%$.

and

$$T_{f_2\overline{X}_R} = \frac{\overline{X}_T - \overline{X}_R - f_2\overline{X}_R}{\hat{\sigma}_W\sqrt{\dfrac{1}{2}\left(\dfrac{1}{n_1} + \dfrac{1}{n_2}\right)}} < -t_{1-\alpha,n_1+n_2-2}.$$

However, this procedure results in random equivalence limits, and hence in a liberal testing procedure, which means that the actual level is greater than the nominal level (Berger and Hsu, 1996). Hauschke (2002) pointed out that from a statistical and regulatory point of view this approach should not be used because it does not control the consumer risk, that is the probability of erroneously concluding bioequivalence.

5.3 Exact power and sample size calculation

Based on fundamental pharmacokinetic relationships, a multiplicative model is commonly used in bioequivalence trials for all concentration-related pharmacokinetic characteristics.

This traditionally implies the assumption of a lognormal distribution for the underlying pharmacokinetic characteristic,

$$X_{ijk} = \exp(\mu_h + s_{ij} + \pi_k + e_{ijk}),$$

where i denotes the sequence, $i = 1, 2$, j denotes the subjects within sequence i, $j = 1, \ldots n_i$, π_k is the effect of the kth period, $k = 1, 2$, with the side condition $\pi_1 + \pi_2 = 0$, and μ_h is the effect of formulation, with $h = R$ if $i = k$ and $h = T$ if $i \neq k$. Taking logarithms of the pharmacokinetic characteristics transforms the multiplicative model on the original scale to the corresponding additive model on the logarithmic scale

$$Y_{ijk} = \ln X_{ijk} = \mu_h + s_{ij} + \pi_k + e_{ijk}.$$

The subject effects s_{ij} are independent normally distributed with expected mean 0 and between-subject variance σ_B^2. The random errors e_{ijk} are independent and normally distributed with expected mean 0 and variances σ_W^2. The random error terms s_{ij} and e_{ijk} are assumed to be mutually independent. Let the ratio of the expected mean values of the test and the reference formulation on the original scale be denoted by $\theta = \exp(\mu_T)/\exp(\mu_R) = \exp(\mu_T - \mu_R)$ and let the interval (θ_1, θ_2) be the equivalence range, where $0 < \theta_1 < 1 < \theta_2$. Then, the following test problem of equivalence is considered:

$$H_0 : \exp(\mu_T - \mu_R) \leq \theta_1 \text{ or } \exp(\mu_T - \mu_R) \geq \theta_2$$

vs.

$$H_1 : \theta_1 < \exp(\mu_T - \mu_R) < \theta_2.$$

After logarithmic transformation and a split into two one-sided hypotheses, the corresponding test problem on the logarithmic scale becomes:

$$H_{01} : \mu_T - \mu_R \leq \ln \theta_1 \quad \text{vs.} \quad H_{11} : \mu_T - \mu_R > \ln \theta_1$$

and

$$H_{02} : \mu_T - \mu_R \geq \ln \theta_2 \quad \text{vs.} \quad H_{12} : \mu_T - \mu_R < \ln \theta_2.$$

Assuming a balanced design, the null hypothesis H_0 can be rejected at significance level α, if the following two conditions hold true:

$$T_{\ln \theta_1} = \frac{\overline{Y}_T - \overline{Y}_R - \ln \theta_1}{\hat{\sigma}_W \sqrt{\dfrac{2}{n}}} > t_{1-\alpha, n-2}$$

and

$$T_{\ln \theta_2} = \frac{\overline{Y}_T - \overline{Y}_R - \ln \theta_2}{\hat{\sigma}_W \sqrt{\dfrac{2}{n}}} < -t_{1-\alpha, n-2}.$$

The power of the testing procedure can be calculated as

$$P(T_{\ln \theta_1} > t_{1-\alpha, n-2} \quad \text{and} \quad T_{\ln \theta_2} < -t_{1-\alpha, n-2} \,|\, \ln \theta_1 < \mu_T - \mu_R < \ln \theta_2 \,, \sigma_W).$$

The random vector $(T_{\ln \theta_1}, T_{\ln \theta_2})$ has a bivariate noncentral t-distribution with $n-2$ degrees of freedom and noncentrality parameters

$$\Theta_1 = \frac{\mu_T - \mu_R - \ln \theta_1}{\sigma_W \sqrt{\dfrac{2}{n}}} \quad \text{and} \quad \Theta_2 = \frac{\mu_T - \mu_R - \ln \theta_2}{\sigma_W \sqrt{\dfrac{2}{n}}}.$$

Since $Corr(T_{\ln \theta_1}, T_{\ln \theta_2}) = 1$, Diletti *et al.* (1991, 1992) applied the methodology of Owen (1965) for the multiplicative model and the corresponding algorithm is applied in this chapter to create the figures and tables (see Appendix at end of chapter).

The noncentrality parameters Θ_1 and Θ_2 depend on the ratio of expected means $\theta = \exp(\mu_T)/\exp(\mu_R) = \exp(\mu_T - \mu_R)$, the within-subject variability σ_W^2 and the bioequivalence range (θ_1, θ_2). In order to facilitate the tabulation and graphical presentations, the within-subject coefficient of variation $CV_W = \sqrt{\exp(\sigma_W^2) - 1}$ is used (Hauschke *et al.*, 1994), and this leads to the following presentation of the noncentrality parameters:

$$\Theta_1 = \frac{\mu_T - \mu_R - \ln \theta_1}{\sigma_W \sqrt{\dfrac{2}{n}}} = \frac{\mu_T - \mu_R - \ln \theta_1}{\sqrt{\dfrac{2\ln(1 + CV_W^2)}{n}}}$$

and

$$\Theta_2 = \frac{\mu_T - \mu_R - \ln \theta_2}{\sigma_W \sqrt{\dfrac{2}{n}}} = \frac{\mu_T - \mu_R - \ln \theta_2}{\sqrt{\dfrac{2\ln(1 + CV_W^2)}{n}}}.$$

With regard to the choice of the bioequivalence range, Hauschke *et al.* (1992) have shown that an equivalence range of the form $(\theta_1, 1/\theta_1)$ should be preferred because it can be shown that, only for equivalence limits so defined, does the power curve have its maximum at $\theta = \exp(\mu_T)/\exp(\mu_R) = 1$, the point of equality.

This is illustrated in Figure 5.2 where it is shown that in contrast to the traditional (0.80, 1.20) bioequivalence range, the (0.80, 1.25) range results in a power curve that attains its maximum at $\theta = 1$ and is symmetric about $\ln 1 = 0$ on the logarithmic scale. In other words, for $\theta > 0$ and a range of the form $(\theta_1, 1/\theta_1)$, the power at $\ln \theta$ is the same as at $-\ln \theta = \ln 1/\theta$ on the logarithmic scale or equivalently, at $\theta = \exp(\mu_T)/\exp(\mu_R)$ and $1/\theta = \exp(\mu_R)/\exp(\mu_T)$ on the original scale. This implies that the test problem and the decision for intervals of the form $(\theta_1, 1/\theta_1)$ are invariant with respect to taking the reciprocal of the ratio of expected means $\exp(\mu_T)/\exp(\mu_R)$.

Figure 5.3 shows the attained power curves for commonly used sample sizes assuming a CV_W of 20% and a range of $(\theta_1, 1/\theta_1) = (0.80, 1.25)$. As the sample size decreases

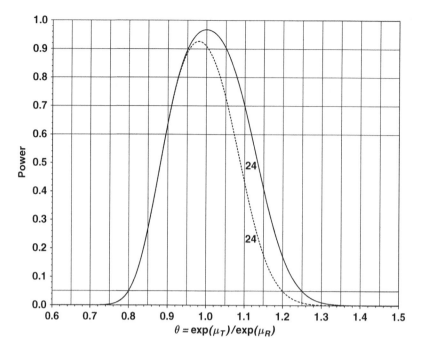

Figure 5.2 Probability of correctly concluding equivalence (power) as a function of the ratio $\theta = \exp(\mu_T)/\exp(\mu_R)$ calculated over the acceptance ranges (0.80, 1.20) (dotted line) and (0.80, 1.25) (solid line), respectively; power curves refer to a total sample size, n, of 24 subjects, a CV_W of 20 % and $\alpha = 0.05$.

and the specific value from the alternative approaches the limits of the equivalence range, the power decreases dramatically.

Table 5.1 gives the total sample sizes needed to attain a power of at least 0.80 and 0.90, respectively, for a significance level $\alpha = 0.05$, $\theta = 0.85, \ldots, 1.20$ from the alternative, and various within-subject coefficients of variation. As an even number of subjects is needed in a balanced crossover design, calculated odd sample sizes have been rounded up.

5.4 Modified acceptance ranges

According to the CPMP (2001) and FDA (1992, 2001) guidelines, equivalence can be concluded for the relative bioavailability measure *AUC* if the 90 % confidence interval lies within the acceptance range of $(\theta_1, 1/\theta_1) = (0.80, 1.25)$. This is also the case for the rate characteristic C_{max}, but in certain cases a wider interval for C_{max} may be acceptable in Europe (see below). However, any use of a wider equivalence acceptance range than (0.80, 1.25) should be justified addressing any safety or efficacy concerns.

With regard to the rate characteristic C_{max}, the acceptance range $(\theta_1, 1/\theta_1) = (0.70, 1/0.70)$ had been discussed in earlier drafts of the CPMP (1991) guidance.

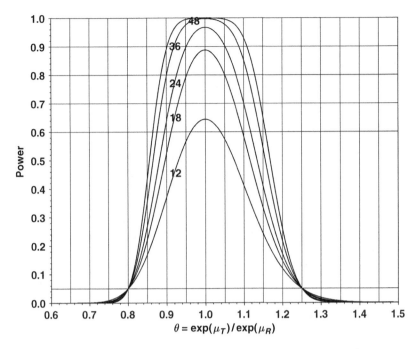

Figure 5.3 Probability of correctly concluding equivalence (power) as a function of the ratio $\theta = \exp(\mu_T)/\exp(\mu_R)$ calculated over the acceptance range $(\theta_1, 1/\theta_1) = (0.80, 1.25)$; power curves refer to a total sample size of $n = 12, 18, 24, 36, 48$ subjects, $\alpha = 0.05$ and $CV_W = 20\%$.

Table 5.1 Total sample sizes, n, needed to attain a power of 0.80, 0.90 for the multiplicative model, for an acceptance range $(\theta_1, 1/\theta_1) = (0.80, 1.25)$, $\theta = \exp(\mu_T)/\exp(\mu_R)$, $\alpha = 0.05$ and various CV_W.

Power	$CV_W(\%)$	θ 0.85	0.90	0.95	1.00	1.05	1.10	1.15	1.20
0.80	10.0	36	12	8	6	8	10	20	76
	12.5	54	16	10	8	10	14	30	118
	15.0	78	22	12	10	12	20	42	168
	17.5	104	30	16	14	16	26	56	226
	20.0	134	38	20	16	18	32	72	294
	22.5	168	46	24	20	24	40	90	368
	25.0	206	56	28	24	28	48	110	452
	27.5	248	68	34	28	34	58	132	544
	30.0	292	80	40	32	38	68	156	642
	32.5	340	92	46	36	44	78	180	748
	35.0	392	106	52	42	50	90	208	860

Table 5.1   Continued.

Power	CV_W (%)	0.85	0.90	0.95	1.00	1.05	1.10	1.15	1.20
	37.5	446	120	58	48	58	102	236	978
	40.0	502	134	66	54	64	114	266	1104
0.90	10.0	48	14	8	8	8	14	26	104
	12.5	74	22	12	10	12	18	40	162
	15.0	106	30	16	12	16	26	58	232
	17.5	142	40	20	16	20	34	76	312
	20.0	186	50	26	20	24	44	100	406
	22.5	232	64	32	24	30	54	124	510
	25.0	284	78	38	28	36	66	152	626
	27.5	342	92	44	34	44	78	182	752
	30.0	404	108	52	40	52	92	214	888
	32.5	470	126	60	46	60	108	250	1034
	35.0	540	146	70	52	68	124	288	1190
	37.5	616	164	80	60	78	140	326	1354
	40.0	694	186	88	66	86	158	368	1528

This concession reflects the experience that single concentrations, in particular extreme concentrations like C_{max}, have a larger within-subject coefficient of variation than integrated characteristics like AUC. The CPMP (2001) guidance again states that for C_{max} a wider bioequivalence range than for AUC may be acceptable in certain cases. Instead of the previous range $(\theta_1, 1/\theta_1) = (0.70, 1/0.70)$ the smaller range of $(\theta_1, 1/\theta_1) = (0.75, 1/0.75) = (0.75, 1.3333)$ is now recommended where a wider interval can be justified. In Figure 5.4, the power curves are shown for $CV_W = 30.0\%$ and values from the alternative as a function of the sample size. Table 5.2 gives the total sample sizes needed to attain a power of at least 0.80 and 0.90 for a significance level $\alpha = 0.05, CV_W = 10.0\%, 12.5\%, \ldots, 40\%$ and values of the ratio from the alternative $\theta = 0.80, \ldots, 1.25$.

In general, the choice of the appropriate bioequivalence range should be based on clinical grounds. Thus, for a drug with a narrow therapeutic range, tighter limits may have to be considered (CPMP, 2001), e.g., $(\theta_1, 1/\theta_1) = (0.90, 1/0.90)$. As shown in Figure 5.5 and Table 5.3, sufficient power can be reached for commonly used sample sizes only for drugs with a small within-subject coefficient of variation.

5.5   Approximate formulas for sample size calculation

The calculation of the exact power is mathematically complex and requires evaluation of the bivariate noncentral t-distribution, which might not be accessible to practitioners. For that reason, Hauschke *et al.* (1992) developed the following approximate

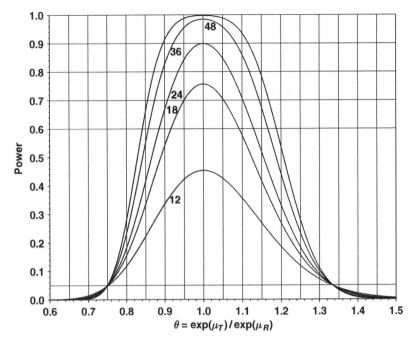

Figure 5.4 Probability of correctly concluding bioequivalence (power) as a function of the ratio $\theta = \exp(\mu_T)/\exp(\mu_R)$ calculated over the acceptance range $(\theta_1, 1/\theta_1) = (0.75, 1.3333)$; power curves refer to a total sample size of $n = 12, 18, 24, 36, 48$ subjects, $\alpha = 0.05$ and $CV_W = 30\%$.

Table 5.2 Total sample sizes, n, needed to attain a power of 0.80, 0.90 for the multiplicative model, for of an acceptance range $(\theta_1, 1/\theta_1) = (0.75, 1.3333)$, $\theta = \exp(\mu_T)/\exp(\mu_R)$, $\alpha = 0.05$ and various CV_W.

Power	$CV_W(\%)$	0.80	0.85	0.90	0.95	1.00	1.05	1.10	1.15	1.20	1.25
0.80	15.0	68	20	10	8	8	8	10	16	28	68
	17.5	92	26	14	10	10	10	12	20	36	92
	20.0	118	34	18	12	10	12	16	24	46	118
	22.5	148	42	20	14	12	14	20	30	58	150
	25.0	182	50	26	16	16	16	22	36	70	182
	27.5	218	60	30	20	18	20	26	44	84	218
	30.0	258	70	34	22	20	22	32	52	98	258
	32.5	300	82	40	26	24	26	36	60	114	300
	35.0	346	94	46	30	26	30	42	68	132	346
	37.5	392	106	52	34	30	34	46	76	150	394

Table 5.2 Continued.

Power	CV_W(%)	θ 0.80	0.85	0.90	0.95	1.00	1.05	1.10	1.15	1.20	1.25
	40.0	442	120	58	38	34	36	52	86	168	444
	42.5	496	134	64	42	36	42	58	96	188	496
	45.0	550	148	72	46	40	46	64	106	208	550
0.90	15.0	94	26	14	10	8	10	12	20	36	94
	17.5	126	36	18	12	10	12	16	26	48	126
	20.0	164	46	22	14	12	14	20	34	62	164
	22.5	206	56	28	18	16	18	26	42	78	206
	25.0	252	68	34	22	18	22	30	50	96	252
	27.5	302	82	40	26	22	24	36	60	114	302
	30.0	356	96	46	30	26	28	42	70	136	358
	32.5	416	112	54	34	28	34	48	82	158	416
	35.0	478	128	62	38	32	38	56	92	180	478
	37.5	544	146	70	44	36	42	64	106	206	544
	40.0	612	164	78	48	42	48	72	118	232	614
	42.5	686	184	88	54	46	54	80	132	258	686
	45.0	760	204	98	60	50	60	88	146	288	762

formulas for sample size determination for the multiplicative model. The total number of subjects, n, needed to achieve a power of $1 - \beta$ at significance level α for a value of the ratio of expected means $\theta = \exp(\mu_T)/\exp(\mu_R) = \exp(\mu_T - \mu_R)$ from the equivalence range $(\theta_1, 1/\theta_1)$ and a within-subject coefficient of variation CV_W is:

$$n \geq 2\left(\frac{CV_W}{\ln \theta_1}\right)^2 (t_{1-\alpha,n-2} + t_{1-\beta/2,n-2})^2 \qquad \text{if } \theta = 1$$

$$n \geq 2\left(\frac{CV_W}{-\ln \theta_1 - \ln \theta}\right)^2 (t_{1-\alpha,n-2} + t_{1-\beta,n-2})^2 \qquad \text{if } 1 < \theta < 1/\theta_1$$

$$n \geq 2\left(\frac{CV_W}{\ln \theta_1 - \ln \theta}\right)^2 (t_{1-\alpha,n-2} + t_{1-\beta,n-2})^2 \qquad \text{and if } \theta_1 < \theta < 1.$$

Table 5.4 gives the total sample sizes n needed to attain a power of at least 0.80 and 0.90, respectively, for a significance level $\alpha = 0.05$, $\theta = 0.85, \ldots, 1.20$ and various within-subject coefficients of variation. For each combination, the exact sample sizes are given in the first line and the approximate ones in the second line, the latter only if they deviate from the exact ones.

The sample sizes based on the approximate formulas are generally greater than the exact ones. Notwithstanding this, the proportional differences from the exact values are very small. Thus, the approximate formulas can be considered as suitable for sample size

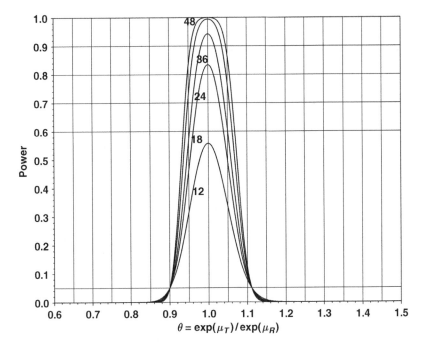

Figure 5.5 Probability of correctly concluding bioequivalence (power) as a function of the ratio $\theta = \exp(\mu_T)/\exp(\mu_R)$ calculated over the acceptance range $(\theta_1, 1/\theta_1) = (0.90, 1.1111)$; power curves refer to a total sample size of $n = 12, 18, 24, 36, 48$ subjects, $\alpha = 0.05$ and $CV_W = 10\%$.

calculation in the case of the multiplicative model. It should be noted that for values of $\theta = \exp(\mu_T)/\exp(\mu_R)$ very near to the point of equality, for example $\theta = 1.01$, the sample size determination by the approximate formula leads to smaller sample sizes than for $\theta = 1$, where the minimum sample size is to be expected for theoretical reasons. This irregularity is due to the discrete step from $t_{1-\beta,n-2}$ for $\theta \neq 1$ to $t_{1-\beta/2,n-2}$ for $\theta = 1$ (Hauschke and Steinijans, 1997). In this case, the exact formula should be used.

5.6   Exact power and sample size calculation by nQuery®

A commonly used software package in the pharmaceutical industry is nQuery Advisor® (Elashoff, 2005), which assists in the choice of an appropriate sample size for a planned clinical study. One feature of this program is power and sample size determination for the proof of equivalence for the ratio of expected means in the balanced two-period, two-sequence crossover design under the assumption of a lognormal distribution. The corresponding algorithm is the one provided by Diletti *et al.* (1991).

Table 5.3 Total sample sizes, n, needed to attain a power of 0.80, 0.90 for the multiplicative model, for an acceptance range $(\theta_1, 1/\theta_1) = (0.90, 1.1111), \theta = \exp(\mu_T)/\exp(\mu_R)$, $\alpha = 0.05$ and various CV_W.

Power	CV_W (%)	θ						
		0.925	0.950	0.975	1.000	1.025	1.050	1.075
0.80	5.0	44	14	8	6	8	12	30
	7.5	94	26	14	12	14	24	66
	10.0	166	44	22	18	22	40	116
	12.5	258	68	32	26	32	62	178
	15.0	368	96	46	36	46	88	254
	17.5	500	130	62	48	62	118	344
	20.0	648	168	80	62	78	154	446
	22.5	816	212	100	78	98	194	562
	25.0	1000	258	122	96	120	236	690
0.90	5.0	60	18	10	8	10	16	42
	7.5	130	36	18	14	18	32	90
	10.0	230	60	30	22	28	56	158
	12.5	356	94	44	32	44	86	246
	15.0	510	132	62	46	62	122	352
	17.5	690	180	84	62	82	164	476
	20.0	898	232	108	78	106	212	618
	22.5	1130	292	134	98	132	266	778
	25.0	1386	358	164	120	162	326	954

For example, a within-subject coefficient of variation of $CV_W = 25\%$ corresponds to the standard deviation

$$\sigma_W = \sqrt{\ln(1 + CV_W^2)} = \sqrt{\ln(1 + 0.0625)} = 0.246.$$

For a significance level of $\alpha = 0.05$, an equivalence range of $(0.80, 1.25)$, and an expected ratio of means of 0.95, a sample size of 28 in total, i.e., 14 per sequence, is necessary to limit the type II error to at most 0.20. It can be seen from Table 5.5 that under the above combination a total sample size of 28 is sufficient for the expected ratios

$$0.95 \leq \theta \leq 1.05, \ \theta = \frac{\exp(\mu_T)}{\exp(\mu_R)}$$

to attain a power of at least 0.80.

It is worthwhile to note that nQuery Advisor® offers a statement feature to produce a paragraph explaining the sample size determination. For example, the following text is given in Table 5.5,

'When the sample size in each sequence group is 14 (and the total sample size is 28), a crossover design will have 80 % power to reject both the null hypothesis that the ratio of the test mean to the standard mean is below 0.800

Table 5.4 Exact (first line) and approximate (second line) total sample sizes needed to attain a power of 0.80 and 0.90; approximate values are only printed if they deviate from the exact ones; $\theta = \exp(\mu_T)/\exp(\mu_R)$, $\alpha = 0.05$, $(\theta_1, 1/\theta_1) = (0.80, 1.25)$ and various CV_W.

Power	CV_W (%)	θ							
		0.85	0.90	0.95	1.00	1.05	1.10	1.15	1.20
0.80	10.0	36	12	8	6	8	10	20	76
		–	–	–	–	–	–	–	–
	15.0	78	22	12	10	12	20	42	168
		–	–	–	–	–	–	–	170
	20.0	134	38	20	16	18	32	72	294
		138	–	–	–	–	–	74	300
	25.0	206	56	28	24	28	48	110	452
		212	58	–	–	–	50	114	466
	30.0	292	80	40	32	38	68	156	642
		306	82	–	34	40	70	162	670
	35.0	392	106	52	42	50	90	208	860
		414	112	54	44	52	96	220	912
	40.0	502	134	66	54	64	114	266	1104
		540	146	70	58	68	124	288	1190
0.90	10.0	48	14	8	8	8	14	26	104
		50	16	–	–	–	–	28	106
	15.0	106	30	16	12	16	26	58	232
		108	–	–	–	–	–	–	234
	20.0	186	50	26	20	24	44	100	406
		190	52	–	–	26	–	102	414
	25.0	284	78	38	28	36	66	152	626
		294	80	–	30	38	68	156	646
	30.0	404	108	52	40	52	92	214	888
		422	114	54	42	54	96	224	928
	35.0	540	146	70	52	68	124	288	1190
		574	154	74	56	72	132	304	1262
	40.0	694	186	88	66	86	158	368	1528
		748	200	96	72	92	170	396	1648

and the null hypothesis that the ratio of test mean to the standard mean is above 1.250; i.e., that the test and standard are not equivalent, in favor of the alternative hypothesis that the means of the two treatments are equivalent, assuming that the expected ratio of means is 0.950, the Crossover ANOVA, $\sqrt{MSE}$ (ln scale) is 0.246 (the SD differences, σ_d(ln scale) is 0.348), that data will be analyzed in the natural log scale using t-tests for differences in means, and that each t-test is made at the 5.0 % level.'

Table 5.5 Screenshot from nQuery Advisor®. Power and sample size determination for the proof of equivalence for the ratio of expected means in the *RT/TR* crossover under the assumption of a lognormal distribution. Reproduced by permission of Elashoff (2005).

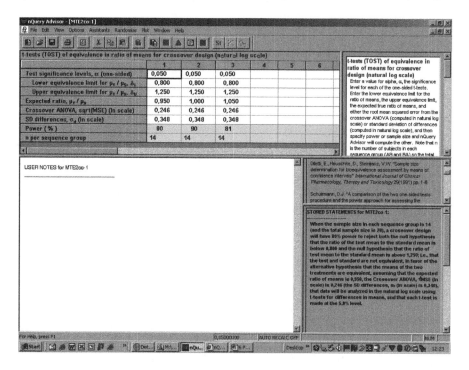

Appendix

In the additive model under a normality assumption, the power can be calculated as follows (Owen, 1965):

$$P(T_{f_1\mu_R} > t_{1-\alpha,n-2} \quad \text{and} \quad T_{f_2\mu_R} < -t_{1-\alpha,n-2} \,|\, f_1\mu_R < \mu_T - \mu_R < f_2\mu_R \,, \sigma_W)$$
$$= Q(-t_{1-\alpha,n-2}, \Delta_2, 0, R) - Q(t_{1-\alpha,n-2}, \Delta_1, 0, R),$$

where

$$Q(t, \Delta, 0, R) = \frac{\sqrt{2\pi}}{\Gamma\left(\frac{n}{2}-1\right) 2^{(n/2)-2}} \int_0^R \Phi\left(\frac{tx}{\sqrt{n-2}} - \Delta\right) x^{n-3} \Phi'(x)dx,$$

$$\Phi'(x) = \frac{1}{\sqrt{2\pi}} \exp\left(-\frac{x^2}{2}\right), \Phi(x) = \int_{-\infty}^x \Phi'(t)dt,$$

$$R = \frac{\Delta_1 - \Delta_2}{A_1 - A_2}, \ A_1 = \frac{t_{1-\alpha,n-2}}{\sqrt{n-2}}, \ A_2 = \frac{-t_{1-\alpha,n-2}}{\sqrt{n-2}},$$

and

$$\Delta_1 = \frac{\dfrac{\mu_T - \mu_R}{\mu_R} - f_1}{CV_R\sqrt{\dfrac{2}{n}}}, \quad \Delta_2 = \frac{\dfrac{\mu_T - \mu_R}{\mu_R} - f_2}{CV_R\sqrt{\dfrac{2}{n}}}.$$

In analogy, the power calculation for the multiplicative model under the assumption of a lognormal distribution is:

$$P(T_{\ln\theta_1} > t_{1-\alpha,n-2} \quad \text{and} \quad T_{\ln\theta_2} < -t_{1-\alpha,n-2} \mid \ln\theta_1 < \mu_T - \mu_R < \ln\theta_2\,, \sigma_W)$$
$$= Q(-t_{1-\alpha,n-2}, \Theta_2, 0, S) - Q(t_{1-\alpha,n-2}, \Theta_1, 0, S),$$

where

$$S = \frac{\Theta_1 - \Theta_2}{A_1 - A_2}, \quad A_1 = \frac{t_{1-\alpha,n-2}}{\sqrt{n-2}}, \quad A_2 = \frac{-t_{1-\alpha,n-2}}{\sqrt{n-2}},$$

and

$$\Theta_1 = \frac{\mu_T - \mu_R - \ln\theta_1}{\sqrt{\dfrac{2\ln(1 + CV_W^2)}{n}}}, \quad \Theta_2 = \frac{\mu_T - \mu_R - \ln\theta_2}{\sqrt{\dfrac{2\ln(1 + CV_W^2)}{n}}}.$$

References

Berger, R.L. and Hsu, J.C. (1996) Bioequivalence trials, intersection-union tests and equivalence confidence sets. *Statistical Science* **11**, 283–319.

Chow, S-C. and Liu, J-P. (2000) *Design and analysis of bioavailability and bioequivalence studies* (2nd edition). Marcel Dekker, New York.

Committee for Proprietary Medicinal Products (1991) *Note for guidance on the investigation of bioavailability and bioequivalence*. EMEA, London.

Committee for Proprietary Medicinal Products (2001) *Note for guidance on the investigation of bioavailability and bioequivalence*. EMEA, London.

Diletti, E., Hauschke, D. and Steinijans, V.W. (1991) Sample size determination for bioequivalence assessment by means of confidence intervals. *International Journal of Clinical Pharmacology, Therapy and Toxicology* **29**, 1–8.

Diletti, E., Hauschke, D. and Steinijans, V.W. (1992) Sample size determination: extended tables for the multiplicative model and bioequivalence ranges of 0.9 to 1.11 and 0.7 to 1.43. *International Journal of Clinical Pharmacology, Therapy and Toxicology* **30**, 287–90.

Elashoff, J.D. (2005) nQuery Advisor® Version 6.0. Los Angeles, CA.

Food and Drug Administration (1992) *Guidance on statistical procedures for bioequivalence studies using a standard two-treatment crossover design*. Division of Bioequivalence, Rockville, MD.

Food and Drug Administration (2001) *Guidance for industry. Statistical approaches to establishing bioequivalence*. Center for Drug Evaluation and Research, Rockville, MD.

Hauschke, D. (2002) A note on sample size determination in bioequivalence trials. *Journal of Pharmacokinetics and Pharmacodynamics* **29**, 89–94.

Hauschke, D. and Steinijans, V.W. (1997) Crossover trials in bioequivalence assessment. In: Vollmar, J. and Hothorn, L. (eds) *Biometrics in the Pharmaceutical Industry*, 27–40, Gustav Fischer, Stuttgart.

Hauschke, D., Steinijans, V.W., Diletti, E. and Burke, M. (1992) Sample size determination for bioequivalence assessment using a multiplicative model. *Journal of Pharmacokinetics and Biopharmaceutics* **20**, 557–61.

Hauschke, D., Steinijans, V.W., Diletti, E., Schall, R., Luus, H.G., Elze, M. and Blume, H. (1994) Presentation of the intrasubject coefficient of variation for sample size planning in bioequivalence studies. *International Journal of Clinical Pharmacology and Therapeutics* **32**, 376–8.

Liu, J-P. and Chow, S-C. (1992) Sample size determination for the two one-sided tests procedure in bioequivalence. *Journal of Pharmacokinetics and Biopharmaceutics* **20**, 101–4.

Owen, D.B. (1965) A special case of a bivariate non-central *t*-distribution. *Biometrika* **52**, 437–46.

Patterson, S. and Jones, B. (2006) *Bioequivalence and statistics in clinical pharmacology*. Chapman & Hall/CRC, Boca Raton.

Phillips, K.F. (1990) Power of the two one-sided tests procedure in bioequivalence. *Journal of Pharmacokinetics and Biopharmaceutics* **18**, 137–44.

6

Presentation of bioequivalence studies

6.1 Introduction

Data on bioequivalence studies are presented in clinical pharmacological journals in different styles and degree of completeness. This depends not only on the authors' willingness to submit individual data, but also on the policy of certain journals to allow only a limited number of figures and/or tables per paper. In the best case, pertinent pharmacokinetic characteristics for each treatment together with the sequences of administration are given. Usually, however, neither individual concentration-time data, nor the sequence of administration, nor the individual values of the pertinent pharmacokinetic characteristics of rate and extent of absorption are provided.

The presentation of results for bioequivalence studies should be in line with the far-reaching international consensus on the design, planning, performance and data analysis of average bioequivalence studies (CPMP, 2001; FDA, 2003), including data transformation and decision procedure. The primary pharmacokinetic characteristics of rate and extent of absorption, the proposed model (multiplicative or additive), the bioequivalence range, the statistical method and the sample size determination, which have to be specified in the study protocol prior to the start of the bioequivalence study, should be recalled when presenting results.

This chapter deals with the appropriate presentation of results from single- and multiple-dose bioequivalence studies. It is based on the pioneering paper by Sauter *et al.* (1992). The single-dose study serves to illustrate the AUC extrapolation and the various single-dose pharmacokinetic characteristics. The multiple-dose study demonstrates the presentation of results for the steady-state characteristics of rate and extent. Since steady-state bioequivalence studies are of particular relevance for modified release formulations

Bioequivalence Studies in Drug Development: Methods and Applications   D. Hauschke, V. Steinijans and I. Pigeot
© 2007 John Wiley & Sons, Ltd

(CPMP, 2001; FDA, 2003), examples involving controlled release formulations have been chosen.

6.2   Results from a single-dose study

In this single-dose, randomized, two-period, two-sequence crossover study in $n = 18$ healthy volunteers, two controlled release theophylline formulations were compared with regard to rate and extent of absorption. The test product (Euphylong®) has pH-independent release characteristics (Dietrich *et al.*, 1988) and shows no relevant food effects (Schulz *et al.*, 1987; Steinijans and Sauter, 1993). It is available in various dose strengths. Different capsule sizes contain different amounts of pellets (beads), which constitute the controlled release mechanism. The dose strength was a 300 mg capsule. The pharmacokinetics and pharmacodynamics of the test formulation have been thoroughly investigated with particular emphasis on once-daily nighttime dosing and nocturnal asthma (Steinijans *et al.*, 1988; D'Alonzo *et al.*, 1990). The reference product was also available as 300 mg capsules containing beads. Its release characteristics show a pronounced pH-dependency (Benedikt *et al.*, 1988), and relevant food and time dependencies have been reported (Hendeles *et al.*, 1985; Jonkman, 1989; Smolensky *et al.*, 1987). Two capsules of either formulation, i.e., 600 mg theophylline, were given with 200 ml of mineral water at 8 p.m., half an hour after a standardized evening meal with a composition of 36 g fat, 42 g protein and 69 g carbohydrates. Xanthine-containing food or beverages were not allowed for two days before and during the entire study. The two treatment periods were one week apart.

The demographic data of the 18 study participants, all of them nonsmokers, are given in Table 6.3, together with the randomized sequence of treatments. Prior to the study, the healthy volunteers underwent physical and laboratory examination, and written informed consent was given by each subject. Twenty-four blood samples for determination of serum theophylline concentrations (STCs) were taken before and up to 72 hours after dosing. They were taken at hourly intervals for the first 8 hours, then at two-hourly intervals up to 24 hours after dosing. Serum theophylline concentrations were measured by HPLC (Schulz *et al.*, 1984); each sample was analyzed in duplicate and the arithmetic mean of the two determinations was used for further evaluation. The individual STCs are given in Table 6.1a for the reference formulation and in Table 6.1b for the test formulation. In addition to the time after dose, the clock time is also given in these tables. Values below the lower limit of quantification, which in this study was 0.06 mg/L, are marked as <0.06. Due to the very low concentrations 60 and 72 hours after dosing, which in the majority of subjects were below the limit of quantification, all graphical presentations have been truncated at 48 hours.

There are three types of standard plots of the concentration-time curves that should be routinely produced for each bioavailability/bioequivalence study. Closed symbols are used for the test product while open symbols indicate the reference product. The medians may be presented as standard plot 2 as an alternative to the geometric means, which may not be unambiguously calculable at early and very late time points with values below the LLoQ (Lower Limit of Quantification).

Table 6.1a Serum theophylline concentrations (mg/L) following a single oral dose of 600 mg theophylline (Reference) at 8 p.m. Concentrations below the lower limit of quantification of 0.06 mg/L are marked as <0.06.

Subject number	Time after dose (h)																							
	0	1	2	3	4	5	6	7	8	10	12	14	16	18	20	22	24	28	36	40	44	48	60	72
Clock time	20	21	22	23	24	1	2	3	4	6	8	10	12	14	16	18	20	24	8	12	16	20	8	20
1	<0.06	<0.06	0.34	0.98	1.44	1.81	2.38	3.22	4.21	6.07	7.94	9.05	8.45	7.23	6.81	5.47	4.79	3.32	1.70	1.35	0.87	0.63	0.23	<0.06
2	<0.06	<0.06	0.42	0.81	1.44	2.15	2.53	3.74	5.38	7.94	7.90	6.59	5.46	4.65	3.38	2.47	2.02	1.16	0.53	0.29	0.15	0.07	<0.06	<0.06
3	<0.06	<0.06	0.48	1.13	1.85	3.56	5.99	8.08	8.71	10.36	11.49	11.49	9.72	9.30	8.00	6.53	5.64	3.57	2.22	1.61	1.15	0.76	0.26	<0.06
4	<0.06	0.19	0.53	1.13	2.03	3.99	6.99	7.16	10.51	10.30	10.32	8.23	7.42	6.09	4.86	4.04	3.44	1.89	1.06	0.70	0.48	0.31	<0.06	<0.06
5	<0.06	<0.06	<0.06	0.36	0.65	0.99	1.22	1.60	2.09	6.70	11.17	9.44	8.62	6.65	5.45	4.39	3.34	1.74	0.73	0.29	0.12	<0.06	<0.06	<0.06
6	<0.06	<0.06	0.25	0.52	0.84	1.43	2.42	4.48	6.15	7.73	7.70	6.67	5.78	4.68	4.32	3.42	2.59	1.61	0.60	0.40	0.16	<0.06	<0.06	<0.06
7	<0.06	<0.06	0.60	0.93	1.36	1.89	2.59	3.29	3.59	5.26	6.46	10.83	9.56	7.31	5.82	4.51	3.44	1.76	0.82	0.52	0.29	0.21	<0.06	<0.06
8	<0.06	<0.06	0.11	0.28	0.58	0.93	1.59	2.08	2.67	3.56	3.34	3.12	2.74	2.32	1.91	1.46	1.30	0.74	0.25	0.15	<0.06	<0.06	<0.06	<0.06
9	<0.06	<0.06	<0.06	0.20	0.83	1.18	1.47	1.84	2.23	3.72	8.92	5.72	5.21	4.81	4.02	3.33	2.63	1.58	0.71	0.58	0.40	0.29	<0.06	<0.06
10	<0.06	<0.06	0.50	1.09	1.71	2.55	3.72	5.41	8.17	10.06	8.38	7.33	5.48	4.43	3.33	2.36	1.70	0.98	0.39	0.25	0.14	0.18	<0.06	<0.06
11	<0.06	<0.06	0.57	0.94	1.39	2.32	4.01	5.51	6.71	6.60	6.82	6.00	5.15	4.24	3.46	2.87	2.17	1.12	0.51	0.38	0.24	0.95	0.41	<0.06
12	<0.06	<0.06	0.66	1.27	2.58	4.50	6.65	8.61	9.39	10.38	10.63	10.47	9.22	8.12	6.65	5.86	4.79	3.66	2.19	1.68	1.27	0.95	0.41	0.14
13	<0.06	0.14	0.60	1.12	1.45	2.34	3.57	4.66	5.57	7.76	8.14	7.79	7.53	6.34	5.39	4.67	3.86	2.61	1.29	1.01	0.67	0.42	0.14	<0.06
14	<0.06	<0.06	0.30	1.06	1.54	2.03	3.18	4.61	5.57	8.53	9.28	9.27	7.90	6.84	6.30	5.37	4.47	3.07	1.64	1.16	0.66	0.36	0.09	<0.06
15	<0.06	<0.06	<0.06	<0.06	0.15	0.38	2.16	5.52	8.99	10.86	9.95	8.65	8.60	7.27	6.11	5.79	5.01	3.49	2.01	1.52	1.09	0.77	0.16	<0.06
16	<0.06	0.25	0.65	1.24	1.89	2.77	3.56	4.85	5.54	7.93	8.91	8.90	7.07	5.87	4.64	3.85	2.97	1.67	0.61	0.36	0.22	0.12	<0.06	<0.06
17	<0.06	<0.06	0.43	0.95	2.01	3.31	4.61	5.91	7.90	11.53	10.44	10.05	8.33	6.95	5.69	4.52	3.77	2.25	1.11	0.79	0.49	0.36	0.09	<0.06
18	<0.06	<0.06	0.45	1.13	1.61	2.39	3.18	4.10	4.85	5.47	5.67	5.87	5.46	4.56	3.97	3.62	3.18	2.10	1.07	0.71	0.44	0.21	<0.06	<0.06

Table 6.1b Serum theophylline concentrations (mg/L) following a single oral dose of 600 mg theophylline (Test) at 8 p.m. Concentrations below the lower limit of quantification of 0.06 mg/L are marked as <0.06.

Subject number	Time after dose (h)																							
	0	1	2	3	4	5	6	7	8	10	12	14	16	18	20	22	24	28	36	40	44	48	60	72
	Clock time																							
	20	21	22	23	24	1	2	3	4	6	8	10	12	14	16	18	20	24	8	12	16	20	8	20
1	<0.06	0.31	1.46	4.53	7.19	8.86	9.07	10.20	9.26	8.79	8.66	8.16	7.42	6.43	5.51	4.70	3.97	2.99	1.47	1.28	0.74	0.56	0.22	<0.06
2	<0.06	<0.06	0.21	0.61	1.13	2.05	2.97	3.83	4.12	4.60	4.72	4.40	4.21	3.47	3.11	2.77	2.22	1.60	0.90	0.64	0.36	0.18	<0.06	<0.06
3	<0.06	0.34	2.52	5.84	8.50	8.98	9.72	9.78	9.82	9.71	9.57	8.60	7.95	7.18	5.85	5.19	4.51	2.88	1.66	1.31	0.91	0.61	0.18	<0.06
4	<0.06	<0.06	2.75	5.49	6.64	7.55	8.51	8.25	8.99	8.21	7.52	7.31	6.76	5.68	4.62	4.02	3.45	2.22	1.28	1.07	0.66	0.35	<0.06	<0.06
5	<0.06	<0.06	0.88	3.49	6.48	6.36	7.33	7.35	7.64	7.19	6.47	5.84	5.57	4.68	3.94	3.01	2.59	1.59	0.83	0.68	0.45	0.23	<0.06	<0.06
6	<0.06	0.23	2.34	4.18	5.17	5.50	5.93	5.59	4.85	4.46	4.22	3.44	3.37	2.63	2.23	1.82	1.70	1.01	0.42	0.29	0.22	0.08	<0.06	<0.06
7	<0.06	1.05	2.02	3.09	3.82	4.41	4.93	5.48	5.85	6.17	6.23	5.84	5.16	4.48	4.00	3.16	2.69	1.78	0.95	0.77	0.49	0.30	0.12	<0.06
8	<0.06	0.19	1.27	2.75	3.23	3.36	3.29	3.89	3.25	2.73	2.12	1.53	1.21	0.95	0.68	0.54	0.42	0.19	0.15	0.10	<0.06	<0.06	<0.06	<0.06
9	<0.06	0.38	2.01	4.73	5.79	6.50	6.71	6.87	6.57	6.10	6.03	5.29	4.53	3.87	3.69	2.77	2.31	1.39	0.89	0.66	0.53	0.37	0.17	<0.06
10	<0.06	0.12	1.29	3.98	5.18	6.61	8.22	8.23	7.79	6.92	6.51	5.36	4.21	3.42	2.76	2.15	1.51	0.77	0.29	0.18	<0.06	<0.06	<0.06	<0.06
11	<0.06	0.50	1.75	3.52	4.37	4.73	4.88	5.04	4.80	4.51	3.96	3.71	3.15	2.51	2.08	1.66	1.36	0.89	0.43	0.38	0.28	0.18	<0.06	0.18
12	<0.06	0.39	1.23	2.89	3.74	5.18	6.24	7.62	7.68	9.34	9.69	9.18	8.27	6.94	6.41	5.72	4.75	3.37	2.38	1.92	1.32	1.00	0.45	<0.06
13	<0.06	0.20	1.29	2.04	3.03	3.56	4.38	4.60	4.97	5.33	5.94	6.01	5.63	4.88	4.29	3.77	3.38	2.47	1.45	1.13	0.73	0.49	0.14	<0.06
14	<0.06	0.08	1.96	4.07	6.71	8.21	8.61	7.98	7.78	7.66	7.20	6.62	6.17	4.89	4.26	3.87	3.21	2.20	1.35	1.12	0.81	0.66	0.25	<0.06
15	<0.06	0.89	2.45	2.99	4.08	5.57	5.69	5.86	5.85	5.88	5.96	5.53	5.12	4.74	4.20	3.71	3.50	2.70	1.91	1.70	1.26	1.01	0.45	0.18
16	<0.06	<0.06	2.55	5.16	7.55	8.46	9.03	8.72	8.38	7.66	6.60	5.58	4.89	4.17	3.36	2.85	2.18	1.33	0.42	0.20	0.04	<0.06	<0.06	<0.06
17	<0.06	0.24	1.80	4.08	6.01	7.77	8.93	9.02	8.59	8.34	7.91	7.06	6.46	5.54	5.15	4.36	3.58	2.55	1.49	1.11	0.85	0.57	0.08	<0.06
18	<0.06	<0.06	0.23	1.24	2.97	3.55	3.78	4.40	4.67	5.25	5.21	5.32	4.53	3.89	3.40	2.85	2.41	1.58	0.93	0.79	0.55	0.43	0.13	<0.06

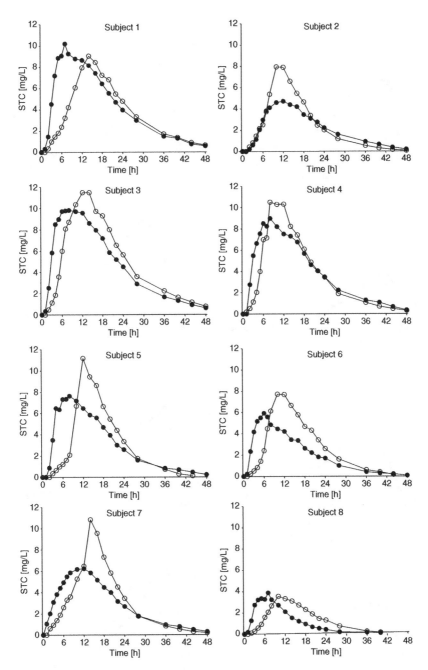

Figure 6.1 Pairwise presentation of individual serum theophylline concentration (STC) versus time curves following a single dose of 600 mg theophylline at 8 p.m. (○ = Reference, ● = Test).

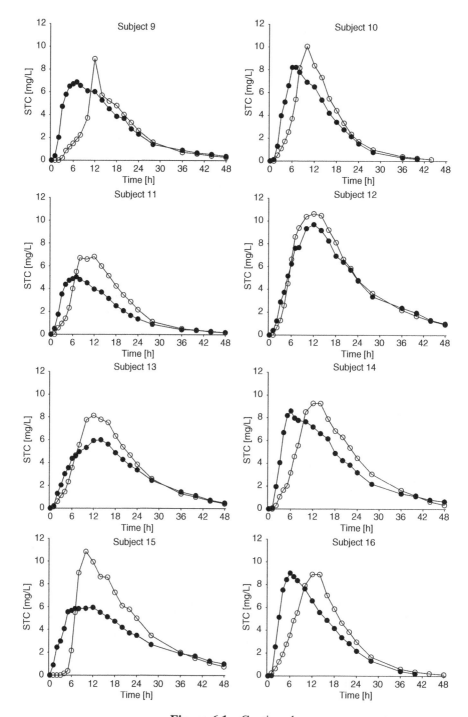

Figure 6.1   Continued.

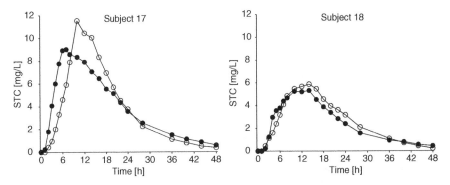

Figure 6.1   Continued.

- Standard plot 1: pairwise, intraindividual comparisons of the concentration-time profiles of the reference and test product (see Figure 6.1)

- Standard plot 2: geometric means of the concentration-time profiles of the reference and test product (see Figure 6.2)

- Standard plot 3: sets of 18 individual concentration-time curves for the reference and test product (see Figure 6.3 a,b)

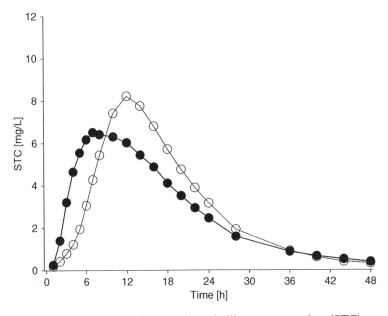

Figure 6.2   Geometric means of serum theophylline concentration (STC) versus time curves following a single dose of 600 mg theophylline at 8 p.m. (o = Reference, • = Test).

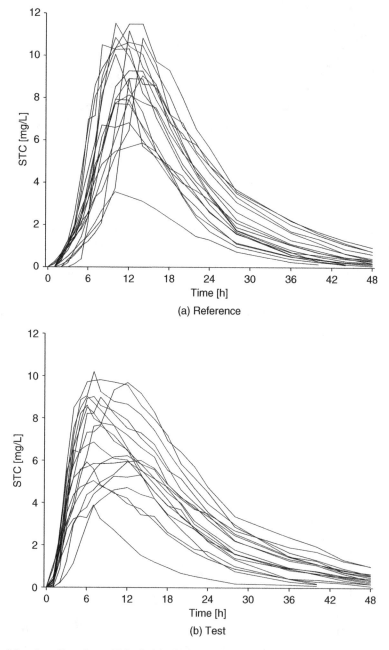

Figure 6.3 a, b   Set of $n = 18$ individual serum theophylline concentration (STC) versus time curves following a single dose of 600 mg theophylline at 8 p.m. (a = Reference, b = Test).

The choice of the appropriate pharmacokinetic characteristics of rate and extent of absorption was the subject of great controversy (Ahr and Schäfer, 1991; Steinijans *et al.*, 1987; Steinijans, 1990). An overview of pharmacokinetic characteristics of rate and extent of absorption in single- and multiple-dose studies is given in Chapter 2.

In the case of controlled release formulations, $AUC(0 - \infty)$ and plateau time $T75\%C_{max}$ have been suggested as primary characteristics of extent and rate of absorption (Schulz and Steinijans, 1991). In order to enable a verification of the AUC calculation from time zero to infinity, the following information is given for each individual in Tables 6.2a and 6.2b for the reference and test product, respectively:

- the time interval used for the estimation of the terminal rate constant λ_z and its estimate $\hat{\lambda}_z$, where t_z denotes the last time point of this interval;

- the estimate of the apparent half-life $t_{1/2} = \ln 2 / \hat{\lambda}_z$;

- the measured concentration C_z at t_z and its estimate $\hat{C}_z$;

- the extrapolated $AUC(t_z - \infty) = \hat{C}_z / \hat{\lambda}_z$, the partial $AUC(0 - t_z)$, the total $AUC(0 - \infty) = AUC(0 - t_z) + \hat{C}_z / \hat{\lambda}_z$, and the ratio $AUC(0 - t_z) / AUC(0 - \infty)$.

It can be seen from Tables 6.2a and b that the extrapolated fraction of the AUC accounted for 2 % of the total AUC on average and for at most 5 % in individual cases.

Since the serum theophylline concentrations 72 hours post dose were below the limit of quantification in 33 out of 36 profiles, the $AUC(0 - \infty)$ was approximated in these cases by $AUC(0 - 72h)$, which was then calculated by the trapezoidal formula after the STCs below the limit of quantification of 0.06 mg/L had been equated to zero. The minor deviations of these approximated values from those given in Tables 6.2a and b show that rather robust estimates of $AUC(0 - \infty)$ were obtained due to frequent and sufficiently long sampling.

In Figure 6.4 the sequence-by-period plot for the primary extent characteristic $AUC(0 - \infty)$ is shown. The results are presented for each sequence in each period as geometric mean and the geometric 68 % range on the original scale, which corresponds to ±1 standard deviation in the logarithmically transformed domain. Figure 6.4 reveals that the AUC values in the group with the treatment sequence reference/test are somewhat higher than those in the other group, irrespective of the treatment. This may reflect clearance differences between the subjects in the two sequences. This is not surprising in the case of theophylline, which is known for its interindividual differences in clearance.

The detailed bioequivalence analysis for $AUC(0 - \infty)$ is given in Table 6.3. This includes the analysis of variance after logarithmic transformation, the corresponding geometric means, as well as the parametric and nonparametric point estimates and 90 % confidence intervals for the ratio of expected means $\exp(\mu_T) / \exp(\mu_R)$. The parametric point estimate of $\exp(\mu_T) / \exp(\mu_R)$ is 0.95, and the corresponding parametric 90 % confidence interval ranges from 0.91 to 1.00. As this is well within the bioequivalence range of 0.80 to 1.25, equivalence with respect to extent of absorption can be concluded. The corresponding nonparametric point estimate is 0.95 and the nonparametric 90 % confidence interval ranges from 0.90 to 1.00. Thus, the results for both statistical methods are nearly identical.

Table 6.2a Pertinent information on the calculation of $AUC(0-\infty)$ including the estimate $\hat{\lambda}_z$ of the terminal rate constant and the extrapolated AUC fraction. Results refer to the data in Table 6.1a (Reference).

Subject number	Interval for estimation of λ_z (h)	$\hat{\lambda}_z$ (1/h)	$t_{1/2}$ (h)	C_z (mg/L)	$\hat{C}_z$ (mg/L)	$AUC(t_z-\infty)$ (mg/L·h)	$AUC(0-t_z)$ (mg/L·h)	$AUC(0-\infty)$ (mg/L·h)	$\dfrac{AUC(0-t_z)}{AUC(0-\infty)}$
1	20–60	0.08391	8.3	0.23	0.23203	2.77	178.33	181.09	0.98
2	36–48	0.16831	4.1	0.07	0.07301	0.43	114.05	114.48	1.00
3	40–60	0.09167	7.6	0.26	0.25888	2.82	238.27	241.09	0.99
4	18–48	0.09756	7.1	0.31	0.31569	3.24	173.68	176.91	0.98
5	36–44	0.22569	3.1	0.12	0.11919	0.53	139.03	139.56	1.00
6	20–40	0.12022	5.8	0.40	0.38535	3.21	121.57	124.77	0.97
7	20–48	0.11915	5.8	0.21	0.19402	1.63	144.97	146.60	0.99
8	24–40	0.13510	5.1	0.15	0.14788	1.09	56.61	57.71	0.98
9	18–48	0.09522	7.3	0.29	0.26578	2.79	106.41	109.20	0.97
10	14–44	0.13111	5.3	0.14	0.13700	1.04	124.57	125.61	0.99
11	28–48	0.09218	7.5	0.18	0.17462	1.89	114.20	116.10	0.98
12	18–72	0.07240	9.6	0.14	0.15857	2.19	235.76	237.95	0.99
13	16–60	0.08997	7.7	0.14	0.14932	1.66	163.43	165.09	0.99
14	40–60	0.12688	5.5	0.09	0.08658	0.68	180.40	181.09	1.00
15	22–48	0.07618	9.1	0.77	0.79547	10.44	196.22	206.66	0.95
16	18–48	0.12962	5.3	0.12	0.12663	0.98	143.02	144.00	0.99
17	18–60	0.10140	6.8	0.09	0.09715	0.96	184.14	185.10	0.99
18	24–48	0.10709	6.5	0.21	0.26185	2.45	123.06	125.50	0.98

Table 6.2b Pertinent information on the calculation of $AUC(0-\infty)$ including the estimate $\hat{\lambda}_z$ of the terminal rate constant and the extrapolated AUC fraction. Results refer to the data in Table 6.1b (Test).

Subject number	Interval for estimation of λ_z (h)	$\hat{\lambda}_z$ (1/h)	$t_{1/2}$ (h)	C_z (mg/L)	$\hat{C}_z$ (mg/L)	$AUC(t_z-\infty)$ (mg/L·h)	$AUC(0-t_z)$ (mg/L·h)	$AUC(0-\infty)$ (mg/L·h)	$\dfrac{AUC(0-t_z)}{AUC(0-\infty)}$
1	16–60	0.08050	8.6	0.22	0.22027	2.74	207.40	210.14	0.99
2	40–48	0.15856	4.4	0.18	0.18357	1.16	97.57	98.72	0.99
3	40–60	0.09982	6.9	0.18	0.18155	1.82	224.13	225.95	0.99
4	18–44	0.07942	8.7	0.66	0.69275	8.72	177.93	186.65	0.95
5	16–48	0.09397	7.4	0.23	0.27304	2.91	144.11	147.01	0.98
6	16–48	0.10821	6.4	0.08	0.11155	1.03	96.50	97.53	0.99
7	20–60	0.08696	8.0	0.12	0.11839	1.36	136.26	137.62	0.99
8	10–28	0.14300	4.8	0.19	0.21596	1.51	44.07	45.58	0.97
9	28–60	0.06664	10.4	0.17	0.17277	2.59	136.77	139.36	0.98
10	20–40	0.13764	5.0	0.18	0.16932	1.23	119.20	120.43	0.99
11	18–48	0.08535	8.1	0.18	0.18023	2.11	90.15	92.26	0.98
12	40–72	0.07223	9.6	0.18	0.18203	2.52	226.11	228.63	0.99
13	40–60	0.10407	6.7	0.14	0.13990	1.34	144.11	145.46	0.99
14	18–60	0.06938	10.0	0.25	0.26462	3.81	176.15	179.96	0.98
15	40–72	0.06943	10.0	0.18	0.18611	2.68	171.18	173.86	0.98
16	22–40	0.14552	4.8	0.20	0.21693	1.49	141.76	143.25	0.99
17	20–48	0.07590	9.1	0.57	0.59466	7.84	184.38	192.22	0.96
18	14–60	0.07761	8.9	0.13	0.14952	1.93	116.06	117.99	0.98

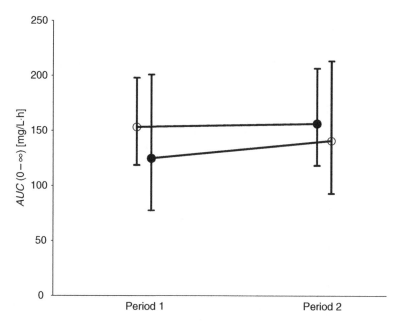

Figure 6.4 Sequence-by-period plot for the primary extent characteristic $AUC(0-\infty)$. The results are given separately for each sequence in each period as geometric mean and the range corresponding to ± 1 standard deviation in the logarithmically transformed domain, i.e., $\exp(\text{mean}(\ln AUC) - \text{sd}(\ln AUC))$, $\exp(\text{mean}(\ln AUC) + \text{sd}(\ln AUC))$ ($\circ$ = Reference, $\bullet$ = Test).

The detailed bioequivalence analysis for the primary rate characteristic plateau time $T75\%C_{max}$ under the assumption of an additive model is given in Table 6.4. This table includes the complete analysis of variance for the untransformed data, the corresponding arithmetic means, as well as the parametric and nonparametric 90 % confidence interval for the difference of expected means $\mu_T - \mu_R$. The parametric point estimate of the difference $\mu_T - \mu_R$ is 2.65 hours and thus outside the stipulated bioequivalence range of ± 1.8 hours. Hence, equivalence with respect to rate of absorption cannot be concluded.

In conclusion, the test and reference product are equivalent with respect to the extent of absorption, but not with respect to the rate of absorption. The plateau time for the test formulation is 10.65 hours and thus 2.65 hours longer than that for the reference product (8 hours). The parametric 90 % confidence interval for the difference in plateau times ranges from 1.43 to 3.87 hours. The results obtained by the corresponding nonparametric analysis are in line with the parametric ones, which therefore can be considered as robust.

The differences between the two products with regard to plateau time are shown in Figure 6.5, which reflects the consistently higher values for the test product, irrespective of the sequence of administration.

These results together with those of the exploratory analysis of the secondary pharmacokinetic characteristics are summarized in Tables 6.5 and 6.6. Table 6.5 gives the geometric mean and the range corresponding to mean ± 1 standard deviation in the

Table 6.3 Bioequivalence analysis for the primary extent characteristic $AUC(0 - \infty)$ based on a multiplicative model, i.e., logarithmic transformation prior to data analysis. The demographic data of the study participants are presented together with the individual *AUCs* for the first and second period. The analysis of variance, geometric means, as well as the parametric and nonparametric point estimates and 90 % confidence intervals for the ratio of expected means $\exp(\mu_T)/\exp(\mu_R)$ are presented subsequently.

Subject number	Age (y)	Weight (kg)	Height (cm)	Sequence	Period 1 (mg/L·h)	Period 2 (mg/L·h)
1	25	66	183	RT	181.09	210.14
2	21	67	183	RT	114.48	98.72
3	25	68	181	TR	225.95	241.09
4	22	70	177	RT	176.91	186.65
5	30	83	191	TR	147.01	139.56
6	22	74	186	TR	97.53	124.77
7	27	70	181	RT	146.60	137.62
8	22	77	182	TR	45.58	57.71
9	39	78	190	RT	109.20	139.36
10	29	65	180	RT	125.61	120.43
11	25	78	179	TR	92.26	116.10
12	37	70	183	RT	237.95	228.63
13	26	70	179	TR	145.46	165.09
14	23	67	177	TR	179.96	181.09
15	27	80	186	TR	173.86	206.66
16	22	68	180	RT	144.00	143.25
17	22	68	176	RT	185.10	192.22
18	28	73	177	TR	117.99	125.50

Analysis of variance after logarithmic transformation of the individual *AUCs*.

Source of variation	Degrees of freedom	Sum of squares	Mean square	F-test	p-value
Between-subject					
Sequence	1	0.21836	0.21836	0.82	0.3778
Subject(Sequence)	16	4.24539	0.26534	41.49	<0.001
Within-subject					
Formulation	1	0.02285	0.02285	3.57	0.0770
Period	1	0.04535	0.04535	7.09	0.0170
Residual	16	0.10233	0.00640		
Total	35	4.63247			

Between-subject $C\hat{V}_B = 37.2$ %, within-subject $C\hat{V}_W = 8.0$ %.

Geometric mean and 68 % range, i.e., [exp(mean(ln AUC) − sd(ln AUC)), exp(mean (ln AUC) + sd(ln AUC))].

	Period 1 Geometric mean	Period 2 Geometric mean	Both periods Geometric mean and 68 % range
Reference	153.31	140.84	146.94 [104.03, 207.56]
Test	124.75	156.50	139.72 [94.56, 206.45]

Point estimate and 90 % confidence interval for the ratio of expected means $\exp(\mu_T)/\exp(\mu_R)$.

Statistical method		Point estimate	Confidence limits		Level of confidence
			Lower	Upper	
Parametric analysis	Two one-sided t-tests	0.95	0.908	0.996	0.9000
Nonparametric analysis	Two one-sided Wilcoxon tests	0.95	0.900	0.996	0.9061

logarithmically transformed domain for the pharmacokinetic characteristics for test and reference, respectively, and, as this is a balanced design, the geometric mean of the individual ratios test/reference as point estimate together with the 90 % confidence interval for the ratio of expected means $\exp(\mu_T)/\exp(\mu_R)$.

If C_{max} or $100\,C_{max}/AUC$ had been taken as rate characteristics, the conclusion would have been the same as with the plateau time. However, for the mean residence time, which only partially reflects the absorption phase, the 90 % confidence interval for $\exp(\mu_T)/\exp(\mu_R)$ is in the bioequivalence range of 0.80 to 1.25.

Table 6.6 gives mean ±1 standard deviation of the pharmacokinetic characteristics for which an additive parametric model is assumed, and the difference between means of test and reference as point estimate together with the 90 % confidence interval for the difference of expected means $\mu_T - \mu_R$. Table 6.6 reveals that in this single-dose study the plateau time and the time above C_{av} (T above C_{av}) show treatment differences in opposite directions. Whereas the values of the plateau time for the test product are fairly similar in the single- and the multiple-dose study, the time above C_{av} almost doubles under steady-state conditions (cf. Table 6.12). This confirms that the time above C_{av} is not a suitable rate characteristic in single-dose studies, at least with regard to the absolute values (Schulz and Steinijans, 1991; see also Table 2.3).

The results of the nonparametric analysis of t_{max} are given in Table 6.7. The median, minimum and maximum are given as summary statistics for t_{max}, the nonparametric point estimate and 90 % confidence interval are given for the difference of expected medians $\mu_T - \mu_R$.

Table 6.4 Bioequivalence analysis for the primary rate characteristic plateau time $T75\% \, C_{max}$ based on an additive model, i.e., data analysis on the original data. The demographic data of the study participants are presented together with the individual plateau times (h) for the first and second period. The analysis of variance for the untransformed data, arithmetic means, as well as the parametric and nonparametric point estimates and 90 % confidence intervals for the difference of expected means $\mu_T - \mu_R$ are presented subsequently.

Subject number	Age (y)	Weight (kg)	Height (cm)	Sequence	Period 1 (h)	Period 2 (h)
1	25	70	183	RT	9.27	11.10
2	21	67	183	RT	6.67	11.15
3	25	68	181	TR	13.95	11.20
4	22	70	177	RT	7.64	11.92
5	30	83	191	TR	11.07	5.50
6	22	74	186	TR	6.83	8.17
7	27	70	181	RT	4.52	11.93
8	22	77	182	TR	5.93	8.33
9	39	78	190	RT	2.25	10.96
10	29	65	180	RT	5.82	7.89
11	25	78	179	TR	10.13	9.34
12	37	70	183	RT	11.53	10.76
13	26	70	179	TR	12.68	10.01
14	23	67	177	TR	10.82	8.83
15	27	80	186	TR	14.74	8.93
16	22	68	180	RT	7.69	8.00
17	22	68	176	RT	7.22	10.55
18	28	73	177	TR	11.35	11.13

Analysis of variance of the untransformed individual $T75\% \, C_{max}$.

Source of variation	Degrees of freedom	Sum of squares	Mean square	F-test	p-value
Between-subject					
Sequence	1	13.530	13.530	2.21	0.1567
Subject(Sequence)	16	98.036	6.127	1.40	0.2553
Within-subject					
Formulation	1	63.229	63.229	14.42	0.0016
Period	1	6.751	6.751	1.54	0.2325
Residual	16	70.136	4.384		
Total	35	251.683			

Between-subject $C\hat{V}_B = 11.7\%$, within-subject $C\hat{V}_W = 26.2\%$.

Arithmetic mean and 68 % range, i.e., mean $\pm$ 1 standard deviation (SD).

	Period 1 Mean	Period 2 Mean	Both periods Mean $\pm$ SD
Reference	6.96	9.05	8.00 ± 2.25
Test	10.83	10.47	10.65 ± 2.34

Point estimate and 90 % confidence interval for the difference of expected means $\mu_T - \mu_R$.

		Point estimate	Confidence limits Lower	Upper	Level of confidence
Statistical method					
Parametric analysis	Two one-sided t-tests	2.65	1.432	3.869	0.9000
Nonparametric analysis	Two one-sided Wilcoxon tests	2.52	1.150	3.820	0.9061

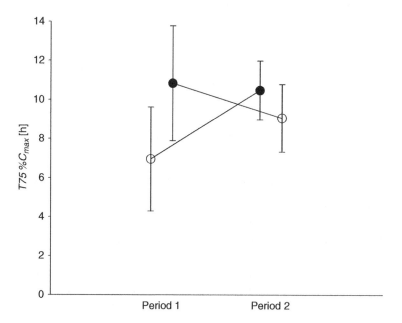

Figure 6.5 Sequence-by-period plot for the primary rate characteristic plateau time $T75\%C_{max}$. The results are given separately for each sequence in each period as mean ± 1 standard deviation ($\circ$ = Reference, $\bullet$ = Test).

Table 6.5 Summary of the statistical analysis of single-dose pharmacokinetic characteristics for which a multiplicative model is assumed. The results are combined for the two periods and are given as geometric mean and the geometric 68 % range, which corresponds to mean ± 1 standard deviation in the logarithmically transformed domain. The results of the bioequivalence analysis are given as the point estimate and 90 % confidence interval for the ratio of expected means $\exp(\mu_T)/\exp(\mu_R)$.

Pharmacokinetic characteristic (P = primary, S = secondary)	Reference Geometric mean and 68 % range	Test Geometric mean and 68 % range	Test/Reference Point estimate and 90 % confidence interval
P: $AUC(0-\infty)$ (mg/L · h)	147 [104, 208]	140 [95, 206]	0.95 [0.91, 1.00]
S: C_{max} (mg/L)	8.8 [6.6, 11.6]	7.0 [5.4, 9.2]	0.80 [0.74, 0.87]
S: $100 C_{max}/AUC$ $(0-\infty)(1/h)$	6.0 [4.9, 7.2]	5.0 [4.1, 6.2]	0.84 [0.77, 0.92]
S: MRT (h)	18.0 [16.1, 20.2]	16.9 [14.0, 20.5]	0.94 [0.89, 0.99]

Table 6.6 Summary of the statistical analysis of single-dose pharmacokinetic characteristics for which an additive model is assumed. The results are combined for the two periods and are given as mean ± 1 standard deviation. The results of the bioequivalence analysis are given as the point estimate and 90 % confidence interval for the difference of expected means $\mu_T - \mu_R$.

Pharmacokinetic characteristic (P = primary, S = secondary)	Reference Mean $\pm$ SD	Test Mean $\pm$ SD	Test – Reference Point estimate and 90 % confidence interval
P: $T75\% C_{max}$ (h)	8.0 ± 2.2	10.7 ± 2.3	2.7 [1.4, 3.9]
S: T above C_{av} (h)	8.4 ± 1.5	6.7 ± 3.4	$-1.7 [-2.8, -0.6]$

Table 6.7 Summary of the statistical analysis of the secondary characteristic t_{max} for which an additive model is assumed. The results are given as median [minimum, maximum]. The results of the bioequivalence analysis are given as the nonparametric point estimate and 90 % confidence interval for the difference of expected medians $\mu_T - \mu_R$.

Pharmacokinetic characteristic (S = secondary)	Reference Median [Min, Max]	Test Median [Min, Max]	Test – Reference Point estimate and 90 % confidence interval
S: t_{max} (h)	12 [8, 14]	7.5 [6, 14]	$-2.5 [-4, -1.5]$

As pointed out in Section 2.2.2, t_{max} is of limited value in characterizing prolonged release formulations with their flat and sometimes multiple peaks. Therefore, no bioequivalence range had been stipulated for t_{max}, and the observed difference given in Table 6.7 has to be assessed on clinical grounds.

6.3   Results from a multiple-dose study

In this multiple-dose, randomized, two-period crossover study in $n = 12$ healthy volunteers, two controlled release theophylline formulations were compared with regard to rate and extent of absorption (Steinijans *et al.*, 1986). The test product was again the Euphylong® pellet formulation. In this study it was available as capsules containing 400 mg anhydrous theophylline. The dose was chosen in order to match the 400 mg strength of the reference tablet, which is also intended for once-daily nighttime dosing. The release characteristics of the reference product show an agitation dependency rather than a pH-dependency (Benedikt *et al.*, 1988). Food effects of the reference product have been described by Karim *et al.* (1985); see also the review by Jonkman (1989). Two capsules of the test formulation or two tablets of the reference formulation were given once daily at 7 p.m., half an hour after the evening meal, with 200 ml of mineral water. On the days of the 24-hour serum theophylline profiles, the evening meals were standardized and had a composition of 36 g fat, 40 g protein and 84 g carbohydrates. The two treatment periods consisted of seven 24-hour intervals each and were separated by a one-week washout period. Only the steady-state profiles after the seventh dose are presented; for further details concerning the complete study design the reader is referred to the original publication (Steinijans *et al.*, 1986).

The demographic data of the 12 study participants, all of them nonsmokers, are given in Table 6.9, together with the randomized sequence of treatments. Prior to the study, the volunteers underwent physical and laboratory examination, and informed consent was given by each subject in writing. Sixteen blood samples for determination of serum theophylline concentrations were taken during the 24-hour steady-state interval, i.e., 144 to 168 hours after the first dose in each treatment period. The samples were taken at hourly intervals for the first 6 hours, thereafter every 2 hours. The individual STCs are given in Table 6.8a for the reference formulation and in Table 6.8b for the test formulation. In addition to the time after first dose, the clock time is also given in these tables.

In multiple-dose studies of controlled-release formulations the % peak-trough fluctuation ($\%PTF = 100(C_{max} - C_{min})/C_{av}$) and the AUC over one steady-state dose interval, in this case 144 to 168 hours after the first dose, have been suggested as primary characteristics of rate and extent of absorption, respectively (Ahr and Schäfer, 1991; APV 1987; Skelly, 1984; Steinijans *et al.*, 1986, 1987, 1989; Steinijans 1989, 1990; Schulz and Steinijans, 1991). The $AUC = AUC(144-168)$ was calculated by the linear trapezoidal rule, and the average steady-state concentration was derived from this as $C_{av} = AUC/24$.

Figure 6.6 gives the pairwise, intraindividual comparisons of the concentration-time profiles for the reference and test product. Figure 6.7 gives the geometric means of the concentration-time profiles of the reference and test product and Figures 6.8a an 6.8b give the sets of 12 individual concentration-time curves for the reference and test product.

Table 6.8a Serum theophylline concentrations (mg/L) following repeated once-daily doses of 800 mg theophylline (Reference) at 7 p.m.

Subject number	Time after first dose (h) 144	145	146	147	148	149	150	152	154	156	158	160	162	164	166	168
Clock time	19	20	21	22	23	24	1	3	5	7	9	11	13	15	17	19
1	3.91	4.95	8.38	11.96	14.70	17.14	16.23	14.30	12.99	11.47	10.89	8.52	7.55	5.67	4.79	3.98
2	7.10	9.53	12.78	16.71	19.54	21.00	19.81	18.26	17.50	13.91	12.97	10.92	9.80	7.86	6.65	5.88
3	4.80	5.09	6.21	9.43	15.17	17.39	16.81	14.63	13.35	11.09	10.80	9.01	7.42	5.74	4.48	3.74
4	4.77	5.84	10.10	15.60	18.76	19.69	19.78	17.59	14.85	13.50	12.52	10.24	8.97	7.58	6.72	5.35
5	7.16	7.14	12.12	14.68	17.61	19.94	20.50	20.91	18.95	16.79	15.97	13.49	11.76	9.26	8.09	7.29
6	1.73	1.67	2.84	2.76	4.89	5.65	11.74	11.28	10.23	8.32	6.95	5.37	3.68	2.65	1.85	1.45
7	11.70	16.08	20.44	22.60	24.10	27.23	25.92	24.65	21.97	19.52	21.04	19.99	18.69	14.14	11.99	9.96
8	2.39	3.53	5.68	6.55	7.80	8.72	10.10	12.85	13.22	11.15	10.39	7.64	5.56	4.20	3.13	2.23
9	1.86	4.01	5.69	8.33	12.85	15.06	13.69	11.53	6.36	5.87	3.36	2.95	2.98	2.45	2.22	1.70
10	3.26	3.15	3.91	10.29	10.70	11.24	12.31	16.09	16.22	13.17	10.68	8.02	5.44	4.16	3.21	2.75
11	6.80	8.60	11.90	14.60	19.40	19.20	20.20	18.50	16.20	15.40	12.60	9.20	8.00	7.70	6.30	5.80
12	4.74	4.75	6.03	6.10	6.19	6.32	6.33	8.75	12.89	13.80	13.91	11.98	10.08	7.91	6.13	4.97

Table 6.8b Serum theophylline concentrations (mg/L) following repeated once-daily doses of 800 mg theophylline (Test) at 7 p.m.

Subject number	Time after first dose (h)															
	144	145	146	147	148	149	150	152	154	156	158	160	162	164	166	168
	Clock time															
	19	20	21	22	23	24	1	3	5	7	9	11	13	15	17	19
1	5.37	4.75	7.53	8.30	9.95	11.70	12.55	11.62	11.14	10.18	9.76	8.77	7.53	6.27	5.20	4.33
2	7.87	9.30	11.52	12.57	12.76	13.52	13.08	13.44	13.27	12.65	11.97	10.94	9.71	8.64	7.26	6.40
3	6.05	7.22	8.97	10.12	11.65	12.29	11.74	12.90	12.71	11.82	12.16	9.94	8.61	7.42	7.17	5.86
4	9.04	7.96	8.67	12.55	14.89	16.11	16.84	17.45	17.24	15.83	15.55	14.43	12.16	10.17	8.55	7.10
5	8.03	7.53	8.78	11.31	13.23	15.83	16.47	16.13	14.95	14.12	14.11	12.14	10.73	8.85	7.38	6.80
6	3.50	3.07	3.53	3.64	4.00	5.04	7.89	10.08	9.72	9.00	8.57	7.42	5.51	3.96	3.32	2.53
7	10.02	9.33	10.45	10.82	12.81	15.23	17.06	18.88	17.81	16.83	16.87	15.27	13.20	10.23	9.61	8.77
8	3.48	3.53	5.95	7.03	8.69	10.58	10.39	10.30	9.65	9.19	9.03	7.83	6.22	4.54	3.78	3.09
9	4.11	3.89	4.54	6.74	9.30	10.94	10.62	10.43	10.07	9.78	9.03	8.13	6.98	5.91	4.69	3.82
10	3.41	3.08	5.37	7.68	8.97	9.81	10.05	10.78	9.47	8.66	8.60	7.11	6.17	4.57	3.92	3.12
11	7.97	7.07	6.47	7.39	8.41	9.17	10.35	12.08	12.68	13.09	13.49	12.81	10.60	9.07	7.51	6.15
12	6.10	6.20	7.10	7.30	8.30	9.00	8.90	10.00	12.30	10.80	13.00	11.50	8.50	7.00	6.40	4.50

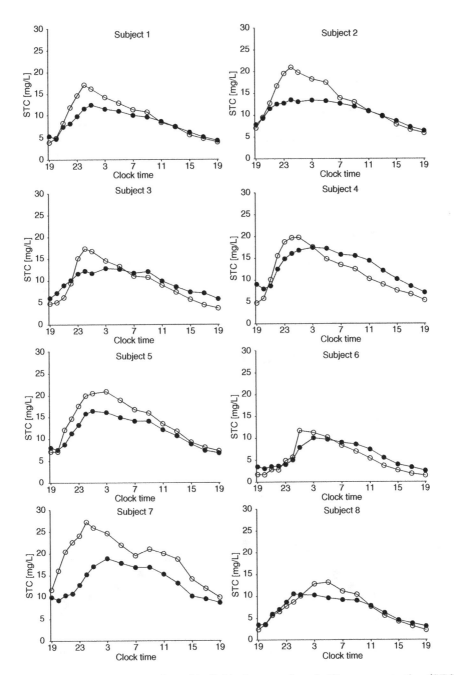

Figure 6.6 Pairwise presentation of individual serum theophylline concentration (STC) versus time curves following repeated once-daily doses of 800 mg theophylline at 7 p.m. (○ = Reference, ● = Test). Time is given as clock time, e.g., 19 corresponds to 7 p.m.

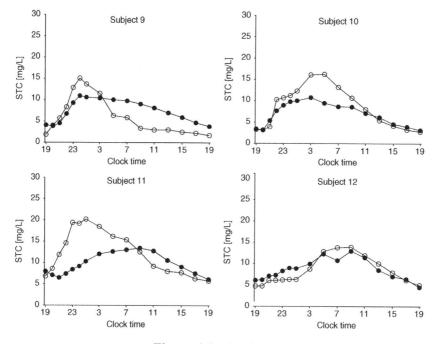

Figure 6.6   Continued.

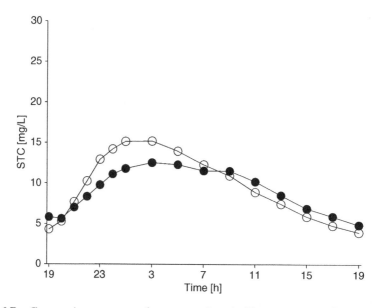

Figure 6.7   Geometric means of serum theophylline concentration-time curves following repeated once-daily doses of 800 mg theophylline at 7 p.m. (○ = Reference, ● = Test). Time is given as clock time, e.g., 19 corresponds to 7 p.m.

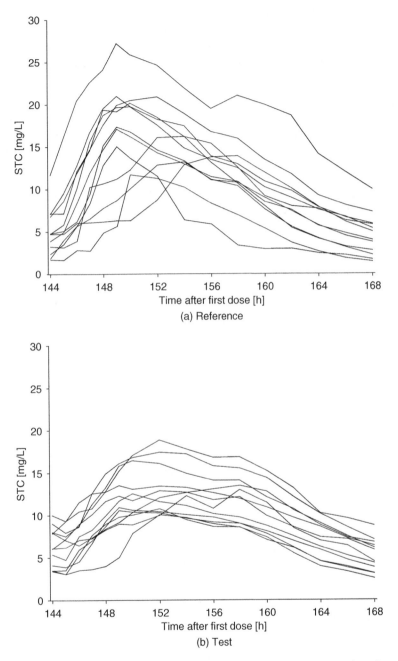

Figure 6.8 a, b   Set of $n = 12$ individual serum theophylline concentration-time curves following repeated once-daily doses of 800 mg theophylline at 7 p.m. (a = Reference, b = Test). Time is given as time after first dose. Due to the evening dosing at 7 p.m., 144 hours corresponds to 7 p.m.

Table 6.9 Bioequivalence analysis for the primary extent characteristic $AUC(144-168)$ based on a multiplicative model, i.e., logarithmic transformation prior to data analysis. The demographic data of the study participants are presented together with the individual $AUCs$ for the first and second period. The analysis of variance, geometric means as well as the parametric and nonparametric point estimates and 90 % confidence intervals for the ratio of expected means $\exp(\mu_T)/\exp(\mu_R)$ are presented subsequently.

Subject number	Age (y)	Weight (kg)	Height (cm)	Sequence	Period 1 (mg/L·h)	Period 2 (mg/L·h)
1	24	73	189	TR	209.01	239.77
2	27	77	188	RT	314.45	265.39
3	24	79	184	RT	237.69	242.20
4	26	72	174	RT	291.34	319.82
5	33	75	184	TR	289.02	343.55
6	28	80	177	RT	138.24	150.56
7	23	80	192	TR	335.41	469.12
8	29	73	186	RT	187.14	177.28
9	24	73	188	TR	187.26	144.55
10	27	72	180	TR	173.37	216.12
11	25	77	193	TR	246.83	301.00
12	24	69	183	RT	217.13	217.80

Analysis of variance after logarithmic transformation of the individual $AUCs$.

Source of variation	Degrees of freedom	Sum of squares	Mean square	F-test	p-value
Between-subject					
Sequence	1	0.08112	0.08112	0.44	0.5237
Subject(Sequence)	10	1.85795	0.18578	14.51	0.0001
Within-subject					
Formulation	1	0.02862	0.02862	2.24	0.1657
Period	1	0.02550	0.02550	1.99	0.1885
Residual	10	0.12802	0.01280		
Total	23	2.12122			

Between-subject $C\hat{V}_B = 30.1$ %, within-subject $C\hat{V}_W = 11.4$ %.

Geometric mean and 68 % range, i.e., $[\exp(\text{mean}(\ln AUC) - \text{sd}(\ln AUC)), \exp(\text{mean}(\ln AUC) + \text{sd}(\ln AUC))]$.

	Period 1 Geometric mean	Period 2 Geometric mean	Both periods Geometric mean and 68 % range
Reference	222.80	267.13	243.96 [170.54, 349.00]
Test	233.57	221.94	227.68 [174.62, 296.86]

Point estimate and 90 % confidence interval for the ratio of expected means $\exp(\mu_T)/\exp(\mu_R)$.

Statistical method		Point estimate	Confidence limits		Level of confidence
			Lower	Upper	
Parametric analysis	Two one-sided t-tests	0.93	0.858	1.015	0.9000
Nonparametric analysis	Two one-sided Wilcoxon tests	0.92	0.858	0.974	0.9069

- Standard plot 1: pairwise, intraindividual comparisons of the concentration-time profiles of the reference and test product (see Figure 6.6)

- Standard plot 2: geometric means of the concentration-time profiles of the reference and the test product (see Figure 6.7)

- Standard plot 3: sets of 12 individual concentration-time curves for the reference and test product (see Figure 6.8 a,b)

In Figure 6.9 the sequence-by-period plot for the primary extent characteristic $AUC(144 - 168)$ is shown. The results are presented for each sequence in each period as geometric mean and the geometric 68 % range on the original scale, which corresponds to ± 1 standard deviation in the logarithmically transformed domain.

The detailed bioequivalence analysis for AUC under the assumption of a multiplicative model is given in Table 6.9. This includes the analysis of variance after logarithmic transformation, geometric means, as well as the parametric and nonparametric point estimates and 90 % confidence intervals for the ratio of expected means $\exp(\mu_T)/\exp(\mu_R)$. The parametric point estimate is 0.93 and the 90 % confidence interval ranges from 0.86 to 1.01. As this is within the bioequivalence range of 0.8 to 1.25, equivalence with respect to extent of absorption can be concluded. The corresponding values according to the nonparametric method are rather similar.

The detailed bioequivalence analysis for the % peak-trough fluctuation ($\%PTF$) under the assumption of a multiplicative model is given in Table 6.10.

The parametric point estimate of the ratio $\exp(\mu_T)/\exp(\mu_R)$ is 0.66 and thus outside the bioequivalence range from 0.80 to 1.25. The 90 % confidence interval ranges from 0.58 to 0.75. The corresponding nonparametric point estimate is 0.67 and the nonparametric 90 % confidence interval ranges from 0.60 to 0.75. Hence, equivalence with respect to rate of absorption cannot be concluded. On the contrary, as the upper limit of the 90 % confidence interval is below the lower limit of the bioequivalence range, a significant difference in the rate of drug release/absorption can be concluded.

The differences between the treatments with regard to the % peak-trough fluctuation are shown in Figure 6.10, which reflects the consistently lower values for the test product, irrespective of the sequence of administration.

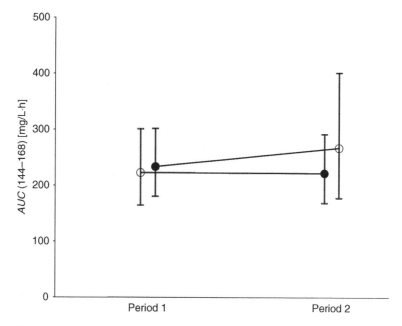

Figure 6.9 Sequence-by-period plot for the primary extent characteristic $AUC(144 - 168)$. The results are given separately for each sequence in each period as geometric mean and the range corresponding to ± 1 standard deviation in the logarithmically transformed domain, i.e., $\exp(\text{mean}(\ln AUC) - \text{sd}(\ln AUC))$, $\exp(\text{mean}(\ln AUC) + \text{sd}(\ln AUC))$ ($\circ = $ Reference, $\bullet = $ Test).

In conclusion, the test and reference product are equivalent with respect to the extent of absorption, but not with respect to the rate of absorption. The % peak-trough fluctuation is 34 % lower for the test formulation than for the reference formulation.

These results together with those of the exploratory analysis of the secondary pharmacokinetic characteristics are summarized in Table 6.11 and 6.12 for the multiplicative and the additive model, respectively.

Table 6.11 gives geometric mean and the range corresponding to mean ± 1 standard deviation in the logarithmically transformed domain for the pharmacokinetic characteristics for test and reference, respectively, and the geometric mean of the individual ratios test/reference as point estimate together with the 90 % confidence interval for the ratio of expected means $\exp(\mu_T)/\exp(\mu_R)$. Table 6.11 reveals that all other rate characteristics such as C_{max}, $100\,C_{max}/AUC$, $\%Swing$ and $\%AUC$ fluctuation (see Section 2.3) lead to the same conclusion as the % peak-trough fluctuation, of not meeting the bioequivalence rate criterion.

Table 6.12 gives means ± 1 standard deviation of the pharmacokinetic characteristics for which an additive parametric model is assumed, and the mean of the differences test – reference as point estimate together with the 90 % confidence interval for the difference of expected means $\mu_T - \mu_R$.

Table 6.10 Bioequivalence analysis for the primary rate characteristic % peak-trough fluctuation (*%PTF*) based on a multiplicative model, i.e., logarithmic transformation prior to data analysis. The demographic data of the study participants are presented together with the individual % peak-trough fluctuations for the first and second period. The analysis of variance, geometric means, as well as the parametric and nonparametric point estimates and 90 % confidence intervals for the ratio of expected means $\exp(\mu_T)/\exp(\mu_R)$ are presented subsequently.

Subject number	Age (y)	Weight (kg)	Height (cm)	Sequence	Period 1 (%)	Period 2 (%)
1	24	73	189	TR	94	132
2	27	77	188	RT	115	64
3	24	79	184	RT	138	70
4	26	72	174	RT	124	78
5	33	75	184	TR	80	96
6	28	80	177	RT	178	120
7	23	80	192	TR	72	88
8	29	73	186	RT	141	101
9	24	73	188	TR	91	222
10	27	72	180	TR	107	150
11	25	77	193	TR	71	115
12	24	69	183	RT	101	94

Analysis of variance after logarithmic transformation of the individual *%PTF*s.

Source of variation	Degrees of freedom	Sum of squares	Mean square	F-test	p-value
Between-subject					
Sequence	1	0.00196	0.00196	0.02	0.8845
Subject(Sequence)	10	0.88436	0.08844	3.11	0.0439
Within-subject					
Formulation	1	1.02611	1.02611	36.08	0.0001
Period	1	0.00037	0.00037	0.01	0.9119
Residual	10	0.28443	0.02844		
Total	23	2.19722			

Between-subject $C\hat{V}_B = 17.5$ %, within-subject $C\hat{V}_W = 17.0$ %.

Geometric mean and 68 % range, i.e., [exp(mean(ln *%PTF*) − sd(ln *%PTF*)), exp(mean(ln *%PTF*) + sd(ln *%PTF*))].

	Period 1 Geometric mean	Period 2 Geometric mean	Both periods Geometric mean and 68 % range
Reference	131	127	129 [98, 170]
Test	85	86	85 [70, 105]

Point estimate and 90 % confidence interval for the ratio of expected means $\exp(\mu_T)/\exp(\mu_R)$.

Statistical method		Point estimate	Confidence limits		Level of confidence
			Lower	Upper	
Parametric analysis	Two one-sided t-tests	0.66	0.584	0.749	0.9000
Nonparametric analysis	Two one-sided Wilcoxon tests	0.67	0.601	0.750	0.9069

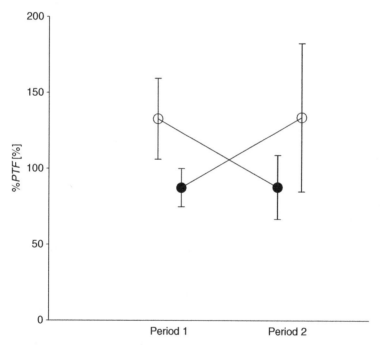

Figure 6.10 Sequence-by-period plot for the primary rate characteristic %*PTF*. The results are given separately for each sequence in each period as geometric mean and the range corresponding to ± 1 standard deviation in the logarithmically transformed domain, i.e., exp(mean(ln %*PTF*) - sd(ln %*PTF*)), exp(mean(ln %*PTF*) + sd(ln %*PTF*)) ($\circ$ = Reference, $\bullet$ = Test).

Table 6.11 Summary of the statistical analysis of multiple-dose pharmacokinetic characteristics for which a multiplicative model is assumed. The results are combined for the two periods and are given as geometric mean and the geometric 68 % range corresponding to mean ± 1 standard deviation in the logarithmically transformed domain. The results of the bioequivalence analysis are given as the point estimate and 90 % confidence interval for the ratio of expected means $\exp(\mu_T)/\exp(\mu_R)$.

Pharmacokinetic characteristic (P = primary, S = secondary)	Reference Geometric mean and 68 % range	Test Geometric mean and 68 % range	Test/Reference Point estimate and 90 % confidence interval
P: $AUC(144–168)$ (mg/L·h)	244 [171, 349]	228 [175, 297]	0.93 [0.86, 1.01]
P: PTF (%)	129 [98, 170]	85 [70, 105]	0.66 [0.58, 0.75]
S: C_{max} (mg/L)	17.4 [13.9, 21.8]	13.1 [10.6, 16.2]	0.76 [0.72, 0.80]
S: $100C_{max}/AUC$ (144–168) (1/h)	7.1 [6.0, 8.4]	5.8 [5.3, 6.2]	0.81 [0.75, 0.88]
S: $Swing$ (%)	337 [199, 571]	167 [117, 237]	0.49 [0.40, 0.60]
S: AUC Fluctuation (%)	35 [26, 48]	24 [19, 30]	0.69 [0.61, 0.77]

Table 6.12 Summary of the statistical analysis of multiple-dose pharmacokinetic characteristics for which an additive model is assumed. The results are combined for the two periods and are given as mean ± 1 standard deviation. The results of the bioequivalence analysis are given as the point estimate and 90 % confidence interval for the difference of expected means $\mu_T - \mu_R$.

Pharmacokinetic characteristic (S = secondary)	Reference Mean $\pm$ SD	Test Mean $\pm$ SD	Test – Reference Point estimate and 90 % confidence interval
S: $T75\%C_{max}$ (h)	7.9 ± 2.0	12.3 ± 1.8	4.4 [3.1, 5.8]
S: T above C_{av}(h)	11.8 ± 1.3	12.8 ± 0.8	1.0 [0.3, 1.8]

The results of the nonparametric analysis of t_{max} are given in Table 6.13. The median, minimum and maximum are given as summary statistics for t_{max}, the nonparametric point estimate and 90 % confidence limits are given for the difference of expected medians $\mu_T - \mu_R$.

Table 6.13 Summary of the statistical analysis of the secondary characteristic t_{max} for which an additive model is assumed. The results are given as median [minimum, maximum]. The results of the bioequivalence analysis are given as the nonparametric point estimate and 90 % confidence interval for the difference of expected medians $\mu_T - \mu_R$.

Pharmacokinetic characteristic (S = secondary)	Reference Median [Min, Max]	Test Median [Min, Max]	Test – Reference Point estimate and 90 % confidence interval
S: t_{max} (h)	6 [5, 14]	8 [5, 14]	0.5 [−1.0, 2.5]

6.4   Conclusions

In this chapter, a detailed presentation of the results of single- and multiple-dose bioequivalence studies is provided. Starting from the individual concentrations based on serial measurements, all calculation steps can be reproduced. Three types of standard concentration-time plots (pairwise intraindividual comparison, geometric mean curves, and sets of individual concentration-time profiles per treatment) together with the sequence-by-period plot, provide fairly complete statistical information on the study results, both from a descriptive and an inferential point of view.

Subtle problems such as the handling of concentrations below the limit of quantification and the AUC extrapolation to infinity in single-dose studies have been dealt with. As pointed out by Schulz and Steinijans (1991), there is an occasional ambiguity in estimating the terminal half-life and its effect on the extrapolated AUC. Presumably, there is no definite answer to this problem, and therefore, it is important to document all steps of analysis in detail as has been done in Tables 6.2a and 6.2b. This will facilitate independent verification of results by a third party such as quality assurance, licensees, reviewers of journals or health authorities.

The tables and graphs presented in this chapter provide a fairly complete analysis of bioequivalence studies. They may be further supplemented by residual plots (Steinijans and Hauschke, 1990). In the case of multiple-dose studies both aspects of bioequivalence, i.e., rate and extent of absorption, can be visualized for each subject in a single plot, with the average steady-state concentration, $C_{av} = AUC /$ dose interval, serving as extent characteristic, and the concentration range during that dose interval, $C_{max} - C_{min}$, reflecting the rate of absorption (cf. Figure 2.7).

In routine bioequivalence publications only a selected subset of the information given in this chapter will be printed. The individual values of the primary characteristics of rate and extent of absorption should be given together with the sequence of administration (Tables 6.3 and 6.4 (single-dose study) and 6.9 and 6.10 (multiple-dose study)). The results of the bioequivalence analysis should be summarized as in Tables 6.5, 6.6, 6.7 (single-dose study) and 6.11, 6.12, 6.13 (multiple-dose study). Although the full analysis of variance as presented within Tables 6.3 and 6.4 (single-dose study) and 6.9 and

6.10 (multiple-dose study) may not be published, it should be made available to the reviewers.

The nonparametric procedure is an alternative to the parametric approach and should be performed routinely for the sake of robustness. With regard to the additive model, the nonparametric procedure has the general advantage of not requiring the symmetry that is assumed in the parametric approach. Thus, for the additive model, the presentation of the results from the nonparametric procedure could even be first choice. In this case, the summary presentations given in Tables 6.6 and 6.12 would be analogous to those in Tables 6.7 and 6.13, respectively. Note that the nonparametric approach is generally recommended for the analysis of t_{max} (CPMP, 2001).

Apart from the geometric mean plots of the concentration-time curves (Figure 6.2, single-dose study and Figure 6.7, multiple-dose study), the pairwise individual plots (Figure 6.1, single-dose study and Figure 6.6, multiple-dose study) should be given routinely. In addition, the presentation for a single-dose study should provide some information on the extrapolated AUC, at least the time intervals used for the estimation of the terminal rate constant and the extrapolated AUC as a fraction of the total AUC (Tables 6.2a and 6.2b).

For the successful publication of a bioequivalence study in a clinical pharmacological journal, Hitzenberger and Steinijans (1994) alluded, from an editorial point of view, to the following points that should be carefully considered

- crossover design or justification for deviation there from;

- specification of primary characteristics of rate and extent of absorption;

- logarithmic transformation of AUC, C_{max}, etc. or justification for deviation there from;

- sample size planning;

- demographic data of study participants;

- individual treatment sequences;

- drug administration under fasting or fed conditions (timing and composition of meals);

- times of blood sampling;

- analytical method and lower limit of quantification;

- description of AUC extrapolation to infinity (method and fraction of total AUC);

- point estimate and 90 % confidence limits for test/reference ratio;

- correct interpretation of results in abstract and conclusion.

In conclusion, the standards set in this chapter for the presentation of results from bioequivalence studies together with the concept of 'Good Biometrical Practice' (Schulz and Steinijans, 1991, Steinijans *et al.*, 1992) will improve the quality and the credibility of bioequivalence studies.

References

Ahr, G. and Schäfer, H.G. (1991) Design and pharmacokinetic characteristics of controlled/modified release products. In: Blume, H., Gundert-Remy, U. and Müller, H. (eds) *Controlled/Modified Release Products*, 85–98, Wissenschaftliche Verlagsgesellschaft, Stuttgart.

APV (1987) Studies on bioavailability and bioequivalence (APV guideline). *Drugs made in Germany* **30**, 161–6.

Benedikt, G., Steinijans, V.W. and Dietrich, R. (1988) Galenical development of a new sustained-release theophylline pellet formulation for once-daily administration. *Arzneimittel-Forschung/Drug Research* **38**, 1203–9.

Committee for Proprietary Medicinal Products (2001) *Note for guidance on the investigation of bioavailability and bioequivalence*. EMEA, London.

D'Alonzo, G.E., Smolensky, M.H., Feldman, S., Gianotti, L.A., Emerson, M.B., Staudinger, H.W. and Steinijans, V.W. (1990) Twenty-four-hour lung function in adult patients with asthma – chronoptimized theophylline therapy once-daily dosing in the evening versus conventional twice-daily dosing. *American Review of Respiratory Disease* **142**, 84–90.

Dietrich, R., Brausse, R., Bautz, A. and Diletti, E. (1988) Validation of the in-vivo dissolution method used for a new sustained-release theophylline pellet formulation. *Arzneimittel-Forschung/Drug Research* **38**, 1220–8.

Food and Drug Administration (2003) *Guidance for Industry: bioavailability and bioequivalence studies for orally administered drug product – general considerations*. Center for Drug Evaluation and Research, Rockville, MD.

Hendeles, L., Weinberger, M., Milavetz, G., Hill, M. and Vaughan, L. (1985) Food-induced 'dose-dumping' from a once-a-day theophylline product as a cause of theophylline toxicity. *Chest* **87**, 758–65.

Hitzenberger, G. and Steinijans, V.W. (1994) From the editors – to reject or not to reject – recent experience with bioequivalence papers. *International Journal of Clinical Pharmacology, Therapy and Toxicology* **32**, 161–4.

Jonkman, J.H.G. (1989) Food interactions with sustained-release theophylline preparations – a review. *Clinical Pharmacokinetics* **16**, 162–79.

Karim, A., Burns, T., Wearley, L., Streicher, J. and Palmer, M. (1985) Food-induced changes in theophylline absorption from controlled release formulations, part I: substantial increased and decreased absorption with Uniphyl tablets and Theo-Dur Sprinkle. *Clinical Pharmacology and Therapeutics* **38**, 77–83.

Sauter, R., Steinijans, V.W., Böhm, A., Diletti, E. and Schulz, H.-U. (1992) Presentation of results from bioequivalence studies. *International Journal of Clinical Pharmacology, Therapy and Toxicology* **30**, 233–56.

Schulz, H.-U. and Steinijans, V.W. (1991) Striving for standards in bioequivalence assessment: a review. *International Journal of Clinical Pharmacology, Therapy and Toxicology* **29**, 293–8.

Schulz, H.-U., Steinijans, V.W. and Gabel, H. (1984) Differences in steady-state plasma levels between aminophylline and theophylline sustained-release micropellets after repeated circadian dosing. *International Journal of Clinical Pharmacology, Therapy and Toxicology* **22**, 621–5.

Schulz, H.-U., Karlsson, S., Sahner-Ahrens, I., Steinijans, V.W. and Beier, W. (1987) Effect of drug intake prior to or after meals on serum theophylline concentrations: Single dose studies with Euphylong. *International Journal of Clinical Pharmacology, Therapy and Toxicology* **25**, 222–8.

Skelly, J.P. (1984) *Guidance for conducting studies on theophylline controlled release products.* Food and Drug Administration, Division of Biopharmaceutics (0928X-4/84).

Smolensky, M.H., Scott, P.H., Harrist, R.B., Hiatt, P.H., Wong, T.K., Baenziger, J.C., Klank, B.J., Marbella, A., Meltzer, A. (1987) Administration-time-dependency of the pharmacokinetic behavior and therapeutic effect of a once-day theophylline in asthmatic children. *Chronobiology International* **4**, 435–47.

Steinijans, V.W. (1989) Pharmacokinetic characteristics of controlled release products and their biostatistical analysis. In: Gundert-Remy, U. and Moeller, H. (eds) *Oral Controlled Release Products – Therapeutic and Biopharmaceutic Assessment*, 99–115, APV Band 22, Wissenschaftliche Verlagsgesellschaft mbH, Stuttgart.

Steinijans, V.W. (1990) Pharmacokinetic characterization of controlled-release formulations. *European Journal of Drug Metabolism and Pharmacokinetics* **15**, 173–81.

Steinijans, V.W. and Hauschke, D. (1990) Update on the statistical analysis of bioequivalence studies. *International Journal of Clinical Pharmacology, Therapy and Toxicology* **28**, 105–10.

Steinijans, V.W. and Sauter, R. (1993) Food studies: acceptance criteria and statistics. In: Midha, K.K. and Blume, H.H. (eds) *Bio-International: bioavailability, bioequivalence and pharmacokinetics. International conference of F.I.P. "Bio-International '92", Bad Homburg, Germany*, 235–50. Medpharm Scientific Publishers, Stuttgart.

Steinijans, V.W., Hauschke, D. and Jonkman, J.H.G. (1992) Controversies in bioequivalence studies. *Clinical Pharmacokinetics* **22**, 247–53.

Steinijans, V.W., Schulz, H.-U., Beier, W. and Radtke, H.W. (1986) Once daily theophylline: multiple-dose comparison of an encapsulated micro-osmotic system (Euphylong pellets) with a tablet. *International Journal of Clinical Pharmacology, Therapy and Toxicology* **24**, 438–47.

Steinijans, V.W., Sauter, R., Böhm, A. and Staudinger, H. (1988) Pharmacokinetic profile of a new sustained-release theophylline pellet formulation for once-daily evening administration. *Arzneimittel-Forschung/Drug Research* **38**, 1241–50.

Steinijans, V.W., Trautmann, H., Johnson, E. and Beier, W. (1987) Theophylline steady-state pharmacokinetics: Recent concepts and their application in chronotherapy of reactive airway diseases. *Chronobiology International* **4**, 331–47.

Steinijans, V.W., Sauter, R., Jonkman, J.H.G., Schulz, H.-U., Stricker, H. and Blume, H. (1989) Bioequivalence studies: Single vs multiple dose. *International Journal of Clinical Pharmacology, Therapy and Toxicology* **27**, 261–6.

7

Designs with more than two formulations

7.1 Introduction

The two-period, two-sequence crossover is the design of choice when assessing the following objectives:

- Bioequivalence of a generic formulation, which serves as test, with the innovator's product or another licensed product, which serves as reference.

- Bioequivalence of two pharmaceutical formulations with a marketed formulation as test and the phase III formulation as reference.

- Lack of drug-drug interaction with a new, potentially interacting drug administered concomitantly with the substrate of interest as test, and the substrate alone as reference (see Chapter 8).

- Lack of food-drug interaction where the investigational drug with food serves as test and the investigational drug fasted as reference (see Chapter 8).

- Time invariance where steady state is the test situation and single dose represents the reference.

There are also situations in drug development where a design for more than two formulations is needed. These include:

- Modified release formulations, which have to be investigated under fasting and nonfasting conditions. Thus, there are two tests, namely the new pharmaceutical formulation, with and without food, and in analogy two references, the current formulation with and without food.

Bioequivalence Studies in Drug Development: Methods and Applications   D. Hauschke, V. Steinijans and I. Pigeot
© 2007 John Wiley & Sons, Ltd

- Dose linearity studies where a predefined dose strength, e.g., the medium or the high dose, serves as reference and the other doses serve as tests (see Section 7.3).

To address these objectives, a Williams design is the most commonly applied crossover design. The purpose of this chapter is to illustrate the application of this special design. Furthermore, due to the investigation of more than one test formulation, simultaneous comparisons might increase the consumer risk. Hence, the issue of multiplicity is discussed at the end of the chapter.

7.2 Williams designs

Under the constraint of the number of formulations being equal to the number of periods, balanced crossover designs according to Williams (1949) are commonly used. A design is balanced if it satisfies the combinatorial properties that each formulation is administered once per subject, occurs the same number of times in each period, and any formulation is preceded equally often by each of the other formulations (Jones and Kenward, 2003). Williams (1949) has shown that if the number of treatments (formulations) is even, balance can be achieved by a single Latin square, but when the number of treatments is odd, two Latin squares are required. Tables 7.1 and 7.2 list recommended balanced designs with three and four formulations (Wagner, 1975).

A crossover design including more than four formulations is rarely used because it may be difficult drawing so many blood samples. Other concerns include potential

Table 7.1 Williams Design with a reference R and two test formulations T_1 and T_2.

Sequence	Period 1	Period 2	Period 3
1	R	T_1	T_2
2	T_1	T_2	R
3	T_2	R	T_1
4	R	T_2	T_1
5	T_1	R	T_2
6	T_2	T_1	R

Table 7.2 Williams Design with a reference R and three test formulations T_1, T_2 and T_3.

Sequence	Period 1	Period 2	Period 3	Period 4
1	R	T_1	T_3	T_2
2	T_1	T_2	R	T_3
3	T_2	T_3	T_1	R
4	T_3	R	T_2	T_1

intraindividual changes in clearance over the prolonged study period, potentially higher dropout rates, and the fact that these investigations are more time consuming and costly.

The parametric statistical analysis is essentially the same as for the classical *RT/TR* design described in Chapter 4. Based on empirical evidence and on theoretical arguments (Senn *et al.* 2004), in general no carryover effects are included in the model for analyzing bioequivalence studies provided that the conditions described in Section 4.3.1 hold true. An example of a Williams design with four formulations is given below in the dose linearity study where the use of a simple carryover model would lead to logical contradictions (Senn *et al.*, 2004). For mathematical approaches to handle carryover effects we refer the reader to Senn (2002). Finally, it should be noted that Duchateau *et al.* (2002) developed a nonparametric method for a Williams design with three formulations.

7.3   Example: Dose linearity study

In pharmacokinetic trials on dose linearity, a minimum of three different doses is administered to each individual subject. The following example refers to a dose linearity study of the pharmacokinetics of pantoprazole after single intravenous administration. Pantoprazole (INN), a substituted benzimidazole sulphoxide, is a selective and long acting inhibitor of the gastric H + /K+-ATPase (Simon *et al.*, 1990). Omeprazole, the first registered substance of this class, is associated with nonlinear pharmacokinetic data following oral (Andersson *et al.*, 1990) and intravenous (Jansen *et al.*, 1988) administration. The more than dose proportional increases in *AUC* are thought to be caused by the interaction of omeprazole with the cytochrome P450 enzyme system (Jansen *et al.*, 1988). These results with omeprazole, and the general discussion about the interaction of an imidazole ring with liver microsomal enzymes (Wilkinson *et al.*, 1974) have drawn particular attention to the pharmacokinetic dose dependency of pantoprazole in man.

The aim of this study in healthy subjects was to investigate the influence of different intravenous doses of pantoprazole on its pharmacokinetic characteristics, namely area under the concentration-time curve $AUC(0 - \infty)$, maximum serum concentration C_{max}, clearance Cl, apparent volume of distribution $V_{d\,area}$ and terminal elimination half-life $t_{1/2}$. It is important to establish whether or not pantoprazole shows linear pharmacokinetics, especially for conditions where higher than normal therapeutic doses are indicated, for example in patients presenting with Zollinger–Ellison syndrome. For illustrative purposes only the results for $AUC(0 - \infty)$ and C_{max} are presented. For further details of this investigation we refer the reader to Bliesath *et al.* (1994).

The study followed a single blind, randomized, four-period, four-sequence crossover design (see Table 7.2). The treatment days were separated by washout periods of at least 1 week. Each of the 12 volunteers participated in four identical study-days and received all doses in randomized order. The study medication was administered to subjects in the fasting state by intravenous infusion for 15 minutes. The doses given were 10, 20, 40 and 80 mg, diluted in commercially available 0.9 % NaCl solution.

The 80 mg pantoprazole dose served as the reference (R), and the other doses as tests, i.e., $T_1 = 10\,\text{mg}$, $T_2 = 20\,\text{mg}$, $T_3 = 40\,\text{mg}$. The individual values of the extent and rate characteristics $AUC(0 - \infty)$ and C_{max}, as well as the randomized sequence of doses are given in Table 7.3.

Table 7.3 Subject number, sequence and individual values of the characteristic $AUC(0 - \infty)$ (μg/ml · h) (first line) and C_{max} (μg/ml) (second line). Reference: 80 mg, Tests: $T_1 = 10\,\text{mg}$, $T_2 = 20\,\text{mg}$, $T_3 = 40\,\text{mg}$.

Subject number	Sequence	Period 1	Period 2	Period 3	Period 4
1	T_3, R, T_2, T_1	5.10	9.61	2.41	1.11
		5.56	10.38	2.09	1.22
2	R, T_1, T_3, T_2	8.21	0.72	2.99	1.37
		8.71	0.75	3.59	1.99
3	T_2, T_3, T_1, R	3.96	7.89	2.13	14.43
		2.89	5.51	1.22	10.79
4	T_3, R, T_2, T_1	6.17	15.68	3.36	1.66
		5.99	15.03	3.04	1.66
5	T_1, T_2, R, T_3	0.74	1.63	6.77	3.25
		1.08	1.71	8.66	4.52
6	R, T_1, T_3, T_2	12.58	0.95	4.84	1.98
		13.91	1.13	5.85	2.26
7	T_2, T_3, T_1, R	2.49	4.11	0.93	7.32
		2.96	4.54	1.12	5.26
8	T_1, T_2, R, T_3	1.31	2.46	12.71	6.56
		1.03	2.10	11.36	5.02
9	T_3, R, T_2, T_1	5.83	11.03	2.86	1.26
		5.27	8.81	2.95	1.30
10	T_2, T_3, T_1, R	3.40	5.93	1.24	14.65
		4.40	5.97	1.29	10.73
11	R, T_1, T_3, T_2	11.95	0.99	6.80	3.13
		11.36	0.89	6.40	3.01
12	T_1, T_2, R, T_3	1.31	2.26	8.93	5.56
		1.60	3.46	11.08	8.08

Table 7.4 Geometric mean and 68% range, i.e., $[\exp(\mathrm{mean}(\ln^*) - \mathrm{sd}(\ln^*)),$
$\exp(\mathrm{mean}(\ln^*) + \mathrm{sd}(\ln^*))]$ where $*$ is AUC or C_{max}.

	10 mg	20 mg	40 mg	80 mg
$AUC(0-\infty)$	1.14	2.50	5.22	10.77
(μg/ml·h)	[0.83, 1.56]	[1.83, 3.42]	[3.89, 7.01]	[8.13, 14.27]
C_{max}	1.16	2.65	5.42	10.19
(μg/ml)	[0.93, 1.45]	[2.02, 3.47]	[4.43, 6.64]	[7.79, 13.33]

Table 7.4 shows the geometric means and the 68 % ranges for $AUC(0-\infty)$ and C_{max}. The dose linearity plots were made on an individual basis and are presented in Figure 7.1.

In order to formally demonstrate dose linearity, the procedure of equivalence assessment was applied to the dose adjusted primary characteristics $AUC(0-\infty)$ and C_{max}. The following SAS® code for the procedure 'proc glm' was used:

```
proc glm data= dose_linearity;
        class subject sequence period formulation;
        model logAUC=sequence subject(sequence) period formulation;
        random subject(sequence) / test;
        lsmeans formulation/pdiff cl alpha=0.1;
        run;
```

and the corresponding output is provided in Table 7.5.

Reversing the signs of the above given differences between treatment means after logarithmic transformation ensures that the first 3 differences are formed versus the reference, which has treatment index 1. Exponential transformation of the results yields the point estimate and 90 % confidence limits for the corresponding ratio test/reference (Table 7.6.)

For the $AUCs$ of the 10 mg dose, the lower limit of the confidence interval, i.e., 0.78, just missed the lower limit of the equivalence range (0.80, 1.25). This was attributed to the greater variation coefficient of results for the lowest dose compared to the other doses. For C_{max} the equivalence criteria were met over the whole dose range.

In conclusion, dose linearity was demonstrated between the doses of pantoprazole for the primary pharmacokinetic characteristics $AUC(0-\infty)$ and C_{max}. The secondary characteristics, clearance, apparent volume of distribution and terminal elimination half-life, were consistently not influenced by the different doses. These favorable pharmacokinetic properties of pantoprazole may be of therapeutic importance, particularly when high doses have to be administered.

7.4 Multiplicity

When comparing the bioavailability of two formulations, multiple comparisons are usually made because rate and extent of bioavailability have to be investigated. Hence, corresponding pharmacokinetic characteristics, for example $AUC(0-\infty)$ and C_{max} are

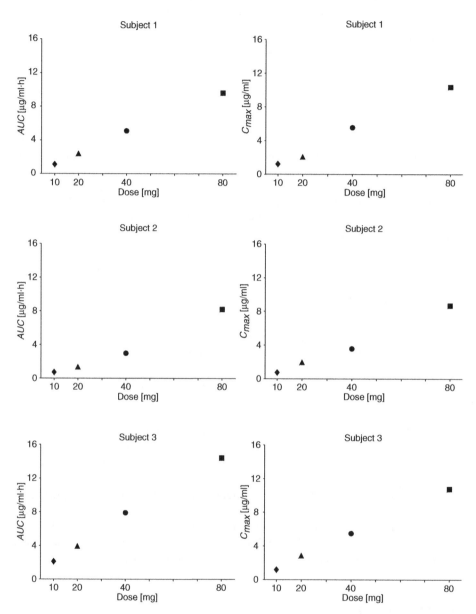

Figure 7.1 Individual values for $AUC\,(0-\infty)$ and C_{max} versus dose in twelve healthy volunteers after 10, 20, 40 and 80 mg pantoprazole i.v.

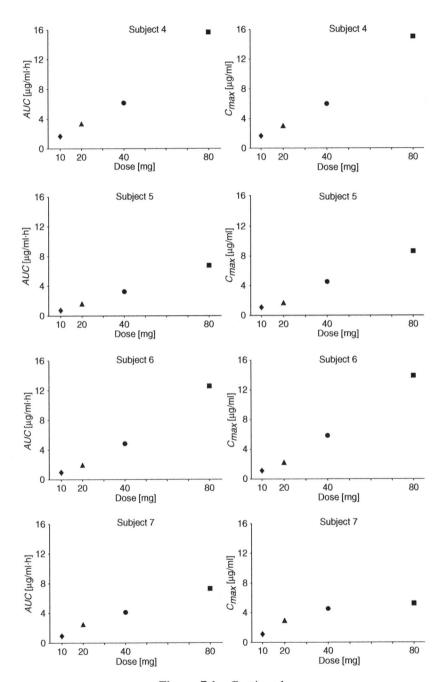

Figure 7.1   Continued.

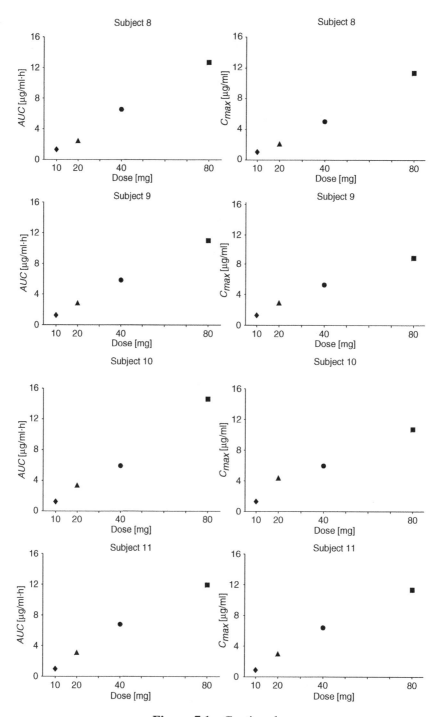

Figure 7.1   Continued.

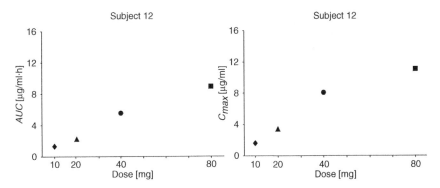

Figure 7.1 Continued.

simultaneously assessed. However, no multiplicity adjustment is needed in this situation because the bioequivalence requirement is equivalence for both rate and extent of bioavailability, i.e., for $AUC(0 - \infty)$ and C_{max} (see Section 7.4.1). Different multiple comparisons arise when more than two formulations are compared in a single study. For example, when comparing the four doses in the above dose linearity study, there are a total of six comparisons, namely 10 mg versus 20, 40 and 80 mg, 20 mg versus 40 and 80 mg, and 40 mg versus 80 mg for $AUC(0 - \infty)$ and C_{max}, respectively. Only three of these comparisons are of interest with regard to dose linearity, namely, 10, 20 and 40 mg versus 80 mg.

Multiple comparisons, if not properly handled, result in an inflated rate of false positive conclusions. This effect is referred to in the literature as 'multiplicity'. An excellent discussion of this issue in drug development was provided by Senn (1997). In the following, consideration is given to controlling the familywise type I error rate to at most $\alpha = 0.05$. In other words, the probability of erroneously rejecting at least one null hypothesis is a maximum of 5 %, regardless of which subset of null hypotheses is true (CPMP, 2002).

7.4.1 Joint decision rule

Bioequivalence of a test and a reference formulation of the same drug substance comprises equivalence with respect to rate and extent of bioavailability. Hence, from a regulatory point of view, this is a simultaneous requirement and both criteria have to be fulfilled for a successful approval of the test formulation. Hauck *et al.* (1995) called this a joint decision rule. From a statistical point of view, this refers to the evaluation of multiple primary endpoints. Bioequivalence can be concluded if equivalence has been demonstrated for all stipulated primary endpoints. Let us consider as primary endpoints $AUC(0 - \infty)$ and C_{max}. This results in the two test problems for equivalence

Table 7.5   SAS® proc glm for the dose linearity study.

```
data dose_linearity;
  input subject sequence $ formulation $ period AUC;

  select (formulation);
    when ('T1') auc=auc*8;
    when ('T2') auc=auc*4;
    when ('T3') auc=auc*2;
    otherwise;
  end;

  logAUC=log(AUC);
  datalines;
1 CDBA T3 1 5.1
1 CDBA R 2 9.61
1 CDBA T2 3 2.41
1 CDBA T1 4 1.11
2 DACB R 1 8.21
2 DACB T1 2 0.72
2 DACB T3 3 2.99
2 DACB T2 4 1.37
3 BCAD T2 1 3.96
3 BCAD T3 2 7.89
3 BCAD T1 3 2.13
3 BCAD R 4 14.43
4 CDBA T3 1 6.17
4 CDBA R 2 15.68
4 CDBA T2 3 3.36
4 CDBA T1 4 1.66
5 ABDC T1 1 0.74
5 ABDC T2 2 1.63
5 ABDC R 3 6.77
5 ABDC T3 4 3.25
6 DACB R 1 12.58
6 DACB T1 2 0.95
6 DACB T3 3 4.84
6 DACB T2 4 1.98
7 BCAD T2 1 2.49
7 BCAD T3 2 4.11
7 BCAD T1 3 0.93
7 BCAD R 4 7.32
8 ABDC T1 1 1.31
8 ABDC T2 2 2.46
8 ABDC R 3 12.71
8 ABDC T3 4 6.56
9 CDBA T3 1 5.83
9 CDBA R 2 11.03
9 CDBA T2 3 2.86
9 CDBA T1 4 1.26
10 BCAD T2 1 3.4
10 BCAD T3 2 5.93
10 BCAD T1 3 1.24
```

```
10 BCAD R 4 14.65
11 DACB R 1 11.95
11 DACB T1 2 0.99
11 DACB T3 3 6.8
11 DACB T2 4 3.13
12 ABDC T1 1 1.31
12 ABDC T2 2 2.26
12 ABDC R 3 8.93
12 ABDC T3 4 5.56
;
run;

proc glm data=dose_linearity;
  class subject sequence period formulation;
  model logauc=sequence subject(sequence) period formulation;
  random subject(sequence)/test;
  lsmeans formulation/pdiff cl alpha=0.1;
run;
quit;
```

              The GLM Procedure
          Class Level Information

Class	Levels	Values
subject	12	1 2 3 4 5 6 7 8 9 10 11 12
sequence	4	ABDC BCAD CDBA DACB
period	4	1 2 3 4
formulation	4	R T1 T2 T3

Number of observations 48

The GLM Procedure

Dependent Variable: logAUC

Source	DF	Sum of Squares	Mean Square	F Value	Pr>F
Model	17	3.70041546	0.21767150	14.16	<.0001
Error	30	0.46110734	0.01537024		
Corrected Total	47	4.16152280			

R-Square	Coeff Var	Root MSE	logAUC Mean
0.889197	5.368296	0.123977	2.309425

Source	DF	Type I SS	Mean Square	F Value	Pr > F
sequence	3	0.84253279	0.28084426	18.27	<.0001
subject(sequence)	8	2.56488306	0.32061038	20.86	<.0001
period	3	0.10769115	0.03589705	2.34	0.0938
formulation	3	0.18530847	0.06176949	4.02	0.0162

Source	DF	Type III SS	Mean Square	F Value	Pr > F
sequence	3	0.84253279	0.28084426	18.27	<.0001
subject(sequence)	8	2.56488306	0.32061038	20.86	<.0001

Table 7.5 Continued.

| period | 3 | 0.10769115 | 0.03589705 | 2.34 | 0.0938 |
| formulation | 3 | 0.18530847 | 0.06176949 | 4.02 | 0.0162 |

The GLM Procedure

Source	Type III Expected Mean Square
sequence	Var(Error) + 4 Var(subject(sequence)) + Q(sequence)
subject(sequence)	Var(Error) + 4 Var(subject(sequence))
period	Var(Error) + Q(period)
formulation	Var(Error) + Q(formulation)

The GLM Procedure

Tests of Hypotheses for Mixed Model Analysis of Variance

Dependent Variable: logAUC

Source	DF	Type III SS	Mean Square	F Value	Pr > F
sequence	3	0.842533	0.280844	0.88	0.4929
Error	8	2.564883	0.320610		

Error: MS(subject(sequence))

Source	DF	Type III SS	Mean Square	F Value	Pr > F
subject(sequence)	8	2.564883	0.320610	20.86	<.0001
period	3	0.107691	0.035897	2.34	0.0938
formulation	3	0.185308	0.061769	4.02	0.0162
Error: MS(Error)	30	0.461107	0.015370		

Least Squares Means

formulation	logAUC LSMEAN	LSMEAN Number
R	2.37688901	1
T1	2.21194600	2
T2	2.30277255	3
T3	2.34609336	4

Least Squares Means for effect formulation
Pr > |t| for H0: LSMean(i) = LSMean(j)

Dependent Variable: logAUC

i/j	1	2	3	4
1		0.0028	0.1535	0.5475
2	0.0028		0.0828	0.0127
3	0.1535	0.0828		0.3988
4	0.5475	0.0127	0.3988	

	logAUC		
formulation	LSMEAN	90% Confidence Limits	
R	2.376889	2.316146	2.437632
T1	2.211946	2.151203	2.272689
T2	2.302773	2.242029	2.363516
T3	2.346093	2.285350	2.406837

Least Squares Means for Effect formulation

		Difference Between Means	90% Confidence Limits for LSMean(i)-LSMean(j)	
i	j			
1	2	0.164943	0.079039	0.250847
1	3	0.074116	− 0.011788	0.160020
1	4	0.030796	− 0.055108	0.116700
2	3	− 0.090827	− 0.176731	− 0.004923
2	4	− 0.134147	− 0.220051	− 0.048243
3	4	− 0.043321	− 0.129225	0.042583

NOTE: To ensure overall protection level, only probabilities associated with pre-planned comparisons should be used.

Table 7.6 Point estimate and 90% confidence limits for dose adjusted $AUC(0 - \infty)$ and C_{max} after 10, 20 and 40 mg, Reference: 80 mg pantoprazole.

	Dose		
	10 mg	20 mg	40 mg
$AUC(0 - \infty)$	0.85	0.93	0.97
	[0.78, 0.92]	[0.85, 1.01]	[0.89, 1.06]
C_{max}	0.91	1.04	1.06
	[0.81, 1.03]	[0.92, 1.17]	[0.94, 1.20]

$$H_0^{extent} : \text{inequivalence for } AUC(0 - \infty)$$

vs.

$$H_1^{extent} : \text{equivalence for } AUC(0 - \infty)$$

and

$$H_0^{rate} : \text{inequivalence for } C_{max}$$

vs.

$$H_1^{rate} : \text{equivalence for } C_{max}.$$

Hence, the test problem for bioequivalence can be formulated as

$$H_0^{joint\ decision\ rule} : H_0^{extent} \cup H_0^{rate}$$

vs.

$$H_1^{joint\ decision\ rule} : H_1^{extent} \cap H_1^{rate}.$$

The statistical analysis can be performed according to the intersection-union principle (Berger and Hsu, 1996), that is, bioequivalence is concluded at a familywise level of $\alpha = 0.05$, if equivalence in extent and rate can be concluded each at level $\alpha = 0.05$. This decision rule is equivalent to the inclusion of the corresponding 90 % confidence intervals for $AUC(0 - \infty)$ and C_{max} in the stipulated equivalence acceptance ranges.

This principle can also be applied to the above example; in order to demonstrate dose linearity, equivalence to 80 mg has to be shown for the dosage strengths 10, 20, and 40 mg based on the dose adjusted pharmacokinetic characteristics $AUC(0 - \infty)$ and C_{max}:

$$H_0^{dose\ adjusted\ characteristics\ for\ 10\,mg} : \text{inequivalence between 10 and 80 mg}$$

vs.

$$H_1^{dose\ adjusted\ characteristics\ for\ 10\,mg} : \text{equivalence between 10 and 80 mg}$$

and

$$H_0^{dose\ adjusted\ characteristics\ for\ 20\,mg} : \text{inequivalence between 20 and 80 mg}$$

vs.

$$H_1^{dose\ adjusted\ characteristics\ for\ 20\,mg} : \text{equivalence between 20 and 80 mg}$$

and

$$H_0^{dose\ adjusted\ characteristics\ for\ 40\,mg} : \text{inequivalence between 40 and 80 mg}$$

vs.

$$H_1^{dose\ adjusted\ characteristics\ for\ 40\,mg} : \text{equivalence between 40 and 80 mg}$$

and hence

$$H_0^{joint\ decision\ rule} : \bigcup_{i=1}^{3} H_0^{dose\ adjusted\ characteristics\ for\ T_i}$$

vs.

$$H_1^{joint\ decision\ rule} : \bigcap_{i=1}^{3} H_1^{dose\ adjusted\ characteristics\ for\ T_i},$$

where $T_1 = 10\,mg$, $T_2 = 20\,mg$, $T_3 = 40\,mg$. Hence, for a joint decision rule where all requirements must be fulfilled, no adjustment of the comparisonwise type I error is needed to keep the familywise type I error under control. However, this intersection-union testing procedure inflates the type II error, that is the probability of erroneously failing to reject at least one null hypothesis (CPMP, 2002). This inflation has to be taken into account by an adequate sample size determination.

7.4.2 Multiple decision rule

Let us consider a bioequivalence trial with a current formulation as reference (R) and two tests, a new (T_1) and an alternative (T_2) pharmaceutical development. The objective of the study is to choose any one of the test formulations for further development.

It is important to distinguish between the multiple decision rule, addressed here, and the joint decision rule. A joint decision rule refers to the situation where the aim of the study would be to show that both T_1 and T_2 are bioequivalent with regard to R. Where we have the option to choose either one of the test formulations T_1 and T_2, the multiple decision rule is indicated and the test problem is formulated as:

$$H_0^{T_1} \; : \; \text{bioinequivalence between } T_1 \text{ and } R$$

$$\text{vs.}$$

$$H_1^{T_1} \; : \; \text{bioequivalence between } T_1 \text{ and } R$$

or

$$H_0^{T_2} \; : \; \text{bioinequivalence between } T_2 \text{ and } R$$

$$\text{vs.}$$

$$H_1^{T_2} \; : \; \text{bioequivalence between } T_2 \text{ and } R$$

and hence,

$$H_0^{multiple\ decision\ rule} \; : \; H_0^{T_1} \cap H_0^{T_2}$$

$$\text{vs.}$$

$$H_1^{multiple\ decision\ rule} \; : \; H_1^{T_1} \cup H_1^{T_2}.$$

This is the union-intersection principle according to Roy (1953), that is, $H_0^{multiple\ decision\ rule}$ is rejected if at least one of the individual hypotheses $H_0^{T_1}$ and $H_0^{T_2}$ is rejected. In contrast to the joint decision rule, the familywise level of $\alpha = 0.05$ has to be split, and the two individual null hypotheses have to be tested at a comparisonwise type I error which is a fraction of α. In the literature, this procedure is called adjusting the type I error (α-spending). A well-known but conservative method is the Bonferroni procedure, which simply tests the individual hypotheses $H_0^{T_1}$ and $H_0^{T_2}$ each at a reduced significance level of $\alpha/2 = 0.025$. Improvements of the Bonferroni procedure have been developed by Holm (1979), Hochberg (1988) and Hommel (1988).

An important feature of bioequivalence trials is that there is at least one reference and the comparisons between the test formulations and the reference are of primary interest. In the literature, these are called many-to-one comparisons. For such comparisons Dunnett (1955) provided a testing procedure and simultaneous confidence intervals. This procedure controls the familywise error (see also Hochberg and Tamhane, 1987) and reflects the underlying design of a bioequivalence study. Therefore, this method should be used when comparing more than one test formulation with a reference. Furthermore, it is worthwhile to note that the Dunnett procedure is implemented in SAS® and can be easily performed.

7.5 Conclusions

This chapter addressed the problem of proving bioequivalence when several test formulations are compared with a reference, for example the above dose linearity study. If the objective of the study is to claim bioequivalence for all tests under investigation with the reference, the concept of a joint decision rule applies and no adjustment of the type I error is necessary.

If it is sufficient to claim bioequivalence of at least one of the test formulations, the familywise error must be controlled (CPMP, 2002) by adjusting the type I error. In this situation the multiple comparison procedure according to Dunnett (1955) should be used.

References

Andersson, T., Cederberg, C., Regårdh, C.G. and Skånberg, I. (1990) Pharmacokinetics of various single intravenous and oral doses of omeprazole. *European Journal of Clinical Pharmacology* **19**, 195–7.

Berger, R.L. and Hsu, J.C. (1996) Bioequivalence trials, intersection union tests and equivalence confidence sets. *Statistical Science* **11**, 283–319.

Bliesath, H., Huber, R., Hartmann, M., Lühmann, R. and Wurst, W. (1994) Dose linearity of the pharmacokinetics of the new H+/K+-ATPase inhibitor pantoprazole after single intravenous administration.*International Journal of Clinical Pharmacology and Therapeutics* **32**, 44–50.

Committee for Proprietary Medicinal Products (2002) *Points to consider on multiplicity issues in clinical trials.* EMEA, London.

Duchateau, L., Janssen, P., Straetemans, R. and Otoul, C. (2002) Adjusting pairwise nonparametric equivalence hypothesis tests and confidence intervals for period effects in 3×3 crossover trials. *Journal of Biopharmaceutical Statistics* **12**, 149–60.

Dunnett, C.W. (1955) A multiple comparison procedure for comparing several treatments with a control. *Journal of the American Statistical Association* **50**, 1096–1121.

Hauck, W.W., Hyslop, T., Anderson, S., Bois, F.Y. and Tozer, T.N. (1995) Statistical and regulatory considerations for multiple measures in bioequivalence testing. *Clinical Research and Regulatory Affairs* **12**, 249–65.

Hochberg, Y. (1988) A sharper Bonferroni procedure for multiple tests of significance. *Biometrika* **75**, 800–2.

Hochberg, Y. and Tamhane, A.C. (1987) *Multiple comparison procedures.* John Wiley & Sons, Inc., Chichester, New York.

Holm, S. (1979) A simple sequentially rejective multiple test procedure. *Scandinavian Journal of Statistics* **6**, 65–70.

Hommel, G. (1988) A stagewise rejective multiple test procedure based on a modified Bonferroni test. *Biometrika* **75**, 383–6.

Jansen, J.B.M.J., Lundborg, P., Baak, L.C., Greve, J., Ohman, M., Stöver, C., Röhss, K. and Lamers, C.B.H.W. (1988) Effect of single and repeated intravenous doses of omeprazole on pentagastrin stimulated gastric acid secretion and pharmacokinetics in man.*Gut* **29**, 75–80.

Jones, B. and Kenward, M.G. (2003) *Design and analysis of cross-over trials* (2nd edition). Chapman & Hall, Boca Raton.

Roy, S.N. (1953) On a heuristic method of test construction and its use in multivariate analysis. *Annals of Mathematical Statistics* **24**, 220–38.

Senn, S. (1997) *Statistical issues in drug development.* John Wiley & Sons, Inc., Chichester, New York.

Senn, S. (2002) *Cross-over trials in clinical research* (2nd edition). John Wiley & Sons, Inc., Chichester, New York.

Senn, S., D'Angelo, G. And Potvin, D. (2004) Carry-over in cross-over trials in bioequivalence: theoretical concerns and empirical evidence. *Journal of Pharmaceutical Statistics* **3**, 13–142.

Simon, W.A., Keeling, D.J., Laing, S.M., Fallowfield, C. and Taylor, A.G. (1990) Pantoprazole BY1023/SK&F96022: Biochemistry of a novel H+/K+-ATPase. *Biochemical Pharmacology* **39**, 1799–1806.

Wagner, J.G. (1975) *Fundamentals of clinical pharmacokinetics.* Drug Intelligence Publications, Inc., Hamilton.

Williams, E.J. (1949) Experimental designs balanced for the estimation of residual effects of treatments. *Australian Journal of Scientific Research* **2**, 149–68.

Wilkinson, C.F., Hetnarski, C.F. and Hicks, L.J. (1974) Substituted benzimidazoles as inhibitors of microsomal oxidation and insecticide synergists. *Pesticide Biochemestry and Physiology* **4**, 299.

8

Analysis of pharmacokinetic interactions

8.1 Introduction

The desirable and undesirable effects of a drug are usually related to the blood/plasma concentrations, which are affected by the absorption, distribution, metabolism and/or excretion (ADME) of the drug. Moreover, the ADME processes, particularly the absorption, are not only characteristics of the drug itself, but may be strongly affected by the specific pharmaceutical formulation. This chapter will focus on pharmacokinetic (PK) interactions as assessed by the modification of the blood/plasma concentration-time profile rather than on pharmacodynamic (PD) interactions as assessed by clinical endpoints including efficacy variables and adverse drug reactions. We have to distinguish between drug–drug and food–drug interactions. In the context of this chapter the focus is on clinical pharmacological studies *in vivo*. *In vitro* studies will be discussed only briefly as a tool to identify potential metabolic interactions to be followed up by *in vivo* drug–drug interaction studies, and in the context of *in vitro/in vivo* association in the case of food–drug interaction studies. The term drug–drug interaction is used if the concentration-time profile of a particular drug, in the following denoted by substrate S, is affected by a concomitantly administered potentially interacting drug I. In the Test/Reference terminology of bioequivalence studies, Test corresponds to S + I, i.e., substrate S plus interacting drug I, while Reference corresponds to S, i.e., the substrate alone. For blinding purposes substrate S may be administered together with a placebo that matches drug I in appearance. When S and I are metabolized by the same CYP450 enzyme, the effect of S on I may also be of interest. The term food–drug interaction is used if changes induced by concomitant food intake are investigated. In this case, Test refers to drug intake with food, while Reference refers to drug intake without food. While food–drug

Bioequivalence Studies in Drug Development: Methods and Applications   D. Hauschke, V. Steinijans and I. Pigeot
© 2007 John Wiley & Sons, Ltd

interactions primarily affect the absorption of a drug, drug–drug interactions may affect both the absorption of the substrate S and/or its metabolism and excretion.

Elimination of a drug usually occurs by metabolism, followed by excretion via the hepatobiliary system into the gut, and/or by renal excretion. Metabolism occurs by the cytochrome P450 family of enzymes located in the hepatic endoplasmic reticulum and the gastrointestinal mucosa, but may also occur by non-P450 enzyme systems, such as N-acetyl and glucuronosyl transferases. Many factors can alter hepatic and intestinal drug metabolism, including the presence or absence of disease and/or variation in social habits such as consumption of food, alcohol or tobacco. While such factors may be relatively stable over time, concomitant medications can alter metabolic routes of absorption and elimination abruptly, and therefore are of concern, particularly for substrates with a narrow therapeutic range of plasma concentrations such as digoxin and theophylline.

With regard to the labeling of a drug in the doctor or patient's information leaflet, three grades of drug–drug or food–drug interactions have to be distinguished. Of real concern are drug interactions that necessitate specific recommendations for a dose adjustment or even safety precautions including a warning in the labeling. Frequently, the marketed formulation allows only dose adjustments by a factor of two, i.e., by halving a tablet or by taking two tablets instead of one. In this case, a decision procedure to support or obviate a dose adjustment is needed. Finally, the claim of 'lack of drug–drug interaction' is gaining importance in view of the polypharmacy seen with most multimorbid patients. It was this most stringent concept of 'lack of interaction' for which the bioequivalence methodology was initially adopted (Steinijans *et al.*, 1991). It was shown that 'lack of interaction' can be handled as an equivalence problem. To this end, administration of the substrate S in the presence of the potentially interacting drug I was considered as the 'Test' situation (S + I), administration of the substrate S alone as the 'Reference' situation. As this 'equivalence' methodology is the only approach that allows control of the consumer risk of erroneously claiming 'lack of interaction', it was adopted in the pertinent guidelines on drug interactions (CPMP, 1997; FDA, 1999; FDA, 2002). The reader should bear in mind that this approach is only acceptable if a pharmacodynamic interaction can be ruled out when drug concentration profiles do not change, i.e., there are no relevant synergistic or antagonist effects of the drugs investigated. A counterexample is the following: digoxin and diuretics may not interact pharmacokinetically, but diuretics can reduce serum potassium and thereby alter the side effect profile of similar concentrations of digoxin.

It is the purpose of pharmacokinetic lack-of-interaction studies to demonstrate that the pharmacokinetics of drug S are not affected by concomitant administration of drug I to a clinically relevant extent. To this end, the range of clinically acceptable variation in the pharmacokinetic characteristics of drug S has to be specified. As an initial default value, the conventional bioequivalence acceptance range of 0.80 to 1.25 is used as equivalence acceptance range for the Test/Reference ratio. The setting of the 'goal posts', which form the lower and upper limits of the acceptance range, is discussed in detail in Section 8.4 on 'Goal Posts for Pharmacokinetic Drug Interactions including No Effect Boundaries'. Once the 'goal posts' are set, we have to show whether or not the effects of concomitant administration of drug I are within this acceptance range. In order to protect the patient, the risk of incorrectly concluding 'lack of interaction' (consumer risk) must be controlled and should be limited to the commonly accepted 5 %. This, however, will not be the case if the classical hypothesis of no difference between concomitant administration of drugs S and I (Test) and administration of drug S alone (Reference) is tested. In this case, a nonsignificant result does not imply that there is no interaction, particularly if the sample size is small and/or the coefficient of variation is large. Instead, it has to be shown that Test and Reference are equivalent, i.e., that they only differ within a clinically accepted range, e.g., 0.80 to 1.25 for the ratio Test/Reference. The underlying decision problem is the same as in bioequivalence assessment if 'bioequivalence' is replaced by 'lack of pharmacokinetic interaction'. Consequently, the entire methodology of bioequivalence analysis including the crossover design, choice of primary pharmacokinetic characteristics, mathematical modeling (log transformation of commonly used primary pharmacokinetic characteristics such as AUC and C_{max}), sample size planning and statistical analysis (ANOVA) can be directly applied to pharmacokinetic lack-of-interaction studies.

However, there is one important difference between 'lack of drug–drug interaction' studies and conventional bioequivalence studies, and this concerns the clearance. As pointed out in Section 2.2.1 'Extent of Bioavailability', clearance can be viewed as the volume of blood from which all drug would appear to be removed per unit time. In bioequivalence studies, the intraindividual invariance of the clearance is a fundamental assumption for the comparison of the exposure characteristic AUC by means of intraindividual ratios (see Section 2.2.1), and thereby also a major motivation for the choice of the crossover design. By the very nature of drug–drug interaction studies the potentially interacting drug I may affect the clearance of the substrate S. Thus, in contrast to conventional bioequivalence studies, where rate and extent of drug absorption are of primary interest, the equivalence of the clearance of the substrate S under Test $(S+I)$ and Reference (S) is of additional interest in drug–drug interaction studies. The approach of Schall and coworkers (1994), who showed how to handle the AUC as a composite characteristic of drug absorption and clearance, will be presented in Section 8.2.6 'Pharmacokinetic Characteristics for Extent of Absorption and Clearance in Drug–Drug Interaction Studies'.

As a consequence of the scientific development within the areas of pharmacokinetics and (bio)equivalence assessment, the focus of interaction studies has changed from ad hoc observational studies to specifically designed studies, which are more and more performed at an early stage of drug development. It is unlikely that population pharmacokinetic studies with their sparse sampling strategy can be used to prove the absence of an interaction. Moreover, such studies may not be randomized and, therefore, can be subject to the usual bias of observational studies. In order to avoid falsely not finding an interaction, it must be ensured that sufficient numbers of patients in population PK studies are taking the potentially interacting drug I.

Instead of population PK studies with the above-mentioned limitations, investigators perform specifically designed interaction studies that allow control of the error probabilities for claims like 'No need for a dose adjustment' or 'Lack of interaction'. As a consequence, the information provided to the prescriber and to the patient has become more extensive and more rigorous (see Section 8.5 'Labeling').

8.2　Pharmacokinetic drug–drug interaction studies

Drug–drug interactions may affect the absorption of the substrate S and/or its distribution, and/or its elimination via metabolism and excretion. Typical modes of interaction for each of the above processes will be briefly described. The presentation closely follows that of the 1997 CPMP Note for guidance: 'The investigation of drug interactions'.

8.2.1　Absorption

A drug given by the oral route of administration could have a direct impact on the gastro-intestinal absorption, or an indirect impact by a pharmacodynamic effect on gastro-intestinal secretion or motility.

P-glycoprotein is gaining increasing recognition for its involvement in the process of drug absorption. P-glycoprotein may contribute to a low drug absorption by decreasing the effective membrane permeability of the drug. It has been reported that many substrates for P-glycoproteins are also substrates for the metabolizing enzyme CYP3A4 (Cummins et al., 2002). Consequently many drugs might first be effluxed by P-glycoproteins and then absorbed again, thus undergoing a local recycling process that might result in an increased presystemic metabolism due to a decreased presentation rate for the CYP3A4 inside the enterocyte. Drug interactions at the intestinal epithelium might therefore affect oral bioavailability by changes in absorption and/or first pass metabolism.

Although gastrointestinal absorption plays a major role in drug–drug interaction studies of orally administered drugs, pulmonary absorption may determine the pharmacokinetic profile of an inhaled drug. Nave et al. (2005) investigated the drug–drug interaction of the inhaled corticosteroid ciclesonide and orally administered erythromycin.

8.2.2　Distribution

Displacement of drug from plasma proteins is the most common explanation for altered distribution in drug interactions. In particular, if the investigation involves a substance with a narrow therapeutic range, a low volume of distribution (e.g., < 2 l/kg body weight) and a high protein binding (e.g., > 85 %), the possibility of relevant changes in free drug concentrations should be considered. However, few displacement interactions result in clinically relevant changes. Conditions for which drug displacement interaction studies should be performed are described in Section 4.2 of the CPMP (1997) guidance.

8.2.3　Elimination

Many known clinically relevant interactions are due to changes in the elimination of drugs. Therefore, information on the relative clearance by metabolic and nonmetabolic routes is of vital interest early in the development of a new drug.

As a consequence of the circulation, clearance of a drug by one organ adds to the clearance by another organ (Rowland and Tozer, 1995). Thus, total clearance is the sum of clearances by each eliminating organ, e.g.,

$$\text{Total clearance} = \text{Renal clearance} + \text{Hepatic clearance.}$$

8.2.3.1 Metabolism

Pharmacokinetic interactions between a substrate S and a potentially interacting drug I may be expected if both drugs are metabolized in the liver via the same enzyme system, e.g., cytochrome P450. Metabolic interaction includes enzyme inhibition and/or induction, which have opposite effects on clearance and whose net effect is of clinical interest. Inhibition may occur after a single dose, whereas induction usually requires multiple dosing; this has to be reflected in the study design.

Examples of substantially changed exposure associated with administration of another drug include (i) increased levels of terfenadine, cisapride, or astemizole with keto-conazole or erythromycin (inhibition of CYP3A4); (ii) increased levels of simvas-tatin and its acid metabolite with mibefradil or itraconazole (inhibition of CYP3A4); (iii) increased levels of desipramine with fluoxetine or paroxetine (inhibition of CYP2D6); and (iv) decreased carbamazepine levels with rifampicin (induction of CYP3A4). Such large changes in exposure can alter the safety and efficacy profile of a drug and/or its active metabolites.

A specific objective of metabolic drug–drug interaction studies is to determine whether the interaction is sufficiently large to necessitate a dose adjustment of the drug itself or the drugs it might be used with, or whether the interaction would require additional therapeutic monitoring.

The cytochrome P450 family (CYP450) includes various major cytochrome P450 subsystems, which are involved in the metabolism of various substrates. In studying an investigational drug as the potentially interacting drug, the choice of substrates (approved drugs) for *in vivo* studies depends on the P450 enzymes affected by the potentially interacting drug. Table 8.1, which is taken from the Appendix of the CPMP (1997) guidance on drug interactions, gives, for each of the major drug metabolizing CYP450 enzymes, examples of substrates, inhibitors, inducers and markers.

'As a general guidance, in vivo metabolic interaction studies should be performed for metabolic pathways responsible for 30 % or more of the total clearance. However, if toxic/active metabolites are formed minor metabolic pathways may also need to be studied' (CPMP, 1997).

8.2.3.1.1 Metabolic induction

Clinically relevant induction occurs during multiple dosing of the inducing drug and is a dose and time dependent phenomenon.

'Points to consider regarding metabolic induction:

- Decide if the relevant enzyme(s), is (are) inducible or not.

- Time is required for the onset and offset of induction.

- When metabolites are pharmacologically active, it should be remembered that the introduction of an inducer may result in an increase in the concentration of the metabolites, possibly resulting in an increased effect.

- The clinical effects of induction might be more serious when the inducer is abruptly withdrawn.

- Many dietary and social habits such as eating charcoal grilled meat or smoking may induce drug metabolism.' (CPMP, 1997.)

Table 8.1 Major drug metabolizing CYP450 enzymes, examples of substrates, inhibitors, inducers and markers.

P450 Enzyme	Substrates	Inhibitors	Inducers	Markers
CYP1A2	Acetaminophen Aromatic amines Caffeine Phenacetin Theophylline	Fluvoxamine Furafylline	Charcoal-grilled beef Cigarette smoke Cruciferous Vegetables	Caffeine
CYP2A6	Coumarin Butadien Nicotine	Diethyldithiocarbamate 8-Methoxypsoralen Tranylcypromine	Barbiturates	Coumarin
CYP2C9	NSAID drugs Phenytoin Tolbutamide S-Warfarin	Sulfaphenazole Sulfinpyrazone	Rifampin Barbiturates	S-Warfarin Tolbutamide
CYP2C19	Citalopram Diazepam Hexobarbital Imipramine Omeprazole Proguanil Propranolol	Tranylcypromine	Rifampin Barbiturates	Mefenytoin Omeprazole
CYP2D6	Several Antidepressants Neuroleptics Beta-blockers Antiarrhythmics Codeine Dextromethorphane Etylmorphine Nicotine	Ajmalicine Chinidin Fluoxetine Paroxetine Quinidine Ritonavir	None known	Debrisoquine Dextromethorphane

CYP2E1	Acetaminophen	Diethyldithiocarbamate	Ethanol	Caffeine
	Alcohols	Dimethyl sulfoxide	Isoniazid	Chlorzoxazone
	Caffeine	Disulfiram		
	Chlorozoxazone			
	Dapsone			
	Enflurane			
	Theophylline			
CYP3A4	Acetaminophen	Clotrimazole	Dexamethasone	Dapsone
	Carbamazepine	Ketoconazole	Phenytoin	Erythromycin
	Cyclosporin	Ritonavir	Rifampin	Ketoconazole
	Digitoxin	Troleandomycin	Troleandomycin	Lidocaine
	Diazepam			
	Erythromycin			
	Felodipine			
	Fluoxetine			
	Nifedipine			
	Quinidine			
	Saquinavir			
	Steroids (e.g., cortisol)			
	Terfenadine			
	Triazolam			
	Verapamil			
	Warfarin			

8.2.3.1.2 Metabolic inhibition

Inhibition is also a dose dependent phenomenon but in contrast to induction, clinically relevant inhibition can occur quickly. In inhibition processes, both the oxidative, the hydrolytic and conjugation pathways may be involved, inhibition of the oxidative enzymes being clinically the most common.

'Points to consider regarding metabolic inhibition:

- Most inhibition is competitive and disappears rather rapidly as soon as the inhibitor is eliminated or decreases after the dose is reduced.

- In contrast to induction, inhibition is often enzyme specific.

- When metabolites are pharmacologically active, it should be remembered that the introduction of an inhibitor may result in a decrease in the concentration of the active metabolites, thereby possibly reducing their effect.

- Some dietary constituents are known inhibitors of specific drug metabolizing enzymes, e.g., grapefruit juice (CYP3A4).' (CPMP, 1997.)

8.2.3.1.3   Change of blood flow

The liver has the greatest metabolic capacity, and the hepatic blood flow is about 90 L/h. Blood clearance and blood flow are related by the following equation:

$$\text{Blood clearance} = \text{Blood flow} \cdot \text{Extraction ratio}.$$

Thus clearance is the product of the extraction ratio of a drug and blood flow, that is volume of blood from which all drug would appear to be removed per unit time. For example, if the extraction of a drug across an organ is 0.5, and the organ blood flow is 1.5 L/min, then each minute 750 ml of the incoming blood is effectively completely cleared of drug as it passes through the organ. The value of the extraction ratio can lie anywhere between zero, when no drug is eliminated, and one, when all drug is eliminated by passage through the organ. A drug with an extraction ratio of less than 0.3 is defined as a 'low extraction drug', a drug with an extraction ratio of 0.3 to 0.7 is defined as an 'intermediate extraction drug', and a drug with an extraction ratio greater than 0.7 is defined as a 'high extraction drug' (Rowland and Tozer, 1995).

For 'high extraction drugs', changes in blood flow produce corresponding changes in clearance, but not in the extraction ratio. Clearance is then said to be *perfusion rate-limited*. For 'low extraction drugs', a change of the blood flow through the liver causes no change in the clearance and hence of the unbound plasma concentration at steady state; however, the extraction ratio will vary inversely with a change in flow (cf. Table 8.2).

8.2.3.2   Renal excretion

Interactions at the level of renal excretion have been reported for many drugs where renal excretion is the dominant route of elimination. The role of renal elimination in the excretion of active metabolites is just as important in the context of such interactions. For drugs where the renal route is a major route of elimination, interactions could occur via changes in protein binding (glomerular filtration rate), urinary pH and/or urinary flow rate (passive reabsorption) and by competition of active secretion in the renal tubule.

Table 8.2   Changes in clearance and extraction ratio with changes in blood flow (modified from Rowland and Tozer, 1995).

Drug with	Blood Flow	Clearance	Extraction Ratio
High extraction ratio	↑	↑	↔
	↓	↓	↔
Low extraction ratio	↑	↔	↓
	↓	↔	↑

Symbols: ↑ = increase; ↔ = little or no change; ↓ = decrease.

8.2.3.3 Hepatic/biliary excretion

For drugs where the biliary route is a major route of elimination, and for which a saturation of the excretory capacity of the liver is possible, interactions caused by competition for hepatic excretion should be considered. The possibility of drugs interfering with enterohepatic circulation should also be considered. Interactions at the level of hepatic excretion have been reported for a few drugs (e.g., rifampicin).

8.2.4 Experimental design of *in vivo* drug–drug interaction studies

Drug development should move early from *in vitro* studies, which will be useful to identify potential metabolic interaction, to definitive, specially designed *in vivo* studies. The best way to study *in vivo* the potential influence of drug I on the pharmacokinetics of a substrate S is to compare the steady-state pharmacokinetics of drugs S and I administered concomitantly (Test) with those of drug S administered alone (Reference). If an interaction is expected primarily at the level of liver metabolism, intravenous studies are adequate; if primarily absorption is to be affected, oral studies are indicated; if absorption, distribution, metabolism and elimination may be affected, intravenous and oral studies will be necessary to differentiate the sites and fractions of the overall interaction. If a competitive mechanism in the metabolism between the substrate and the interacting drug is expected, the interacting drug should ideally be dosed in a fashion that ensures adequate inhibitor drug concentrations during the assessment of the substrate pharmacokinetics.

In order to reduce variability, a crossover design is usually appropriate. Other designs may be chosen in specific situations, but should be justified in the study protocol.

In studies involving simple induction or inhibition, it may be adequate to investigate the effect of the potentially interacting drug I on the pharmacokinetics of the drug serving as substrate S. However, when both drugs S and I are substrates for the same enzyme, it is important to investigate the pharmacokinetics of both drugs administered singly and in combination to the same subjects. In order to enable an intraindividual comparison, an additional concentration-time profile of drug I is taken in the absence of drug S, and a three-period crossover design with randomized treatments S, I and S + I will be appropriate.

In the most commonly used design for orally administered drugs, both S and I are investigated at steady state in a randomized, two-period crossover study. More precisely, repeated oral administration of the substrate S serves as Reference. For example, S may be given twice daily (b.i.d.), possibly with an initial loading dose to shorten the time to reach steady state. Repeated oral administration of drug S until steady state, as under Reference, and then additionally repeated oral administration of drug I, while dosing of drug S is continued, serves as Test. The verification that steady-state conditions have been reached is usually made by comparing the predose levels (sometimes referred to as trough values) during 3 to 4 dosing intervals prior to the steady-state sampling interval.

Although this design is optimal from a theoretical point of view, it may cause logistical difficulties due to the long time required to reach steady-state concentrations for both drugs S and I. Therefore, the following modifications have to be considered in practice. Firstly, the steady states of both drugs are built up in parallel using suitable initial loading doses. Secondly, the steady state of drug I is replaced by a single dose which, however, may have to be higher than the repeated standard dose would be, so that similar maximum concentrations can be expected.

In order to shorten the time to reach steady state, repeated oral administration may be replaced by a two-step infusion to rapidly reach steady-state concentrations. Such designs have been advocated by Steinijans *et al.* (1991) and have been used in the following examples.

8.2.5   Examples to illustrate drug–drug interactions and the lack thereof

The following two examples of pharmacokinetic lack-of-interaction studies with theophylline were selected for two reasons. Firstly, they vividly illustrate the difference in magnitude of a negligible interaction and a pronounced interaction, which in a certain way supports the assay validity, i.e., the ability of the chosen design to pick up a true drug–drug interaction if it exists. Secondly, the chosen two-step infusion is an elegant way of rapidly reaching steady-state concentration without the need for a long build-up by repeated oral administration. The intravenous administration of theophylline allows us only to test for a clearance interaction, which is the primary focus of this investigation. It is not considered as a limitation, since oral formulations are available for which the lack of food–drug interaction has been convincingly demonstrated (Schulz *et al.*, 1987; Steinijans and Sauter, 1993). Theophylline is a widely used bronchodilator with a narrow therapeutic range. Serum concentrations of 8–15 mg/L were considered optimal by some authors (Barnes *et al.*, 1982), while others, particularly in the US, where bronchodilator monotherapy with theophylline was in focus, aimed for 10–20 mg/L (Weinberger, 1984).

Pharmacokinetic drug interactions with theophylline have been summarized by Jonkman and Upton (1984). Theophylline (1,3-dimethylxanthine) is metabolized by hepatic cytochrome P450-dependent enzymes (Campbell *et al.*, 1987; Robson *et al.*, 1988), as are the investigated drugs caffeine (1,3,7-trimethylxanthine) (Campbell *et al.*, 1987) and pantoprazole (Simon *et al.*, 1991).

In the first example (Jonkman *et al.*, 1991), the influence of 300 mg t.i.d. caffeine (drug I) on the steady-state pharmacokinetics of theophylline (substrate S) was investigated in eight healthy male volunteers. The study was an open, randomized, two-period crossover trial with two study periods of eight days each and no washout. On day six of the respective study period (i.e., with or without t.i.d. caffeine) 1200 mg anhydrous theophylline were administered as a rapid-loading infusion of 370 mg during 0.5 h, starting at 8 a.m., followed by a constant-rate infusion of 830 mg during 23.5 h. In this way, theophylline steady-state concentrations of approximately 10 mg/L were obtained for practically 24 h in the caffeine-free Reference session. Twenty-four hours corresponds to one dosing cycle of caffeine in the test period, where 300 mg caffeine were given as 50 mg tablets at 8 a.m., 2 p.m. and 8 p.m. from day one until 2 p.m. on day eight. This caffeine dose corresponds to six to ten cups of brewed coffee per day and was considered as a realistic amount of caffeine to be investigated. Blood samples were taken frequently up to 60 h after the start of the first theophylline infusion.

The median plasma concentrations of theophylline and caffeine are shown in Figure 8.1. The primary characteristic for confirmative analysis was the area under the plasma theophylline concentration-time curve (*AUC*) extrapolated to infinity. The point estimate and

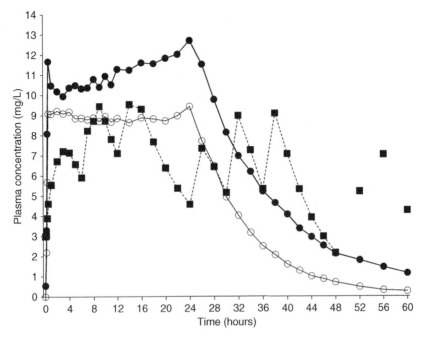

Figure 8.1 Median plasma concentrations ($n = 8$): theophylline (solid lines) with ($\bullet$) and without ($\circ$) caffeine; caffeine (dotted line, ■). Theophylline was administered as a two-step intravenous infusion of 1200 mg during 24 h; 300 mg caffeine t.i.d. were given orally at 6, 6 and 12 h intervals. The last three caffeine concentrations at 52, 56 and 60 h were insufficient to draw a pharmacokinetic profile consistent with dosing at 48 and 54 h. For details, see example 1 (from Jonkman *et al.*, 1991).

non-parametric 90 % confidence limits for the ratio Test/Reference (with/without caffeine) were 1.40 (1.28, 1.54). This means that the *AUC* increased by 40 % and that equivalence, i.e., 'lack of interaction', cannot be claimed. Moreover, as the lower limit of the 90 % confidence interval is 1.28, it exceeds the upper equivalence acceptance limit of 1.25 and a statistically significant interaction can be concluded. In view of the narrow therapeutic range of theophylline, such an interaction may also become clinically relevant.

In the second example (Schulz *et al.*, 1991) the influence of repeated once-daily injections of 30 mg pantoprazole (drug I) on the steady-state pharmacokinetics of theophylline (substrate S) was investigated in eight healthy male volunteers. Pantoprazole is a selective gastric H^+, K^+-ATPase inhibitor from the class of substituted benzimidazoles (Fitton and Wiseman, 1996; Shin *et al.*, 1994). The study was an open, randomized two-period crossover trial with study periods of two days (placebo) and five days (pantoprazole), respectively, and a washout period of at least one week. In each study period approximately 700 mg anhydrous theophylline were administered as a rapid-loading infusion of 351.3 mg theophylline during 0.5 h, starting at 7 a.m. on day one (placebo) or day four (pantoprazole), respectively, followed after a 5 min interval by a constant-rate infusion of 348.4 mg during 9h 55 min. In this way, theophylline steady-state concentrations of approximately 10 mg/L were obtained for practically 10 h, which was long enough to cover the period of measurable serum concentrations of pantoprazole. Daily injections of 30 mg pantoprazole during 2 min on days one to five were given in the Test session; on day four, pantoprazole was injected during the 5 min interval between the short- and long-term theophylline infusions. Although the pharmacokinetic characteristics of pantoprazole do not provide constant serum concentrations over the observational period, the administration regimen used in the study reflects the clinically recommended once-daily dosing, which is well supported by the long duration of action of this proton pump inhibitor due to the covalent binding of its activated form to the gastric H^+/K^+-ATPase in the parietal cells.

In the Reference session, a 2 min injection of placebo was given on day one (between the theophylline infusions) and on day two. Blood samples to determine serum pantoprazole-Na and theophylline concentrations were taken frequently up to 12 and 36 h, respectively, after the start of the first theophylline infusion. An additional pantoprazole profile in the absence of theophylline was taken on day one of the Test session.

The median serum concentrations of theophylline and pantoprazole-Na are shown in Figure 8.2. The primary characteristic for confirmative analysis was the theophylline

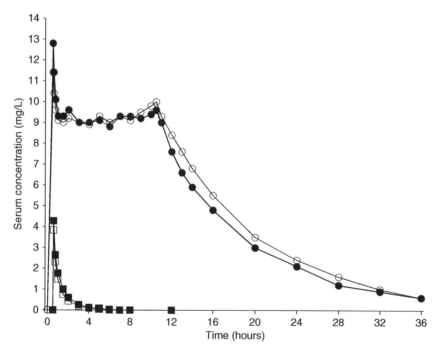

Figure 8.2 Median serum concentrations (n = 8): theophylline with (•) and without (○) pantoprazole; pantoprazole-Na with (■) and without (□) theophylline. Theophylline was administered as a two-step intravenous infusion of 700 mg during 10.5 h; 30 mg pantoprazole were injected during 2 min on days one to five. For details, see example 2 (from Schulz *et al.*, 1991).

AUC extrapolated to infinity. The point estimate and 90 % confidence limits for the ratio Test/Reference (with/without pantoprazole) were 0.94 (0.84, 1.05). This means that the *AUC* decreased by 6 % and that, with a consumer risk of 5 %, equivalence, i.e., 'lack of pharmacokinetic interaction', can be concluded.

A retrospective power analysis based on the confidence interval approach for the primary characteristic theophylline *AUC* showed an observed ratio of the geometric means of 0.944 and an estimated within-subject coefficient of variation,

$$CV_W = \sqrt{\exp(MS_{within}) - 1},$$

of 11.5 %, where MS_{within} denotes the mean square of error in the analysis of variance; hence, $n = 8$ subjects were sufficient to obtain a power of 80 %, i.e., a producer risk of 20 % (see Chapter 5). It is worth noting that these results compare very well with those of the prospective power analysis for sample size planning, for which expected Test/Reference ratios between 0.95 and 1.05 and a within-subject coefficient of variation of 10 % were assumed. These assumptions together with a requested power of 80 % resulted in $n = 8$ subjects (Diletti *et al.*, 1991). The tables in the publication also provide the sample sizes for a power of 90 %.

Further examples of lack of drug–drug interaction studies, involving 14 different substrates representing most of the relevant CYP450 enzymes are given in the updated review paper by Steinijans *et al.* (1996) on the lack of pantoprazole drug interactions in man. This review not only reflects a variety of chosen designs but also presents pharmacodynamic endpoints, such as prothrombin time, in addition to or in lieu of pharmacokinetic endpoints. Utilizing the recommended approach of presenting point estimates and 90 % confidence intervals on the Test/Reference ratio, the results of the 14 drug–drug interaction studies have been summarized in Figure 8.3.

8.2.6 Pharmacokinetic characteristics for extent of absorption and clearance in drug–drug interaction studies

Lack of drug–drug interaction implies equivalent pharmacokinetic concentration-time profiles of the substrate S under Test and Reference conditions, i.e., in the presence and absence of the potentially interacting drug I. The optimum characterization of concentration-time profiles by means of pertinent pharmacokinetic characteristics has been discussed in detail in Chapter 2 'Metrics to characterize concentration-time profiles in single- and multiple-dose bioequivalence studies'. Although the focus in that chapter was on characteristics for rate and extent of absorption, the more general concepts of early, peak and total exposure were also discussed. The recommendations given can be summarized as follows: The area under the concentration-time curve (*AUC*) is universally accepted as characteristic of the extent of drug absorption, that is of total drug exposure. As detailed in Chapter 2, $AUC(0 - \infty)$ serves as characteristic in single-dose studies, while AUC_τ, over one steady-state dosing interval τ, serves as steady-state characteristic. With regard to the rate of drug absorption into the systemic circulation, regulatory authorities favor C_{max}, the observed maximum concentration, as rate characteristic in single-dose studies, and the % peak-trough fluctuation as rate characteristic in multiple-dose studies.

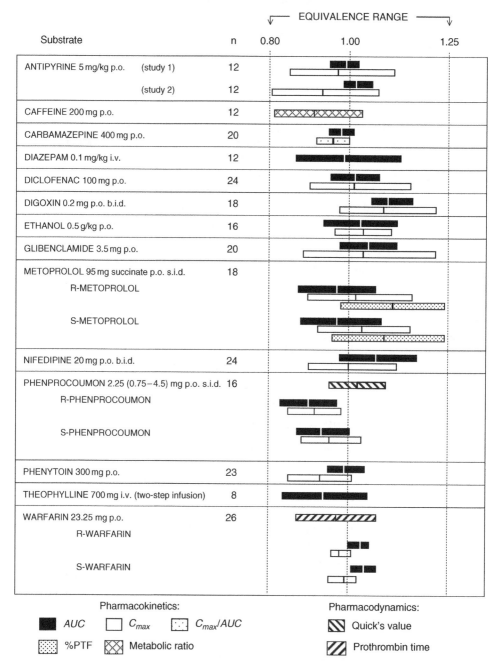

Figure 8.3 Point estimate (geometric mean) and 90 % confidence interval for the ratio Test/Reference = (substrate + pantoprazole)/(substrate + placebo) of population

Scrutiny of the literature indicates that C_{max}/AUC may be a better rate characteristic in single-dose studies, and that the plateau time may be particularly suitable in multiple-dose studies of controlled (prolonged) release formulations (cf. Chapter 2).

However, an important difference between drug–drug interaction studies and bioequivalence studies is that for two formulations of the same drug as considered in bioequivalence studies, generally no difference with respect to the clearance is expected, whereas in drug–drug interaction studies an effect of one drug on the clearance of another drug is not only possible, but may be the likely mechanism of interaction for many classes of drugs.

The area under the drug concentration-time curve (AUC) is, in general, a characteristic of the amount of drug available in the systemic circulation. In bioequivalence studies of oral dosage forms, AUC is conventionally used as a characteristic for the extent of absorption of the drug. Specifically, the ratio of geometric means of the $AUCs$ of the Test and Reference formulation is used as an estimate of the relative bioavailability of the two formulations under investigation. This is justified because in bioequivalence studies one can generally assume that differences between the formulations might affect the absorption, but not the clearance, of the drug. However, while an interaction between two drugs may be caused by one drug affecting the absorption of the other drug, an interaction may also be caused by one drug affecting the clearance of the other drug. Thus, in drug–drug interaction studies the area under the curve is not a pure characteristic of the extent of absorption, but a composite characteristic of extent of absorption and clearance. In particular, when the study results indicate that an interaction is present, one should investigate whether the interaction is due to an effect of drug I on the extent of absorption of drug S, or on the clearance of drug S. For this purpose, the elimination half-life of a drug was suggested as a characteristic for the elimination or clearance,

---

medians are indicated by the vertical line in the centre of the horizontal bars and the bars themselves. Closed bars refer to AUC, the primary characteristic of systemic exposure. In the studies with oral drug administration, AUC reflects the extent of absorption, while C_{max} (open bars), C_{max}/AUC (dotted bar), and at steady state the % peak-trough fluctuation ($\%PTF$; intensely dotted bars) reflect the rate of absorption. The crossed bar refers to the ratio of caffeine metabolites in urine as a marker of CYP1A2 activity. The hatched bars refer to the pharmacodynamic characteristic excess-AUC of the prothrombin time in the case of warfarin, and to Quick's value in the case of phenprocoumon. The excess-$AUC(0 - 168h)$ of the prothrombin time (PTT) above the individual baseline was chosen as primary characteristic because of its greater discriminatory power to detect drug-induced changes in PTT as compared with the total AUC, which is dominated by the AUC below the baseline (about 85 % of the total AUC). Equivalence, i.e., lack of pharmacokinetic or pharmacodynamic interaction, is concluded if the 90 % confidence interval is entirely in the respective equivalence range, which conventionally is 0.80 to 1.25 for pharmacokinetic characteristics.

and the ratio of AUC and the elimination half-life as a characteristic for the extent of absorption (Schall *et al.*, 1994).

8.2.6.1 Theoretical background on AUC as a composite measure of absorption and clearance

The following theoretical derivations are taken from the pioneering paper by Schall *et al.* (1994). In a bioequivalence study of oral dosage forms, with equal doses given under Test and Reference, the Test/Reference ratio of AUC is given by

$$\frac{AUC_T}{AUC_R} = \frac{f_T}{f_R} \cdot \frac{CL_R}{CL_T}$$

where f_T and f_R are the absolute bioavailabilities (fraction of the dose absorbed) of the Test and Reference formulation, respectively. Since, in bioequivalence studies, it is reasonable to assume that Test and Reference do not differ with respect to clearance ($CL_T = CL_R$, but possibly $f_T \neq f_R$), the Test/Reference ratio of AUC is equal to the Test/Reference ratio f_T/f_R of absolute bioavailabilities. This is the rationale for using AUC as a characteristic for the extent of absorption in bioequivalence studies, and, in particular, for using the Test/Reference ratio of AUC as a measure of the extent of absorption of the Test relative to the Reference formulation.

In drug–drug interaction studies, where drug S is given orally, the above equation remains valid, but the assumption that $CL_T = CL_R$ can no longer be made. In general, drug I may affect f, the extent of absorption of drug S (for example, by affecting the rate of stomach emptying), or the clearance of drug S (for example, by affecting the metabolism of drug S). Often, there is a priori knowledge that an interaction, if it should occur, will affect the clearance rather than the absorption of the drug in question. In this case, it is reasonable to assume the reverse of the usual assumption made in bioequivalence studies, namely that $f_T = f_R$ but possibly $CL_R \neq CL_T$, so that the Test/Reference ratio of the AUC is a measure of relative clearance, and not of relative extent of absorption.

In general, however, AUC is a characteristic of both extent of absorption and clearance in drug–drug interaction studies. In the following, we distinguish between the case when an analysis of the characteristic AUC indicates lack of interaction, and the case when such an analysis indicates the presence of an interaction between two drugs.

Case 1: Analysis of AUC indicates lack of interaction

When an analysis of the characteristic AUC in a drug–drug interaction study indicates lack of interaction, the amount of drug S available in the systemic circulation is not affected by concomitant administration of drug I. This would usually imply that drug I neither affects the extent of absorption of drug S (that is, f_T and f_R are essentially the same), nor the clearance of drug S (that is, CL_T and CL_R are essentially the same). This is so because it is unlikely that drug I would affect drug S in such a way as to increase the absorption and decrease the clearance (or vice versa) by approximately equal amounts, leading to a Test/Reference mean ratio of AUC close to unity. Thus, further analysis, specifically of the clearance of drug S, should not be needed.

However, in the interpretation of the result, and in the wording of the conclusion one should take into account that AUC is a characteristic for both extent of absorption and clearance. Based on equivalence with respect to AUC one should, therefore, not merely conclude that 'drug I does not affect the extent of absorption of drug S', but one should conclude that 'the amount of drug S available in the systemic circulation is not affected by concomitant administration of drug I'. In that case one would usually be justified in concluding that 'drug I neither affects the extent of absorption, nor the clearance of drug S'.

Case 2: Analysis of AUC indicates presence of an interaction

When an analysis of the characteristic AUC indicates that there is an interaction, it is of interest to find out whether drug I affects the extent of absorption or the clearance of drug S. Schall et al. (1994) proposed the use of two additional pharmacokinetic characteristics for this purpose: the elimination half-life of drug S, to assess whether drug I affects the clearance of drug S, and the ratio of AUC and the elimination half-life (equivalently the product of AUC and the elimination rate constant), to assess whether drug I affects the extent of absorption of drug S.

The use of these characteristics can be motivated by considering the one-compartment open model for the drug concentrations C as a function of time t, namely

$$C(t) = f \cdot \frac{D}{V} \cdot \frac{k_a}{k_a - k} \left(e^{-kt} - e^{k_a t} \right),$$

where k_a and k are the absorption and elimination rate constants, respectively, f is the absolute bioavailability, D is the dose, and V is the apparent volume of distribution (Ritschel, 1986). It is well known that for the one-compartment open model

$$AUC = f \cdot \frac{D}{V} \cdot \frac{1}{k}$$

In general, $CL = f \cdot D / AUC$, so that for the one-compartment open model

$$CL = k \cdot V.$$

Under the usual assumption that the volume of distribution for the Test and Reference is the same, and noting that $t_{1/2} = \ln 2/k = 0.693/k$ holds for the elimination half-life $t_{1/2}$, we have

$$\frac{CL_T}{CL_R} = \frac{k_T}{k_R} = \frac{t_{1/2,R}}{t_{1/2,T}}.$$

Thus, the Reference/Test ratio of the elimination half-lives, and the Test/Reference ratio of the elimination rate constants, equal the Test/Reference ratio of the clearances.

Furthermore,

$$\frac{AUC_T \cdot k_T}{AUC_R \cdot k_R} = \frac{AUC_T / t_{1/2,T}}{AUC_R / t_{1/2,R}} = \frac{f_T}{f_R},$$

so that the Test/Reference ratio of $AUC/t_{1/2}$ or alternatively the Test/Reference ratio of the product of AUC and k, equals the Test/Reference ratio of absolute bioavailabilities.

Thus, under the one-compartment open model, the elimination half-life $t_{1/2}$ and the ratio of AUC and $t_{1/2}$ are characteristics of the clearance and of the extent of absorption, respectively. Under higher compartment models this remains true if drug I affects only the absolute bioavailability f, or the elimination half-life of drug S, or both (but not, for example, the distribution). These relationships also remain valid with drug concentration-time curves with a lag time, or higher order absorption kinetics, even if the lag time and absorption rates are affected by drug I (Schall *et al.*, 1994).

The ratio of AUC and $t_{1/2}$ or equivalently, the product of AUC and k, has, in a different context, first been proposed as an elimination rate-adjusted characteristic of bioavailability by Upton *et al.* (1982a, b).

8.2.6.2   Examples to illustrate the composite character of AUC

As examples of application, Schall *et al.*, 1994 used an interaction study involving warfarin, and an interaction study between furosemide and ranitidine. In each case the study results were reported as the geometric means of the pharmacokinetic characteristics AUC, $t_{1/2}$ and $AUC/t_{1/2}$ together with the relevant Test/Reference mean ratios and 90 % confidence intervals for these characteristics. The estimates of the mean ratios and 90 % confidence intervals were calculated based on the standard analysis of variance after logarithmic transformation of the data (multiplicative model).

Example 1: Interaction study with warfarin

The first example was taken from a 6-way interaction study where warfarin was administered either with placebo (Reference), or with one of five different drugs known to interact with warfarin. The study was originally conducted to develop a model for the detection of warfarin–drug interactions in man (Duursema *et al.*, 1992). Only the results relating to the drugs rifampicin and cholestyramine are considered here. Rifampicin is a hepatic microsomal enzyme-inducing agent, and is thus expected to increase the clearance of warfarin; in contrast, cholestyramine is an inhibitor of absorption from the gastrointestinal tract, and is thus expected to reduce the absorption of warfarin.

The study results are summarized in Table 8.3. As expected, both rifampicin and cholestyramine decreased the mean AUC of warfarin. If one were unaware of the likely mechanisms of interaction, one might conclude that both drugs decrease the 'extent of absorption' of warfarin. However, as the analysis of the characteristic $AUC/t_{1/2}$ shows, this is only true for cholestyramine. The differences in warfarin AUC between the treatments 'warfarin + rifampicin' and 'warfarin + placebo', however, are solely due to a difference in the elimination half-life, and thus the clearance, of warfarin. Thus, an analysis of the characteristic $AUC/t_{1/2}$ correctly identifies the dominant mechanisms by which rifampicin and cholestyramine affect warfarin kinetics, namely by an effect on clearance in the case of rifampicin, and primarily by an effect on extent of absorption in the case of cholestyramine.

Table 8.3 Warfarin interaction study: results for variables $AUC, t_{1/2}$, and $AUC/t_{1/2}$ ($n = 17$).

Variable		Warfarin + placebo	Warfarin + rifamipicin	Warfarin + cholestyramine
AUC	Geometric mean	106	54.2	68.9
($\mu g \cdot h/ml$)	Mean ratio		0.51	0.65
	90 % confidence interval		0.48–0.54	0.62–0.68
$t_{1/2}$	Geometric mean	35.3	16.8	30.0
(h)	Mean ratio		0.48	0.85
	90 % confidence interval		0.45–0.51	0.79–0.91
$AUC/t_{1/2}$	Geometric mean	3.00	3.22	2.30
($\mu g/ml$)	Mean ratio		1.07	0.77
	90 % confidence interval		0.99–1.16	0.71–0.83

Mean ratio = Ratio of 'warfarin + interacting drug' over 'warfarin + placebo'

Example 2: Furosemide/ranitidine interaction study

The second example refers to an interaction study of ranitidine and oral furosemide. Prior to the study, two possible mechanisms for an interaction of ranitidine with oral furosemide were postulated: firstly, ranitidine increases gastric pH, and thus could affect the absorption of furosemide; secondly, ranitidine could lower liver blood flow and thus decrease the elimination of furosemide.

The study results (Table 8.4) show that the furosemide AUC is increased with concomitant administration of ranitidine compared to placebo. The question of interest is whether this is due to an increase in absorption or a decrease in clearance of furosemide. Since the elimination half-lives of furosemide for the two treatments satisfy the usual bioequivalence criterion, one can conclude that the increase in AUC is due to an increased absorption of furosemide (as indicated by the results for the second-step characteristic $AUC/t_{1/2}$) and not due to a decrease in furosemide clearance (as confirmed by the results for the second-step characteristic $t_{1/2}$).

8.2.6.3   Recommendation for subsequent analyses

In summary, it is recommended that in pharmacokinetic drug–drug interaction studies the characteristic AUC is used as the primary characteristic for the amount of drug available in the systemic circulation. If the analysis of the characteristic AUC indicates equivalence, lack of interaction with respect to extent of absorption and clearance can be concluded. If in the first step of analysis the composite characteristic AUC indicates the presence of an interaction, the characteristics $t_{1/2}$ and $AUC/t_{1/2}$ should be analyzed in an additional second step to identify the source of the interaction, namely whether the interaction is due to a change in clearance or in extent of absorption.

Table 8.4 Furosemide/ranitidine interaction study: results for variables AUC, $t_{1/2}$, and $AUC/t_{1/2}$ ($n = 18$).

Variable		Furosemide + placebo	Furosemide + ranitidine
AUC	Geometric mean	2.015	2.703
($ng \cdot h/ml$)	Mean ratio		1.34
	90 % confidence interval		1.14–1.58
$t_{1/2}$	Geometric mean	1.41	1.34
(h)	Mean ratio		0.96
	90 % confidence interval		0.86–1.07
$AUC/t_{1/2}$	Geometric mean	1.434	2.012
(ng/ml)	Mean ratio		1.40
	90 % confidence interval		1.12–1.75

Mean ratio = Ratio of 'furosemide + ranitidine' over 'furosemide + placebo'

8.3 Pharmacokinetic food–drug interactions

With increasing generic substitution, food–drug interaction studies have gained considerable importance. Food–drug interaction studies focus on the effect of food on the release and absorption of a drug. In view of dramatic and clinically relevant food effects observed with certain theophylline sustained release formulations (Hendeles *et al.*, 1985; Karim *et al.*, 1985a, b; Smolensky *et al.*, 1987), bioequivalence between a Test and a Reference formulation under only one nutritional condition, e.g. fasting, is by no means sufficient to allow generic substitution (Blume, 1991). The reported food effects, with *AUC* increases of 100 % and decreases of 50 % for certain formulations (Karim, 1985a, b), are far beyond the usually accepted 25 % increase and 20 % decrease in bioequivalence studies between formulations. The CPMP (2001) guidance on bioequivalence also addresses this issue with particular emphasis on controlled release formulations. The FDA (2002) guidance recommends a study comparing the bioavailability under fasting and fed conditions for all orally administered modified release drug products. As pointed out in Section 2.2.2, modified release formulations include two essentially different types of release modifications, so-called 'prolonged release' formulations and 'delayed release' formulations.

8.3.1 Classification of food effects

Early characterization of food effect response is important in drug development to provide dosing conditions that will minimize variability in drug absorption during pivotal clinical trials. Food effect studies are also important in testing *in vivo* performance of a dosage form under widely different physiological conditions.

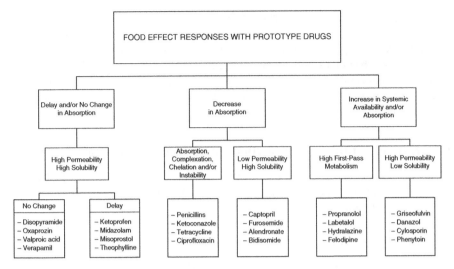

Figure 8.4 Classification of the food effect responses of prototype drugs on the basis of: (i) stability, chelation and/or complexation; (ii) effect on metabolism, and (iii) effect on permeability and/or solubility (Karim, 1996).

The various ways in which food can effect gastrointestinal (GI) physiology, and thereby drug absorption, are summarized in Figure 8.4 (Karim, 1996). Of great importance for the drug absorption process are changes in gastric emptying time, GI motility, splanchnic blood flow, and GI secretion.

The absorption of drugs from the gastro-intestinal tract can be affected considerably by simultaneous intake of meals, particularly meals with a high fat content. In this regard the following factors play an important role: increase in pH in the stomach, intensification of bile secretion, reinforcement of motility, increase of blood-flow and retardation of the gastric transit time. Prior to initiating an *in vivo* food–drug interaction study, some of these factors should be mimicked *in vitro*. Ideally, the *in vitro* release should not be affected by pH value, buffer capacity, surface tension, turbulence of the dissolution medium and agitation by the apparatus. The most recent regulatory requirements on *in vitro* dissolution can be found in the corresponding guidelines. A comprehensive overview of the various *in vitro* dissolution tests together with rather extensive examples was presented by Dietrich *et al.* (1988). The absence of all of the above mentioned *in vitro* factors on the dissolution of the formulation investigated was confirmed *in vivo* by extensive food–drug interaction studies which clearly demonstrated lack of food interaction for this formulation (Schulz *et al.*, 1987; Steinijans and Sauter, 1993).

On the other hand, the ability of the *in vivo* equivalence methodology to detect major *in vitro* modifications was convincingly demonstrated by Steinijans *et al.* (1995). Differences were seen in the *in vivo* pharmacokinetic characteristics for two apparently identical theophylline sustained release products, which were used as reference products in bioequivalence studies in the US and in Europe, respectively. Although both reference formulations were manufactured by the same international group according to the same *in vitro* controlled release principle, their *in vivo* differences in concentration-time profiles could – in this case retrospectively – be explained by different *in vitro* dissolution profiles after 4 hours.

The relevance of a pH-dependency on the *in vitro* dissolution and hence on the *in vivo* bioavailability has been known for a long time, even dramatic effects in the case of some sustained release formulations (Hendeles *et al.*, 1985; Karim *et al.*, 1985b). However, pH dependency still is a cause of significant food interactions with certain marketed modified release formulations (Wonnemann *et al.*, 2006).

8.3.2   Experimental design of food–drug interaction studies

As drug intake with or after meals is quite common, by 1991 Blume had already suggested the following scheme of bioequivalence studies in the case of controlled release formulations (cf. Figure 8.5).

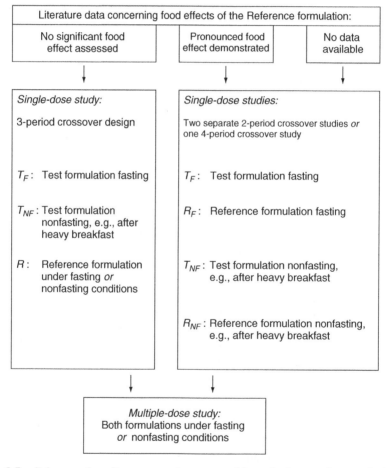

Figure 8.5   Scheme of studies proposed to assess bioequivalence of controlled release dosage forms (with the permission of Professor Henning Blume).

There are no universally accepted standards of meal composition. Detailed information on the composition of a high fat American breakfast can be found in the excellent overview by Karim (1996); further information addressing the composition of breakfast, lunch and evening meals can be found in Steinijans and Sauter (1993).

Similarly to 'lack of drug–drug interaction' as discussed in the previous chapter, 'lack of food–drug interaction' can also be handled as an equivalence problem utilizing the well-established methodology (Schulz *et al.*, 1987; Steinijans and Sauter, 1993; CPMP, 2001; FDA, 2002). If 'lack of food–drug effect' cannot be demonstrated, the resulting food effects (point estimate and 90 % confidence limits), together with the recommended mode of administration, should be clearly stated in the labeling of the particular formulation.

8.3.3   Example: Theophylline food interaction study

The following example from the work of Steinijans and Sauter (1993) illustrates the obvious food–drug interaction with one formulation (lower panel of Figure 8.6), whereas the other formulation appears to be free of any relevant food effect (upper panel).

8.4   Goal posts for pharmacokinetic drug interaction studies including no effect boundaries

Results of pharmacokinetic drug–drug and food–drug interaction studies should be reported as 90 % confidence intervals about the geometric mean ratio of the selected pharmacokinetic characteristics, with (S + I) and without (S) the interacting drug, i.e., Test = S + I = substrate S plus interacting drug I, Reference = S = substrate alone. While the geometric mean ratio serves as a point estimate of the magnitude of the effect, the 90 % confidence interval allows a statistical inference. If the 90 % confidence interval is entirely in the equivalence acceptance range, lack of interaction will be concluded (Steinijans *et al.*, 1991; CPMP, 1997; FDA, 1999; FDA, 2002). The lower and upper limits of the equivalence acceptance range are sometimes called 'goal posts'. In the FDA (1999) guidance the term 'no effect boundaries' is also used. Unless such boundaries have been stipulated on the basis of concentration-response relationships, PK/PD models or other available information for the substrate S, a sponsor may use as default a no-effect boundary of 0.80 to 1.25 for the Test/Reference ratio. In this case,

> 'standard Agency practice is to conclude that no clinically significant differences are present' (FDA, 1999).

In the FDA guidance on food–drug interaction (2002) it is stated that the conventional no-effect boundaries of 0.80 to 1.25 apply to both primary characteristics, AUC and C_{max}. In contrast, the CPMP (2001) guidance on bioavailability and bioequivalence allows an extended acceptance range of 0.75 to 1.33 for C_{max}, if justified.

The thresholds for a clinically relevant drug–drug interaction should be based on clinical relevance and safety considerations. The CPMP (1997) guidance on the investigation of drug interactions states the following:

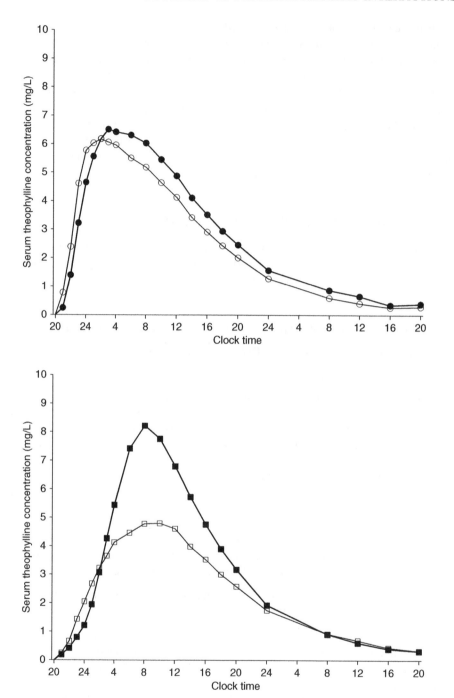

Figure 8.6   Geometric mean value curves ($n = 18$) of serum theophylline concentrations following a single dose of 600 mg theophylline at 8 p.m. of the Test formulation

> 'When considering potential therapeutic consequences of an interaction (dosage reductions or increases), the acceptance range to conclude lack of interaction may be wider (or narrower) than the interval of 0.80 to 1.25 commonly used in establishing bioequivalence.'

Frequently, dose adjustments are only possible by a factor of two, i.e., either half a tablet or two tablets instead of one. The goal posts needed for a formalized decision procedure must be justified on clinical grounds. They have to take into account the dose response and safety profile of the respective substrate.

8.5 Labeling

Both guidances on drug interaction studies (CPMP, 1997 and FDA, 1999) emphasize that the point estimate of the effect size together with the 90 % confidence interval should form the basis for any potential recommendations of dose modifications in the SmPC (Summary of Product Characteristics). The guidances devote very instructive sections on the labeling of relevant drug–drug interaction data, including both positive and important negative findings.

For example, if *in vivo* metabolic drug–drug interaction studies indicate a clinically significant pharmacokinetic interaction, the FDA (1999) guidance considers the following labeling language as appropriate:

> 'The effect of drug I on the pharmacokinetics of substrate S has been studied in ... patients/healthy subjects. The C_{max}, AUC, half-life and clearances of substrate S increased/decreased by ... % (90 % confidence interval: ... to ...) in the presence of drug I. This indicates that drug I can inhibit the metabolism of drugs metabolized by CYP3A4 and can increase blood concentrations of such drugs. (See PRECAUTIONS, WARNINGS, DOSAGE AND ADMINISTRATION, or CONTRAINDICATIONS sections).'

For reasons of consistency the wording 'probe drug' used in the FDA guidance was replaced by 'substrate' in the citation.

In a recent Draft Guidance on Drug Interaction Studies (FDA, 2006), classifications of the magnitude of inhibitors were given. As an example, we will consider the classification that has been proposed for CYP3A as a substrate: If an investigational drug increases the AUC of oral midazolam or other CYP3A substrates by 5-fold or higher ($\geq$ 5-fold), it can be labeled as a *strong* CYP3A inhibitor. If an investigational drug, when given at the highest dose and shortest dosing interval, increases the AUC of oral midazolam or other sensitive CYP3A substrates by between 2- and 5-fold ($\geq$ 2- and < 5-fold), or 1.25- and 2-fold ($\geq$ 1.25- and < 2-fold), respectively, it can be labeled as a *moderate* or *weak* CYP3A inhibitor, respectively.

(upper panel: o =fasting, • = nonfasting) and the Reference formulation (lower panel: □ = fasting, ■ = nonfasting). This intraindividual comparison is based on the respective parts of two separate crossover studies in $n = 18$ subjects each under fasting and nonfasting conditions, respectively.

Even in the case where interaction studies have not been performed, a labeling similar to the following is likely to be requested (CPMP, 1997):

> 'Although interaction studies have not been performed, since the drug is metabolized by CYP3A4, it is expected that ketoconazole, itraconazole, clotrimazole, ritonavir... inhibit its metabolism. On the other hand, inducers of this enzyme such as rifampicin, phenytoin... may reduce the levels of the drug. Since the magnitude of an inducing or inhibiting effect is unknown, such drug combinations should be avoided.'

8.6   Conclusions

The primary purpose of drug–drug and food–drug interaction studies is to quantify and to clinically assess potential interactions. Pertinent guidelines on drug interactions (CPMP, 1997; FDA, 1999; FDA, 2002) request that the results of pharmacokinetic drug–drug and food–drug interaction studies should be reported as 90 % confidence intervals about the geometric mean ratio of recommended pharmacokinetic characteristics such as AUC and C_{max}. In drug–drug interaction studies, the Test treatment refers to the simultaneous administration of substrate S and the interacting drug I, (S + I), while the Reference treatment refers to the administration of the substrate alone, (S). In food–drug interaction studies, the Test treatment refers to the administration of the investigated drug with food, while the Reference treatment refers to the administration of the drug without food.

The geometric mean ratio serves as a point estimate of the magnitude of the effect, and the 90 % confidence interval allows a statistical inference. If the 90 % confidence interval is entirely in the a priori stipulated equivalence acceptance range, lack of interaction will be concluded (Steinijans et al., 1991; CPMP, 1997; FDA, 1999; FDA, 2002). The underlying decision problem in demonstrating lack of drug–drug and lack of food–drug interaction is the same as in bioequivalence assessment, if 'bioequivalence' is replaced by 'lack of pharmacokinetic drug–drug interaction' or 'lack of pharmacokinetic food–drug interaction', respectively. Consequently, the entire methodology of bioequivalence analysis including the crossover design, choice of primary pharmacokinetic characteristics, mathematical modeling (log transformation of commonly used primary pharmacokinetic characteristics such as AUC and C_{max}), sample size planning and statistical analysis (ANOVA) can be directly applied to pharmacokinetic lack of interaction studies.

However, if in drug–drug interaction studies the analysis of the composite characteristic AUC indicates the presence of an interaction, the characteristics $t_{1/2}$ and $AUC/t_{1/2}$ should be analyzed in addition, to identify whether the interaction is due to an effect on clearance or on the extent of absorption.

References

Barnes, P.J., Greening, A.P., Neville, L., Timmers, J. and Poole, G.W. (1982) Single-dose slow-release aminophylline at night prevents nocturnal asthma. *Lancet* **I**, 229–304.

Blume, H. (1991) Influence of food on the bioavailability of controlled/modified release products: are food studies necessary? In Blume, H., Gundert-Remy, U. and Möller, H. (eds) *Controlled/modified release products.* Wissenschaftliche Verlagsgesellschaft mbH, Stuttgart Paperback APV Band **29**, 115–25.

Campbell, M.E., Grant, D.M., Inaba, T. and Kalow, W. (1987) Biotransformation of caffeine, paraxanthine, theophylline and theobromine by polycyclic aromatic hydrocarbon-inducible cytochrome(s) P-450 in human liver microsomes. *Drug Metabolism and Disposition* **15**, 237–49.

Committee for Proprietary Medicinal Products (1997) Note for guidance: The investigation of drug interactions. EMEA, London.

Committee for Proprietary Medicinal Products (2001) Note for guidance: Investigation of bioavailability and bioequivalence. EMEA, London.

Cummins, C.L., Wu. C.Y. and Benet, L.Z. (2002) Sex-related differences in the clearance of cytochrome P450 3A4 substrates may be caused by P-glycoprotein. *Clinical Pharmacology and Therapeutics* **72**, 474–89.

Dietrich, R., Brausse, R., Bautz, A. and Diletti, E. (1988) Validation of the in-vitro dissolution method used for the new sustained-release theophylline pellet formulation. *Arzneimittelforschung/Drug Research* **38**, 1220–8.

Diletti, E., Hauschke, D. and Steinijans, V.W. (1991) Sample size determination for bioequivalence assessment by means of confidence intervals. *International Journal of Clinical Pharmacology, Therapy and Toxicology* **29**, 1–8.

Duursema, L., Müller, F.O., Hundt, H.K.L., Heyns, A. du P., Meyer, B.H. and Luus, H.G. (1992) Model to detect warfarin–drug interactions in man. *Drug Investigation* **4**, 395–402.

Fitton, A. and Wiseman, L. (1996) Pantoprazole – a review of its pharmacological properties and therapeutic use in acid-related disorders. *Drugs* **51**, 460–82.

Food and Drug Administration (1999) Guidance for industry: in vivo drug metabolism/drug interaction studies. Center for Drug Evaluation and Research (CDER) and Center for Biologics Evaluation and Research (CBER), Rockville, MD.

Food and Drug Administration (2002) Food-effect bioavailability and fed bioequivalence studies. Center for Drug Evaluation and Research (CDER), Rockville, MD.

Food and Drug Administration (2006) Draft guidance for industry: drug interaction studies – study design, data analysis, and implications for dosing and labeling. Center for Drug Evaluation and Research (CDER) and Center for Biologics Evaluation and Research (CBER), Rockville, MD.

Hendeles, L., Weinberger, M., Milavetz, G., Hill, M. and Vaughan, L. (1985) Food-induced 'dose-dumping' from a once-a-day theophylline product as a cause of theophylline toxicity. *Chest* **87**, 758–65.

Jonkman, J.H.G. and Upton, R. (1984) Pharmacokinetic drug interactions with theophylline. *Clinical Pharmacokinetics* **9**, 309–34.

Jonkman, J.H.G., Sollie, F.A.E., Sauter, R. and Steinijans, V.W. (1991) The influence of caffeine on the steady-state pharmacokinetics of theophylline. *Clinical Pharmacology and Therapeutics* **49**, 248–55.

Karim, A., Burns, T., Wearley, L., Streicher, J. and Palmer, M. (1985a) Food-induced changes in theophylline absorption from controlled release formulations, part I: substantial increased and decreased absorption with Uniphyl tablets and Theo-Dur Sprinkle. *Clinical Pharmacology and Therapeutics* **38**, 77–83.

Karim, A., Burns, T., Janky, D. and Hurwitz, A. (1985b) Food-induced changes in theophylline absorption from controlled release formulations, part II: importance of meal composition and dosing time relative to meal intake in assessing changes in absorption. *Clinical Pharmacology and Therapeutics* **38**, 642–647.

Karim, A. (1996) Importance of food effect studies early in drug development. In: Midha, K.K. and Nagai, T. (eds)*Bioavailability, bioequivalence and pharmacokinetic studies. International conference of F.I.P. "Bio-International '96", Tokyo, Japan*, 221–9, Business Center of Academic Societies Japan, Tokyo.

Nave, R., Drollmann, A., Steinijans, V.W., Zech, K., Bethke, T.D. (2005) Lack of pharmacokinetic drug–drug interaction between ciclesonide and erythromycin. *International Journal of Clinical Pharmacology and Therapeutics* **43**, 264–70.

Ritschel, W.A. (1986) *Handbook of basic pharmacokinetics* (3rd edition). Drug Intelligence Publications, Hamilton.

Robson, R.A., Miners, J.O., Matthews, A.P., Stupans, I., Meller, D., McManus, M.E. and Birkett, D.J. (1988) Characterization of theophylline metabolism by human liver microsomes. *Biochemical Pharmacology* **37**, 1651–9.

Rowland, M. and Tozer, T.N. (1995) *Clinical pharmacokinetics – concepts and applications* (3rd edition). Lippincott, Williams and Wilkins, Philadelphia.

Schall, R., Hundt, H.K.L. and Luus, H.G. (1994) Pharmacokinetic characteristics for extent of absorption and clearance in drug/drug interaction studies. *International Journal of Clinical Pharmacology and Therapeutics* **32**, 633–7.

Schulz, H.-U., Karlsson, S., Sahner-Ahrens, I., Steinijans, V.W. and Beier, W. (1987) Effect of drug intake prior to or after meals on serum theophylline concentrations: Single dose studies with Euphylong. *International Journal of Clinical Pharmacology, Therapy and Toxicology* **25**, 222–8.

Schulz, H.-U., Hartmann, M., Steinijans, V.W., Huber, R., Lührmann, B., Bliesath, H. and Wurst, W. (1991) Lack of influence of pantoprazole on the disposition kinetics of theophylline in man. *International Journal of Clinical Pharmacology, Therapy and Toxicology* **29**, 369–75.

Shin, J.M., Besancon, M., Prinz, C., Simon, A. and Sachs, G. (1994) Continuing development of acid pump inhibitors: site of action of pantoprazole. *Alimentary Pharmacology and Therapeutics* **8** (Suppl. 1), 11–23.

Simon, W.A., Büdingen, C., Fahr, S., Kinder, B. and Koske, M. (1991) The H^+, K^+-ATPase inhibitor pantoprazole (BY1023/SK&F96022) interacts less with cytochrome P450 than omeprazole and lansoprazole. *Biochemical Pharmacology* **42**, 347–55.

Smolensky, M.H., Scott, P.H., Harrist, R.B., Hiatt, P.H., Wong, T.K., Baenziger, J.C., Klank, B.J., Marbella, A. and Meltzer, A. (1987) Administration-time-dependency of the pharmacokinetic behavior and therapeutic effect of a once-a-day theophylline in asthmatic children. *Chronobiology International* **4**, 435–47.

Steinijans, V.W. and Sauter, R. (1993) Food studies: acceptance criteria and statistics. In: Midha, K.K. and Blume, H.H. (eds) *Bio-International: bioavailability, bioequivalence and pharmacokinetics. International conference of F.I.P. "Bio-International '92", Bad Homburg, Germany*, 235–50, Medpharm Scientific Publishers, Stuttgart.

Steinijans, V.W., Sauter, R. and Diletti, E. (1995) Shape analysis in single- and multiple-dose studies of modified-release products. In: Midha, K.K. and Blume, H.H. (eds) *Bio-International II: bioavailability, bioequivalence and pharmacokinetic studies. International conference of F.I.P. "Bio-International '94", Munich, Germany*, 193–206, Medpharm Scientific Publishers, Stuttgart.

Steinijans, V.W., Hartmann, M., Huber, R. and Radtke, H.W. (1991) Lack of pharmacokinetic interaction as an equivalence problem. *International Journal of Clinical Pharmacology, Therapy and Toxicology* **29**, 323–8.

Steinijans, V.W., Huber, R., Hartmann, M., Zech, K., Bliesath, H., Wurst, W. and Radtke, H.W. (1996) Lack of pantoprazole drug interactions in man: an updated review. *International Journal of Clinical Pharmacology and Therapeutics* **34**, 243–62.

Upton, R.A., Thiercellin, J-F., Guentert, T.W., Wallace, S.M., Powell, J.R., Sansom, L. and Riegelman, S. (1982a) Intraindividual variability in theophylline pharmacokinetics: statistical verification in 39 of 60 healthy young adults. *Journal of Pharmacokinetics and Biopharmaceutics* **10**, 123–34.

Upton, R.A., Thiercellin, J-F., Moore J.K. and Riegelman, S. (1982b) A method for estimating within-individual variability in clearance and volume of distribution from standard bioavailability studies. *Journal of Pharmacokinetics and Biopharmaceutics* **10**, 135–46.

Weinberger, M. (1984) The pharmacology and therapeutic use of theophylline. *Journal of Allergy and Clinical Immunology* **73**, 525–40.

Wonnemann, M., Schug, B., Schmücker, K., Brendel, E., van Zwieten, P.A. and Blume, H. (2006) Significant food interactions with a nifedipine modified-release formulation marketed in the European Union. *International Journal of Clinical Pharmacology and Therapeutics* **44**, 38–48.

9

Population and individual bioequivalence

9.1 Introduction

As seen from the previous chapters, the concept of average bioequivalence is based on the comparison of distances between formulations in terms of mean rate or extent of exposure. Hence, the decision on bioequivalence of two formulations is solely based on a comparison of the means of the pharmacokinetic characteristic (bioavailability metric) of interest, thus ignoring the fact that the distributions of the selected metric may differ between the two formulations in other distributional characteristics, e.g., their variances (see e.g., Anderson and Hauck, 1990; Hauck and Anderson, 1994). For illustration, see Figure 9.1 (Elze and Blume, 1999); it depicts plasma concentration profiles for 18 subjects. Scenario (a) is related to two formulations with similar rates of absorption and variability. Scenario (b) shows more variable plasma concentration profiles under the test formulation. Surprisingly, the average curves of test and reference formulation nearly coincide for both situations. This means that two bioequivalent, but highly variable formulations may lead to rather different effects under one formulation as compared to the other when a patient starts treatment. Since average bioequivalence obviously does not protect against such an effect a new concept of bioequivalence, namely population bioequivalence (PBE) has been introduced by Hauck and Anderson (1992). Measures that address population bioequivalence should therefore not only compare population means under the reference and test formulation but also the between-subject variance in bioavailability.

Another issue arises when an individual patient switches from one formulation to another. Here again it may happen that both formulations, although being on average bioequivalent, may lead to clearly different effects, which could be explained by the presence of a subject-by-formulation interaction (Ekbohm and Melander, 1989). Possible

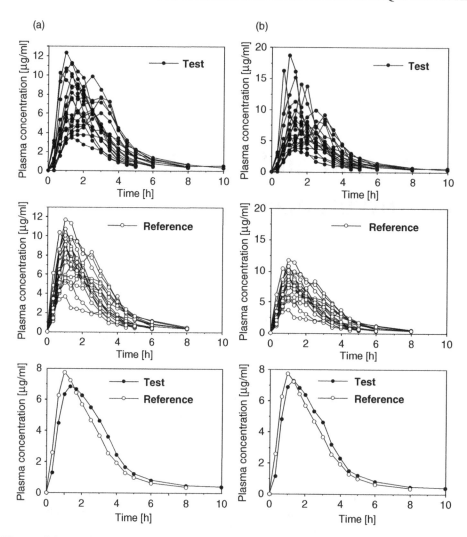

Figure 9.1 Individual plasma concentration profiles for 18 subjects under test and reference formulation and average profiles under both formulations for (a) two formulations with comparable variability and (b) a more variable test formulation (adapted from Elze and Blume, 1999; with the permission of Martina Elze).

sources of a subject-by-formulation interaction are shown in Figure 9.2 (Patterson, 2001, p. 12, 45). Figure 9.2 (a) represents the classical situation where a subject's reaction to one drug (here: the test formulation) is more variable than to the other one (here: the reference formulation). Subject-by-formulation interaction can also occur due to unpredictable reactions to the two formulations (see Figure 9.2 (b)). Another possible scenario for the occurrence of a subject-by-formulation interaction is depicted in Figure 9.2 (c). Here,

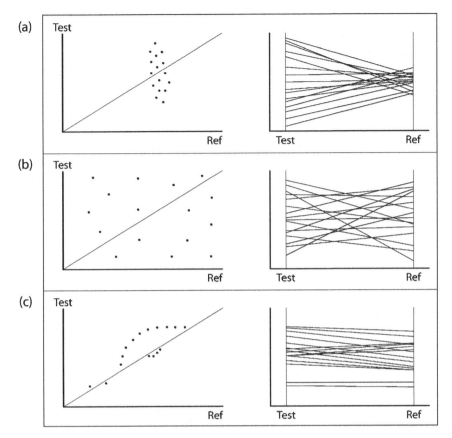

Figure 9.2 Potential sources of subject-by-formulation interactions (adapted from Patterson, 2001; with the permission of Scott Patterson).

subjects can be grouped into subgroups with similar responses to the drug formulation within those subgroups, but highly different responses between them.

Taking potential subject-by-formulation interactions into account has led to the concept of individual bioequivalence (IBE) (Anderson and Hauck, 1990; Wellek, 1993). If IBE holds, pharmacokinetic responses to the reference and test formulation should not differ too much in the majority of patients. Thus, appropriate measures of IBE should also account for the within-subject variances under both formulations.

Summarizing, population and individual bioequivalence can conceptually be distinguished as follows: If PBE is fulfilled, a patient who has not yet received one of the formulations may be safely prescribed either of them, whereas IBE should guarantee that a patient can be safely switched from the reference to the test formulation.

The purpose of this chapter is to provide a comprehensive overview of the most important statistical approaches to test for individual or population bioequivalence. Necessary details to understand the statistical theory behind these techniques are given. This should enable the reader to follow their derivations and to decide on the adequate method in a specific situation. We will first present a brief history of these new bioequivalence concepts. The underlying study design and the corresponding statistical models will then be introduced before the various statistical methods are discussed. Methods that can be used to assess population as well as individual bioequivalence will be derived in detail for population bioequivalence. The major steps and results will then be repeated for individual bioequivalence. These approaches will be complemented by methods that are specific to population or individual bioequivalence, but may be used within the same procedure, e.g., stepwise procedures. Further remarks on the differences between aggregate and disaggregate criteria will help to evaluate their appropriateness. The chapter should, however, not be closed without at least briefly addressing how to assess average bioequivalence in replicate designs. The moment-based approach that has been recommended by the FDA will be illustrated by a practical example.

9.2 Brief history

The introduction of these new bioequivalence concepts has raised a lively and controversial debate on (i) which measures are appropriate to assess population and individual bioequivalence, (ii) how such measures should be statistically evaluated, and (iii) whether population or individual bioequivalence are necessary at all to protect public health. For an overview of regulatory requirements and scientific issues in bioequivalence trials, see for example Chow and Liu (1995), Chinchilli (1996) and Chen (1997).

In 1997, the FDA published a draft guidance on the issue of bioequivalence of drug products, where average bioequivalence was no longer regarded as sufficient to protect public health (FDA Guidance, 1997). Instead, the population or individual bioequivalence approach should be used to assess bioequivalence depending on whether the corresponding proof was to be performed prior or subsequent to the approval of an innovator drug. Based on a classical two-period, two-sequence, randomized crossover design (see Chapter 3) PBE should be assessed to approve bioequivalence of a to-be-marketed formulation and a formulation used in pivotal clinical studies when major formulation and/or manufacturing changes have been made prior to approval of a new drug. A four-period, two-sequence, randomized crossover design ($TRTR/RTRT$) (see Section 9.3.2), a so-called replicate design, was proposed for the assessment of IBE. Assessment of IBE was required for approval of new formulations after the new drug had already been approved for market, thus targeting generic manufacturers but also pharmaceutical companies intending to change the formulation and/or manufacturing of their drug after approval. Further requirements were related e.g., to adequate washout periods so that carryover effects could be neglected. The preferred bioequivalence characteristics, i.e., AUC and C_{max}, remained unchanged. It was proposed to use an aggregate, reference-scaled or constant-scaled, moment-based measure as proposed by Schall and Luus (1993), Schall (1995a), and Schall and Williams (1996), which will be introduced in subsequent sections. Aggregate measures combine the various aspects for assessing PBE or IBE, respectively, within one measure, in contrast to disaggregate measures which assess e.g., the means, variances, and subject-by-formulation interaction separately.

The problem of assessing population or individual bioequivalence was formulated as a statistical test problem with bioequivalence to be claimed if the upper bound of a two-sided 90 % confidence interval of the corresponding aggregate measure was below a predetermined bound. It was proposed to calculate the confidence intervals based on a nonparametric bootstrap percentile interval (Efron and Tibshirani, 1993) as introduced by Schall and Luus (1993), where the FDA recommended at least 2000 bootstrap samples. For more details on this procedure see e.g., Sections 9.4.1.1.1 and 9.5.1.1.1. The guidance considered further aspects such as treatment of unequal carryover effects, outliers and drugs with a narrow therapeutic range.

This draft guidance caused controversial debates on scientific and on practical aspects of the given recommendations (see Midha et al., 1997; Endrenyi et al., 1998). Major concerns came from academia as well as from pharmaceutical industry regarding (i) use of an aggregate measure because of the potential trade-off between variances and differences in means which allows for a nonhierarchical ordering of ABE, PBE and IBE, i.e., it may happen that IBE could be claimed without having demonstrated ABE, (ii) scaling because of a potentially liberal declaration of bioequivalence, and (iii) the additional uncertainty due to the nonparametric bootstrap percentile that is realized via a Monte Carlo algorithm (see Section 9.5.4). It was also commented that in practice it has not been observed that average bioequivalence is not sufficient to protect public health and that the clinical need for more stringent criteria than average bioequivalence has not been demonstrated. Especially criticized was the fact that subject-by-formulation interactions need not be considered for assessing bioequivalence (see Section 9.10). In addition, even the argument that switchability is necessary for registration of a new formulation is doubtful in contrast to prescribablity as has been demonstrated by Senn (2001). The various criticisms will be discussed in more detail below.

As a consequence of the critical comments, in 1998 the FDA established a panel consisting of representatives from academia and industry, the so-called 'Blue Ribbon Panel' to advise the FDA Working Group on individual and population bioequivalence. In 1999, the Pharmaceutical Research and Manufacturers Association (PhRMA) initiated a panel to work on this issue. The whole debate finally led to two new draft guidances in 1999 (FDA Guidance, 1999a, b), where in the first draft guidance advice on the preferred study design was given. In addition, it was suggested that during a period of two years all pharmaceutical companies had to perform a replicate design study to get market access, having the option to decide on the criterion to assess bioequivalence. The second draft guidance (FDA Guidance, 1999b) focused on more statistical aspects including study designs, models and test procedures. Although the aggregate criterion was retained, it was now proposed to replace the nonparametric bootstrap percentile by a parametric approach based on the method of moments exploiting the Cornish–Fisher expansion as introduced by Hyslop et al. (2000). The bootstrap procedure should only be considered as a kind of 'back-up' in case the new approach fails by coming up with misleading results. Furthermore, it was recommended to use the restricted maximum likelihood (REML) estimator for assessing average bioequivalence in studies with a replicate design. For population or individual bioequivalence, however, the REML estimator was only to be used if a substantial amount of missing data occurred in the dataset.

Responses to the 1999 draft guidances were still doubt-filled as to whether the new bioequivalence criteria really provided added value compared to average bioequivalence (Hauschke and Steinijans, 2000; Barrett et al., 2000a, b; Hsuan, 2000; Steinijans, 2001).

Most comments asked for a better ground based on simulations and more extensive data collection to argue for one or the other approach. In addition, it was argued that there was no reported evidence of a clinical failure of a formulation that was shown to be 'average bioequivalent' to a reference drug (see report of the panel formed by PhRMA: Barrett *et al.*, 2000a, b). The 1999 Workshop of FDA/AAPS on 'Individual Bioequivalence' stated that 'little evidence existed to warrant the use of the new bioequivalence methods based on sufficient and adequate safety of patients in the marketplace under average bioequivalence and that subject-by-formulation [interaction] had not been established as a surrogate marker for therapeutic failure . . . '. Population and individual bioequivalence were referred to as a 'theoretical' solution to a 'theoretical' problem (Patterson, 2001, p. 182). In October 2000, it was recommended in a revised FDA guidance (FDA Guidance, 2000) to use replicate designs for highly variable and modified release drugs, where market approval would normally require demonstration of average bioequivalence. PBE or IBE criteria may be applied if justified from a regulatory agency's perspective.

The whole process ended up with the FDA guidance in 2003, where the FDA omitted the IBE and PBE concepts from their guidance in view of a critical FDA review of results from applying these techniques in practice (FDA Guidance, 2003).

It should be mentioned that many more statistical procedures, but also practical strategies for PBE and IBE have been proposed during the process of criticizing average bioequivalence and trying to establish new bioequivalence criteria. Some of these approaches will be briefly addressed in subsequent sections of this chapter. For a more detailed description of the historical background on the development of population and individual bioequivalence we refer the reader to Patterson (2001).

9.3   Study designs and statistical models

9.3.1   Classical two-period, two-sequence crossover design

As discussed in previous chapters a classical two-period, two-sequence crossover design may be used to assess average bioequivalence. Study subjects are randomly allocated to two treatment sequences, where they receive in sequence 1 the reference formulation (R) and test formulation (T) in periods 1 and 2, while in sequence 2, subjects receive the formulations in reverse order with an adequate washout period between periods 1 and 2. This design is referred to as the *RT/TR* design (see Chapter 3, especially Table 3.5). This design is sufficient to estimate the mean response under test and reference formulation but also to estimate the between-subject variances, which implies that this design is also sufficient to assess population bioequivalence.

9.3.2   Replicate designs

The classical two-period, two-sequence crossover design is no longer sufficient when individual bioequivalence needs to be assessed based on the criterion recommended by the FDA (1997), because it is not possible to estimate the within-subject and between-subject variances, each under test and reference formulation separately. This requires a replicate design where, in contrast to the standard crossover study, each study subject receives at least the reference formulation in two periods to enable the estimation of the corresponding within-subject variances. Of the various replicate designs that can be thought of, the FDA recommended in their 1997 and 1999 draft guidances (FDA, 1997, 1999b) a four-period, two-sequence design, where the study subjects are randomly allocated to two treatment sequences: In sequence 1 they receive the test formulation (T) in period 1, the reference formulation (R) in period 2, the test again in period 3 and finally the reference formulation in period 4, while in sequence 2 the formulations are administered in reverse order, i.e., starting with the reference formulation in period 1. Adequate washout periods have to be used between each two periods. This is referred to as the *TRTR/RTRT* design (see Table 9.1).

An example for a four-period design with more than two sequences is given in Table 9.2.

As an alternative to a four-period, two-sequence crossover study, a three-period, two-sequence crossover design as presented in Table 9.3 could be used. It has to be noted, however, that such a design requires a greater sample size than the four-period design given in Table 9.1, to achieve the same statistical power for assessing individual bioequivalence (see FDA, 1999b, Appendix C). Further replicate designs can be envisaged.

It is especially recommended not to use replicate designs with more than two sequences to avoid ambiguities in the estimation of the relevant parameters for assessing bioequivalence. These ambiguities occur because different models can be used in replicate designs with more than two sequences, that neither lead to the same parameter estimators nor to

Table 9.1 The *TRTR/RTRT* design.

Sequence	Period 1	Washout	Period 2	Washout	Period 3	Washout	Period 4
1	T		R		T		R
2	R		T		R		T

Table 9.2 The *TRRT/RTTR/TTRR/RRTT* design.

Sequence	Period 1	Washout	Period 2	Washout	Period 3	Washout	Period 4
1	T		R		R		T
2	R		T		T		R
3	T		T		R		R
4	R		R		T		T

Table 9.3 The *TRT/RTR* design.

Sequence	Period 1	Washout	Period 2	Washout	Period 3
1	T		R		T
2	R		T		R

efficient estimators. To be more precise (see Appendix B of FDA, 1999b), a main effect model for a four-period, two-sequence design, i.e., a model including main effects for treatment, sequence and period with in total five degrees of freedom, is not a saturated model, which means that it does not account for all seven degrees of freedom attributable to the eight cells of this design (see Table 9.1). Introducing, for instance, an effect for sequence-by-period interaction, would lead to a fully saturated model. Both types of models, the main effects model and the saturated model, lead to the same parameter estimators in a replicate design with only two sequences provided there are no missing values and the study is conducted in one group of subjects. This is, however, no longer the case for a replicate crossover trial with more than two sequences (see Table 9.2). Here, main effects models will lead e.g., to different estimators of the treatment effects than saturated models, unless there is the same number of study subjects in each sequence.

However, where unequal carryover effects are to be considered, replicate crossover designs with more than two sequences may be adequate, depending on the type of carryover effects to be accounted for (for more details see Appendix B of FDA, 1999b). According to the FDA guidances (FDA, 1997, 1999b) the occurrence of unequal carryover effects is less likely in a bioequivalence trial that meets all scientific criteria, if the planned trial is a single-dose study with healthy study subjects, where the administered drug is not an endogenous entity and if more than adequate washout periods have been adhered to.

9.3.3   Additive model

As introduced in the *RT/TR* design (see Section 4.2.1) the pharmacokinetic response can be modeled using a multiplicative approach or, taking its logarithm, by an additive model. For the *TRTR/RTRT* replicate design as introduced in Table 9.1 we will focus here on an additive model where carryover effects are neglected. As in Section 4.2.1, let Y_{ijk} denote the logarithm of the pharmacokinetic characteristic of interest with $i = 1, 2$ the number of sequences, $j = 1, \ldots, n_i$ the number of subjects per sequence and $k = 1, \ldots, 4$ the number of periods, then we can assume the following mixed-effect model (see Shao *et al.*, 2000a):

$$Y_{ijk} = \mu + \tau_h + \pi_k + \upsilon_i + \gamma_{hik} + s_{ijh} + e_{ijk},$$

where μ is the overall mean; τ_h is the fixed effect under formulation h, where $h = R$, if $(i, k) = (1, 2), (1, 4), (2, 1), (2, 3)$ and $h = T$ otherwise, and $\tau_R + \tau_T = 0$; μ_R and μ_T as introduced before are then given as $\mu + \tau_R$ and $\mu + \tau_T$, respectively; π_k is the fixed effect of the kth period with $\Sigma_k \pi_k = 0$; υ_i is the fixed effect of the ith sequence with $\Sigma_i \upsilon_i = 0$; γ_{hik} is the fixed effect of interaction between sequence, period and formulation, summing to zero over any index; s_{ijh} is the random effect of the jth subject in the ith sequence under formulation h with (s_{ijT}, s_{ijR}) $(i = 1, 2, j = 1, \ldots, n_i)$ independent identically distributed random vectors with expected mean 0 and unknown covariance matrix

$$\begin{pmatrix} \sigma_{BT}^2 & \rho \sigma_{BT} \sigma_{BR} \\ \rho \sigma_{BT} \sigma_{BR} & \sigma_{BR}^2 \end{pmatrix};$$

Table 9.4 Layout for the *TRTR/RTRT* replicate design on the additive scale.

Sequence	Period 1	Period 2	Period 3	Period 4
1 (TRTR)	$Y_{1j1} = \mu + \tau_T + \pi_1$ $+v_1 + \gamma_{T11}$ $+s_{1jT} + e_{1j1}$ $j = 1, \ldots, n_1$	$Y_{1j2} = \mu + \tau_R + \pi_2$ $+v_1 + \gamma_{R12}$ $+s_{1jR} + e_{1j2}$ $j = 1, \ldots, n_1$	$Y_{1j3} = \mu + \tau_T + \pi_3$ $+v_1 + \gamma_{T13}$ $+s_{1jT} + e_{1j3}$ $j = 1, \ldots, n_1$	$Y_{1j4} = \mu + \tau_R + \pi_4$ $+v_1 + \gamma_{R14}$ $+s_{1jR} + e_{1j4}$ $j = 1, \ldots, n_1$
2 (RTRT)	$Y_{2j1} = \mu + \tau_R + \pi_1$ $+v_2 + \gamma_{R21}$ $+s_{2jR} + e_{2j1}$ $j = 1, \ldots, n_2$	$Y_{2j2} = \mu + \tau_T + \pi_2$ $+v_2 + \gamma_{T22}$ $+s_{2jT} + e_{2j2}$ $j = 1, \ldots, n_2$	$Y_{2j3} = \mu + \tau_R + \pi_3$ $+v_2 + \gamma_{R23}$ $+s_{2jR} + e_{2j3}$ $j = 1, \ldots, n_2$	$Y_{2j4} = \mu + \tau_T + \pi_4$ $+v_2 + \gamma_{T24}$ $+s_{2jT} + e_{2j4}$ $j = 1, \ldots, n_2$

e_{ijk} are independent random errors with expected mean 0 and variances σ^2_{Wh}; and (s_{ijT}, s_{ijR}) and e_{ijk} are assumed to be independent. Let us further define σ^2_D with

$$\sigma^2_D = Var(s_{ijT} - s_{ijR}) = \sigma^2_{BT} + \sigma^2_{BR} - 2\rho\sigma_{BT}\sigma_{BR}.$$

Please note that σ^2_{BT} and σ^2_{BR} are between-subject variances and σ^2_{WT} and σ^2_{WR} are within-subject variances under the test and reference formulation, respectively. In the above model, additional constraints on the interaction effects may be necessary to make them estimable, but this does not affect the derivation and discussion of population or individual bioequivalence criteria. Table 9.4 shows the layout of the above model in the *TRTR/RTRT* design for the two sequences and four periods.

9.3.4 Basic concepts of aggregate measures

Before deriving the aggregate measures for population or individual bioequivalence under the model specified above, let us give a rough idea how these measures can be calculated. Various suggestions can be found in the literature, see for example Ekbohm and Melander (1989), Anderson and Hauck (1990), Sheiner (1992), Holder and Hsuan (1993), Schall und Luus (1993), Endrenyi (1994), Esinhart and Chinchilli (1994), Schall (1995a), Chinchilli (1996), Schall and Williams (1996), Hwang and Wang (1997), and, for an overview, Patnaik *et al.* (1997). Although distinct, these proposed methods exploit essentially similar ideas. Some completely different approaches for measuring and statistically assessing PBE and IBE will be briefly summarized in Section 9.7.

As already mentioned above, the new concepts of PBE and IBE were motivated by the need to consider further distributional characteristics of the pharmacokinetic response of interest than solely the means when assessing bioequivalence of two formulations. The two main approaches of an aggregate measure will be briefly introduced in the following. Let us assume any replicate design with the reference formulation being administered twice. For simplification, let Y_T, Y_R, and Y'_R denote the bioavailabilities following the administration of the test once and the reference formulation twice. Then, the first, so-called moment-based approach, measures the discrepancy of the two formulations by comparing the expected squared differences of the bioavailabilities, where the expectation has to be derived depending on the bioequivalence concept of interest, the chosen crossover design and the statistical model for the bioavailabilities. The two formulations are said to be bioequivalent, if

$$\Theta_{mom} = E(Y_T - Y_R)^2 - E(Y_R - Y'_R)^2 < \theta_{mom}.$$

The second, probability-based approach compares the probabilities of the differences of the bioavailabilities not exceeding a predefined value r, where, of course, these probabilities have to be calculated for each bioequivalence concept assuming a specific statistical model and reflecting the chosen crossover design. Here, two formulations are said to be bioequivalent if

$$\Theta_{prob,d} = P(|Y_T - Y_R| \le r) - P(|Y_R - Y'_R| \le r) > \theta_{prob,d}$$

or analogously, if

$$\Theta_{prob,r} = \frac{P(|Y_T - Y_R| \le r)}{P(|Y_R - Y'_R| \le r)} > \theta_{prob,r}.$$

Please note that the bioequivalence parameters are denoted with Θ and the bounds with θ. To distinguish the moment-based and the probability-based approach a lower index *mom* or *prob* is added, respectively. In addition for the probability-based approach, the index d or r indicates difference or ratio of probabilities, respectively. An upper index *pop* and *ind* will distinguish between population and individual bioequivalence. The bounds θ_{mom} as well as r, $\theta_{prob,d}$, and $\theta_{prob,r}$ are fixed constants that are predetermined by drug regulatory authorities. When deriving the above probabilities and expectations for PBE, it is assumed that when comparing Y_T and Y_R as well as Y_R and Y'_R, test and reference are administered to different subjects (FDA, 2001). Thus, $Y_T - Y_R$ and $Y_R - Y'_R$ represent between-subject differences, where Y_T, Y_R, and Y'_R are assumed to be independent, and Y_R and Y'_R to be identically distributed. For IBE, $Y_T - Y_R$ and $Y_R - Y'_R$ represent within-subject differences, where Y_T, Y_R, and Y'_R are considered to be from the same study subject and thus have to be treated as dependent.

According to the FDA (1997, 1999b) the above criteria should be used in scaled versions where scaling is with respect to the variance of the reference formulation. A decision among the resulting criteria should depend on the within-subject variability and the therapeutic range of the drug under consideration (Schall and Williams, 1996; see also Schall, 1995b), where roughly speaking, the within-subject variability gives an indication of the distribution of an individual's responses to a drug and the therapeutic window gives the distance between the minimum effective exposure and the maximum tolerable exposure for a drug. That is, we have to distinguish between (i) a narrow therapeutic window and a low within-subject variability as for instance for theophylline, (ii) a narrow therapeutic window and a high within-subject variability as for cyclosporine, (iii) a wide therapeutic window and a low-to-medium within-subject variability which is the case for most drugs, and (iv) a wide therapeutic window and a high within-subject variability as e.g., for chlorpromazine. Let us briefly summarize the recommendation regarding a scaled or unscaled version of the above criteria: A scaled approach should be applied to drugs with a narrow therapeutic window and a low within-subject variability to be sure that the test formulation is no more variable than the pioneer's product, and to highly variable drugs to reduce the burden of unnecessary studies; whereas an unscaled approach is appropriate for most drugs. To be more precise, the FDA (1997) recommended for the moment-based approach the following scaling: the reference and test formulation are said to be bioequivalent if $\Theta_{mom} < \theta_{mom}$ with

$$
\Theta_{mom} = \begin{cases} \dfrac{E(Y_R - Y_T)^2 - E(Y_R - Y_R')^2}{\sigma^2} & if\ \sigma^2 \geq \sigma_0^2 \\[3mm] \dfrac{E(Y_R - Y_T)^2 - E(Y_R - Y_R')^2}{\sigma_0^2} & if\ \sigma^2 < \sigma_0^2 \end{cases}
$$

with $\sigma^2 = E(Y_R - Y_R')^2/2$ and σ_0^2 the total variance or within-variance of the reference formulation, respectively, beyond which the scaled criterion has a wider bioequivalence range compared to its unscaled counterpart. This value has to be predetermined by drug regulatory authorities; the FDA (1997) recommended a value of 0.2 for σ_0 (for the reasoning behind this value see Sections 9.4.1 for PBE and 9.5.1 for IBE). Usually, dividing the difference of the expected squared differences of the bioavailabilities by σ_0^2 is referred to as the constant-scaled approach, whereas scaling with σ^2 is called the reference-scaled approach.

For the probability-based approach Schall (1995a) proposed replacing r in

$$
P_{TR} = P(|Y_T - Y_R| \leq r) \text{ and } P_{RR} = P(|Y_R - Y_R'| \leq r)
$$

by $\gamma\sqrt{2}\sigma$ with γ a positive constant. For criteria on how to choose γ we refer the reader to Schall (1995a).

9.3.5 Example: The antihypertensive patch dataset

For illustrative purposes we consider in the following an example given by the FDA at http://www.fda.gov/cder/bioequivdata/index.htm where it is referred to as dataset 17A. The dataset describes a four-period, two-sequence crossover trial where an antihypertensive patch has been administered to a total of 37 subjects. It is stated that these data are considered to have a large subject-by-formulation interaction ($\sigma_D > 0.15$), which would make it necessary to assess individual bioequivalence according to the above concerns. The design and the number of subjects per sequence are summarized in Table 9.5.

Table 9.5 Replicate design to assess individual bioequivalence.

		Period			
Sequence	Number of subjects	1	2	3	4
1	18	T	R	R	T
2	19	R	T	T	R

Table 9.6 Values of AUC and C_{max} for study subjects under T (test formulation) and R (reference formulation) in a four-period, two-sequence crossover bioequivalence study (design and number of subjects as in Table 9.5).

Subject	Sequence	AUC Period 1	2	3	4	Cmax Period 1	2	3	4
1	RTTR	1020.65	1321.23	900.42	1173.61	109	145	106	146
2	TRRT	950.59	1637.71	2076.75	1485.93	96.3	194	341	316
3	RTTR	1188.82	1440.99	1501.20	1481.27	128	155	138	192
4	TRRT	774.44	585.89	801.26	773.51	87.6	56.2	89.1	84.6
5	TRRT	1563.08	1571.75	1917.37	1886.05	161	145	194	178
6	RTTR	1119.22	781.20	800.85	942.50	119	66.9	82	117
7	RTTR	1876.81	1726.01	1653.70	1111.10	232	170	194	135
8	TRRT	2549.54	3738.21	3800.33	5408.38	229	393	395	677
9	TRRT	2291.93	1223.74	1949.10	3184.15	204	126	202	365
10	RTTR	1392.92	826.36	1220	1607.52	222	68.6	112	200
11	RTTR	5239.22	8894.11	7726.47	7451.66	871	1710	1090	1450
12	TRRT	1044.18	1023	1178.20	1155.25	91.1	111	196	104
13	TRRT	744.57	985.58	1721.01	4217.64	80.2	127	215	413
14	RTTR	1629.67	2081.88	1302.65	2805.07	168	263	134	355
15	RTTR	3054.97	3370.78	2644.44	5941.36	323	502	401	630
16	TRRT	3469	1712.59	1680.07	3285.23	449	284	141	405
17	TRRT	3006.95	3063.28	1764.34	2055.51	289	277	162	203
18	RTTR	2323.41	1063.45	960.10	2629.35	344	131	101	718
19	TRRT	4989.43	6439.82	4945.42	2321.03	744	1150	769	263
20	RTTR	2673.38	1686.63	2260.34	4632.96	361	226	538	691
21	TRRT	2081.19	1028.75	758.83	1168.12	295	108	73.2	140
22	RTTR	10843.61	13162.65	13505.79	13575.90	1530	1330	1520	1650
23	TRRT	736.50	947.58	1426.96	681.66	87.4	124	151	75.5
24	RTTR	2747.09	3651.63	2543.63	1056.48	353	480	300	110
25	TRRT	2064.25	2251.24	2228.06	2633.27	253	414	314	470
26	TRRT	1092.48	1141.68	1550.98	996.55	138	118	163	95.5
27	RTTR	2011.28	2109.67	2902.35	2283.60	467	444	512	495
28	RTTR	3793.47	4165.73	4666.95	3274.41	727	454	471	473
29	RTTR	1427.53	1591.38	1909.97	1911.43	139	183	167	164
30	TRRT	2333.74	2878.94	1698.30	1142.33	308	355	156	98.9
31	RTTR	1932.80	1620.69	2279.44	3251.14	334	228	289	528
32	TRRT	1835.61	2760.92	3188.04	2480.39	167	232	321	236
33	TRRT	8330.61	6064.54	8737.60	8353.62	954	873	857	930
34	RTTR	3612.64	2494.45	3153.79	6386.19	491	417	527	1010
35	RTTR	1061.92	987.86	1422.71	1220.58	97.4	94.1	186	103
36	TRRT	2212.39	1438.48	1984.76	2640.43	226	137	237	237
37	RTTR	2252.76	2262.88	1957.66	3084.05	304	255	301	685

Table 9.6 gives the values AUC and C_{max} under the reference and test formulation for each of the 37 subjects involved in this trial. There were no missing values.

This dataset will be analyzed in Section 9.9 where the criteria originally recommended by the FDA (FDA Guidance, 2001) will be applied. The corresponding measures and the resulting criteria will be introduced in Sections 9.4.1.1.2, 9.5.1.1.2, and 9.8.

9.4 Population bioequivalence

9.4.1 Moment-based criteria

To derive the moment-based criterion for assessing PBE the parameter Θ_{mom} introduced in 9.3.4 has to be calculated with

$$\Theta_{mom} = \frac{E(Y_R - Y_T)^2 - E(Y_R - Y_R')^2}{\max\{\sigma_0^2, \sigma^2\}}.$$

Since for assessing PBE $Y_T - Y_R$ and $Y_R - Y_R'$ refer to between-subject differences, Y_T, Y_R and Y_R' can be treated as independent. This yields

$$E(Y_T - Y_R)^2 = E(Y_T^2) - 2E(Y_T Y_R) + E(Y_R^2)$$
$$= \left(E(Y_T^2) - \mu_T^2\right) + \left(E(Y_R^2) - \mu_R^2\right) - 2E(Y_T Y_R) + \mu_T^2 + \mu_R^2$$
$$= \sigma_{BT}^2 + \sigma_{WT}^2 + \sigma_{BR}^2 + \sigma_{WR}^2 - 2\mu_T\mu_R + \mu_T^2 + \mu_R^2$$
$$= (\mu_T - \mu_R)^2 + \sigma_T^2 + \sigma_R^2$$

and $E(Y_R - Y_R')^2 = 2\sigma_R^2$.

Please note that $\sigma_{BR}^2 + \sigma_{WR}^2 = \sigma_R^2$ and $\sigma_{BT}^2 + \sigma_{WT}^2 = \sigma_T^2$ denote the total variances under reference and test formulation, respectively. Thus, a test and a reference formulation can be said to be population bioequivalent if, in the case of the scaled criterion,

$$\Theta_{mom}^{pop} = \frac{(\mu_T - \mu_R)^2 + \sigma_T^2 - \sigma_R^2}{\max\{\sigma_0^2, \sigma_R^2\}} < \theta_{mom}^{pop}.$$

That is, Θ_{mom}^{pop} is a nonlinear function of $\mu_T - \mu_R$ and the variance components and θ_{mom}^{pop} denotes the predetermined bound for the moment-based criterion for assessing PBE. The FDA (1997) fixed 0.02 as maximum difference for the variance under test and reference formulation, i.e., for $\sigma_T^2 - \sigma_R^2$, and, as already mentioned, 0.04 for σ_0^2. The choice of this value for σ_0^2 was motivated by the so-called population difference ratio (PDR) and the corresponding criterion for average bioequivalence. The PDR compares the expected squared difference of the bioavailabilities under test and reference formulation with the expected squared difference of the bioavailabilities under replicated administration of the reference formulation. More precisely, this ratio is defined as:

$$PDR = \sqrt{\frac{E(Y_T - Y_R)^2}{E(Y_R - Y_R')^2}} = \sqrt{\frac{(\mu_T - \mu_R)^2 + \sigma_T^2 + \sigma_R^2}{2\sigma_R^2}}.$$

The FDA gives 1.25 as the largest allowable value of *PDR* in analogy to the average bioequivalence criterion. Obviously, the *PDR* is closely related to the reference-scaled version of the moment-based aggregate measure of PBE:

$$PDR = \sqrt{\Theta_{mom,ref}^{pop}/2 + 1} \quad with \quad \Theta_{mom,ref}^{pop} = \frac{(\mu_T - \mu_R)^2 + \sigma_T^2 - \sigma_R^2}{\sigma_R^2}.$$

Referring to the 80/125 criterion, which means that the ratio of the expected bioavailabilities under test formulation and under reference formulation has to lie, with a certain probability, within a range from 80 % to 125 %, gives ln(1.25) as the upper bound for $\mu_T - \mu_R$. To obtain the limit for σ_0^2, the reference-scaled measure $\Theta_{mom,ref}^{pop}$ is now replaced by $[\ln(1.25)]^2/\sigma_0^2$ with ln(1.25) as the limit for $\mu_T - \mu_R$ again according to the criterion of average bioequivalence and assuming $\sigma_T^2 = \sigma_R^2$. Thus, we get

$$PDR = \sqrt{\frac{[\ln(1.25)]^2}{2\sigma_0^2} + 1} \leq 1.25$$

which results in a value for σ_0^2 of about 0.04. This results in the following value for θ_{mom}^{pop}:

$$\theta_{mom}^{pop} = \frac{[\ln(1.25)]^2 + 0.02}{0.04} \approx 1.74483.$$

The criterion for Θ_{mom}^{pop} cannot be transferred to the original scale, which is the one major criticism against it. For further analyses it may be helpful to rewrite it as follows:

$$(\mu_T - \mu_R)^2 + \sigma_T^2 - \sigma_R^2 - \max\left\{\sigma_0^2, \sigma_R^2\right\} \theta_{mom}^{pop} < 0.$$

Let us now assume that the reason behind the concept of population bioequivalence, that is different variances under test and reference formulations, does not hold, but that the variances are equal. Then, $\sigma_T^2 - \sigma_R^2 = 0$ and θ_{mom}^{pop} is

$$\theta_{mom}^{pop} = \frac{[\ln(1.25)]^2}{0.04},$$

which gives for the linearized criterion above

$$(\mu_T - \mu_R)^2 - 0.04\frac{[\ln(1.25)]^2}{0.04} < 0$$

$$\Leftrightarrow (\mu_T - \mu_R)^2 < [\ln(1.25)]^2$$

$$\Leftrightarrow -\ln(1.25) < \mu_T - \mu_R < \ln(1.25)$$

$$\Leftrightarrow \ln \frac{1}{1.25} < \mu_T - \mu_R < \ln(1.25)$$

$$\Leftrightarrow 0.8 < \frac{\exp(\mu_T)}{\exp(\mu_R)} < 1.25.$$

Thus, if the assumptions related to the concept of PBE do not apply, the moment-based criterion to assess PBE reduces to the well-known criterion to assess ABE.

9.4.1.1 Statistical procedures

For statistical assessment of PBE according to the moment-based criterion an estimator of Θ_{mom}^{pop} has to be derived, where the unknown parameters in the numerator and the denominator can be estimated using an analysis of variance (ANOVA) or the method of restricted maximum likelihood (REML) under mixed effects models. This can be done by using, for instance, the SAS® procedure PROC MIXED. Let us denote the resulting estimator as $\hat{\Theta}_{mom}^{pop}$.

To solve the test problem of population bioequivalence,

$$H_0 : \Theta_{mom}^{pop} \geq \theta_{mom}^{pop} \text{ vs. } H_1 : \Theta_{mom}^{pop} < \theta_{mom}^{pop},$$

an appropriate statistical testing procedure has to be derived where PBE can be claimed if the null hypothesis is rejected at a significance level of 5 %. According to the FDA guidances (1997, 1999b) the statistical test should be based on a two-sided 90 % confidence interval or a one-sided upper 95 % confidence interval for Θ_{mom}^{pop} where the null hypothesis is to be rejected if the upper bound is smaller than θ_{mom}^{pop}. Due to the nonlinearity of the estimator $\hat{\Theta}_{mom}^{pop}$ its exact distribution is difficult to determine analytically. In addition, no distributional assumption has yet been met, so that a nonparametric approach like the bootstrap would be appropriate to derive an approximate confidence interval.

9.4.1.1.1 The bootstrap procedure

In the 1997 draft guidance, the FDA recommended calculating a bootstrap confidence interval based on the proposal by Schall and Luus (1993). The Monte Carlo algorithm for this bootstrap procedure reads as follows:

Step 1: An unbiased estimator of the population bioequivalence parameter Θ_{mom}^{pop} is given as

$$\hat{\Theta}_{mom}^{pop} = \frac{(\hat{\mu}_T - \hat{\mu}_R)^2 - \hat{\sigma}_D^2/n + \hat{\sigma}_T^2 - \hat{\sigma}_R^2}{\max\{\sigma_0^2, \hat{\sigma}_R^2\}}, \quad n = n_1 + n_2,$$

where $\hat{\mu}_T, \hat{\mu}_R, \hat{\sigma}_D^2, \hat{\sigma}_T^2$, and $\hat{\sigma}_R^2$ are obtained from ANOVA or REML.

Step 2: Let $Y_{ij} = (Y_{ij1}, Y_{ij2}, Y_{ij3}, Y_{ij4})'$ and $Y_i = (Y_{i1}, \ldots, Y_{in_i})'$. For each fixed sequence i, draw a simple random sample $Y_i^{*b} = (Y_{i1}^{*b}, \ldots, Y_{in_i}^{*b})'$ with replacement from Y_i. That is, the bootstrap samples are obtained using subjects as sampling units, stratified by sequence. According to the FDA draft guidance (1997), at least $B = 2000$ replications are recommended, i.e., repeat this process for $b = 1, \ldots, B = 2000$ to obtain B bootstrap samples $Y_i^{*1}, \ldots, Y_i^{*B}$, $i = 1, 2$.

Step 3: For each $b = 1, \ldots, B$, compute $\hat{\mu}_T^{*b}, \hat{\mu}_R^{*b}, \hat{\sigma}_D^{*b}, \hat{\sigma}_T^{*b}$, and $\hat{\sigma}_R^{*b}$ by using the same methods as those in Step 1 but with the dataset (Y_1, Y_2) replaced by the bootstrap dataset (Y_1^{*b}, Y_2^{*b}) and let

$$
\tilde{\Theta}_{mom}^{pop*b} = \begin{cases} \dfrac{(\hat{\mu}_T^{*b} - \hat{\mu}_R^{*b})^2 - (\hat{\sigma}_D^{*b})^2/n + (\hat{\sigma}_T^{*b})^2 - (\hat{\sigma}_R^{*b})^2}{(\hat{\sigma}_R^{*b})^2} & if \quad \hat{\sigma}_R^2 \geq \sigma_0^2 \\[4mm] \dfrac{(\hat{\mu}_T^{*b} - \hat{\mu}_R^{*b})^2 - (\hat{\sigma}_D^{*b})^2/n + (\hat{\sigma}_T^{*b})^2 - (\hat{\sigma}_R^{*b})^2}{\sigma_0^2} & if \quad \hat{\sigma}_R^2 < \sigma_0^2. \end{cases}
$$

Step 4: Let $\tilde{\Theta}_{mom,FDA}^{pop}(95)$ denote the 95th percentile of $\tilde{\Theta}_{mom}^{pop*b}$, $b = 1, \ldots, B$. Then, population bioequivalence can be claimed if and only if $\tilde{\Theta}_{mom,FDA}^{pop}(95) < \theta_{mom}^{pop}$.

This procedure will be referred to as the FDA bootstrap procedure. It does not fully coincide with the standard bootstrap percentile method (Efron and Tibshirani, 1993, Chapter 13.3). This can be obtained by replacing $\tilde{\Theta}_{mom}^{pop*b}$ in Step 3 by:

$$
\tilde{\Theta}_{mom}^{pop*b} = \begin{cases} \dfrac{(\hat{\mu}_T^{*b} - \hat{\mu}_R^{*b})^2 - (\hat{\sigma}_D^{*b})^2/n + (\hat{\sigma}_T^{*b})^2 - (\hat{\sigma}_R^{*b})^2}{(\hat{\sigma}_R^{*b})^2} & if \quad (\hat{\sigma}_R^{*b})^2 \geq \sigma_0^2 \\[4mm] \dfrac{(\hat{\mu}_T^{*b} - \hat{\mu}_R^{*b})^2 - (\hat{\sigma}_D^{*b})^2/n + (\hat{\sigma}_T^{*b})^2 - (\hat{\sigma}_R^{*b})^2}{\sigma_0^2} & if \quad (\hat{\sigma}_R^{*b})^2 < \sigma_0^2. \end{cases}
$$

For $\sigma_R^2 \neq \sigma_0^2$ both procedures are consistent, which means that for the 95th percentile of the standard bootstrap percentile, denoted by $\hat{\Theta}_{mom,BP}^{pop}(95)$, and $\tilde{\Theta}_{mom,FDA}^{pop}(95)$ it holds that for n tending to infinity

$$
\lim P(\hat{\Theta}_{mom,BP}^{pop}(95) > \theta_{mom}^{pop}) = 0.95 \text{ and } \lim P(\tilde{\Theta}_{mom,FDA}^{pop}(95) > \theta_{mom}^{pop}) = 0.95.
$$

Both procedures are, however, inconsistent for $\sigma_R^2 = \sigma_0^2$. This was explicitly shown by Shao *et al.* (2000a) for the moment-based criterion to assess IBE, but also holds true for the case considered here. If we use the so-called *m*-out-of-*n* bootstrap procedure (see Shao and Tu, 1995, Chapter 3.6) instead of the bootstrap percentile, we get a bootstrap confidence interval that is consistent regardless of whether $\sigma_R^2 = \sigma_0^2$ or not. But the *m*-out-of-*n* bootstrap is not as efficient as the standard bootstrap if the latter is consistent. In addition, from a practical point of view, the failure of the bootstrap percentile is not that crucial since it occurs only with probability zero.

9.4.1.1.2   A parametric confidence interval

Before the theoretical properties of the bootstrap percentile had been published, the FDA revised its draft. Due to a controversial discussion of the bootstrap that was mainly related to the randomness of the resulting bootstrap confidence interval, FDA (1999b) recommended a parametric approach based on a principle for constructing approximate confidence intervals for linear functions of variance components. For this purpose, Hyslop *et al.* (2000) assumed a normal distribution for the transformed pharmacokinetic characteristic of interest, e.g., the logarithm of AUC, and derived a parametric confidence interval for assessing individual bioequivalence (see Section 9.5.1.1.2). They extended an idea of Graybill and Wang (1980) and Ting *et al.* (1990); see also the method by Howe (1974), which employs a Cornish–Fisher expansion. For a correct application of this approach, the linearized version of the moment-based criterion for assessing PBE has to be reparametrized such that the resulting estimator reads as a function of independent components for which confidence intervals can be computed. It will be seen that this was not fully achieved.

For simplicity, let us focus on the reference-scaled version, as the constant-scaled version can be treated analogously. The linearized version of the reference-scaled PBE criterion

$$(\mu_T - \mu_R)^2 + \sigma_T^2 - \sigma_R^2 - \sigma_R^2 \theta_{mom}^{pop} < 0$$

can be rewritten as follows:

$$\eta_{mom,ref}^{pop} = \delta^2 + \sigma_{UT}^2 + 0.5\,\sigma_{VT}^2 - (1 + \theta_{mom}^{pop})(\sigma_{UR}^2 + 0.5\sigma_{VR}^2) < 0$$

with $\delta = \mu_T - \mu_R$, $\sigma_{Uh}^2 = 0.5(\sigma_h^2 + Cov(Y_{1h}, Y_{2h}))$, $\sigma_{Vh}^2 = \sigma_h^2 - Cov(Y_{1h}, Y_{2h})$, $h = T, R$. Here, Y_{1h} and Y_{2h} denote the bioavailabilities of the first and the second period in which formulation h has been administered. Based on $\eta_{mom,ref}^{pop}$ the test problem of population bioequivalence can be formulated as

$$H_0 : \eta_{mom,ref}^{pop} \geq 0 \text{ vs. } H_1 : \eta_{mom,ref}^{pop} < 0,$$

which again will be solved via a confidence interval. This requires estimators of the components of $\eta_{mom,ref}^{pop}$ and their distributions.

For each subject j in each sequence i let I_{ij} denote the difference of the mean bioavailabilities under test and reference formulation, i.e.,

$$I_{1j} = 0.5\,(Y_{1j1} + Y_{1j3}) - 0.5\,(Y_{1j2} + Y_{1j4}) \text{ and } I_{2j} = 0.5\,(Y_{2j2} + Y_{2j4}) - 0.5\,(Y_{2j1} + Y_{2j3}),$$

where for instance I_{1j} results from the fact that in sequence 1 the test formulation is administered in period 1 and 3, whereas the reference formulation is administered in period 2 and 4 (cf. Table 9.4).

Using these reparametrizations, we get as estimator of δ

$$\hat{\delta} = \frac{1}{2}\sum_{i=1}^{2}\frac{1}{n_i}\sum_{j=1}^{n_i}I_{ij}$$

which, due to the model assumptions above, is normally distributed with

$$E(\hat{\delta}) = \delta \text{ and } Var(\hat{\delta}) = \frac{1}{4}\sum_{i=1}^{2}\frac{1}{n_i}\sigma_I^2.$$

An unbiased estimator of σ_I^2 can be obtained as

$$\hat{\sigma}_I^2 = \frac{1}{n-2} \sum_{i=1}^{2} \sum_{j=1}^{n_i} (I_{ij} - \bar{I}_{i.})^2 \text{ with } n = n_1 + n_2, \bar{I}_{i.} = \frac{1}{n_i} \sum_{j=1}^{n_i} I_{ij},$$

which is then distributed as $(n-2)^{-1} \sigma_I^2 \chi_{n-2}^2$, where χ_{n-2}^2 denotes a χ^2-distribution with $n-2$ degrees of freedom.

Next, the variance components of $\eta_{mom,ref}^{pop}$ have to be estimated. For this purpose, let us introduce, for each subject j in each sequence i, random variables U_{ijh} and V_{ijh} that give the means and the scaled differences of the bioavailabilities under the test formulation and the reference formulation, respectively, i.e.,

$$U_{1jT} = \tfrac{1}{2}(Y_{1j1} + Y_{1j3}), U_{2jT} = \tfrac{1}{2}(Y_{2j2} + Y_{2j4}), U_{1jR} = \tfrac{1}{2}(Y_{1j2} + Y_{1j4}), U_{2jR} = \tfrac{1}{2}(Y_{2j1} + Y_{2j3}),$$

$$V_{1jT} = \tfrac{1}{\sqrt{2}}(Y_{1j1} - Y_{1j3}), V_{2jT} = \tfrac{1}{\sqrt{2}}(Y_{2j2} - Y_{2j4}), V_{1jR} = \tfrac{1}{\sqrt{2}}(Y_{1j2} - Y_{1j4}), V_{2jR} = \tfrac{1}{\sqrt{2}}(Y_{2j1} - Y_{2j3}).$$

Based on

$$\hat{\sigma}_{Uh}^2 = \frac{1}{n-2} \sum_{i=1}^{2} \sum_{j=1}^{n_i} (U_{ijh} - \bar{U}_{i.h})^2$$

$$\hat{\sigma}_{Vh}^2 = \frac{1}{n-2} \sum_{i=1}^{2} \sum_{j=1}^{n_i} (V_{ijh} - \bar{V}_{i.h})^2$$

with

$$\bar{U}_{i.h} = \frac{1}{n_i} \sum_{j=1}^{n_i} U_{ijh} \text{ and } \bar{V}_{i.h} = \frac{1}{n_i} \sum_{j=1}^{n_i} V_{ijh}$$

we get adequate estimators of the variance components of $\eta_{mom,ref}^{pop}$ since

$$E(\hat{\sigma}_{Uh}^2) = Var(U_h) = Var\left(\tfrac{1}{2}(Y_{1h} + Y_{2h})\right) = \tfrac{1}{4}\left(\sigma_h^2 + \sigma_h^2 + 2Cov(Y_{1h}, Y_{2h})\right)$$
$$= \tfrac{1}{2}\left(\sigma_h^2 + Cov(Y_{1h}, Y_{2h})\right)$$

and

$$E(\hat{\sigma}_{Vh}^2) = Var(V_h) = Var\left(\tfrac{1}{\sqrt{2}}(Y_{1h} - Y_{2h})\right) = \tfrac{1}{2}\left(\sigma_h^2 + \sigma_h^2 - 2Cov(Y_{1h}, Y_{2h})\right)$$
$$= \sigma_h^2 - Cov(Y_{1h}, Y_{2h}).$$

Please note that

$$\hat{\sigma}_{Uh}^2 \sim \frac{\sigma_{Uh}^2}{n-2}\chi_{n-2}^2 \text{ and } \hat{\sigma}_{Vh}^2 \sim \frac{\sigma_{Vh}^2}{n-2}\chi_{n-2}^2.$$

Based on theses point estimators and their distributions an upper confidence limit for $\eta_{mom,ref}^{pop}$ can be calculated. For convenience, let us briefly recall the basic idea for constructing confidence intervals for linear functions of variance components. Let $\hat{\varsigma}$ be an estimator of a real-valued parameter ς which is approximately normally distributed, then the upper limit of an approximate two-sided $(1\text{-}2\alpha)100\,\%$ confidence interval for ς, based on $\hat{\varsigma}$, may be obtained as

$$\hat{\varsigma} + z_{1-\alpha}\sqrt{\widehat{Var}(\hat{\varsigma})} = \hat{\varsigma} + \sqrt{z_{1-\alpha}^2 \widehat{Var}(\hat{\varsigma})}$$

with $z_{1-\alpha}$ denoting the $(1-\alpha)$ quantile of a standard normal distribution and $\widehat{Var}(\hat{\varsigma})$ an estimator of $Var(\hat{\varsigma})$. Where $\hat{\varsigma}$ is an estimated variance component which follows a χ^2-distribution with ν degrees of freedom, it is known that an exact $(1\text{-}2\alpha)100\,\%$ confidence interval is given by

$$\left[\frac{\nu\hat{\varsigma}}{\chi_{1-\alpha,\nu}^2} ; \frac{\nu\hat{\varsigma}}{\chi_{\alpha,\nu}^2} \right].$$

Comparing both upper confidence limits we see

$$\hat{\varsigma} + \sqrt{z_{1-\alpha}^2 \widehat{Var}(\hat{\varsigma})} \approx \frac{\nu\hat{\varsigma}}{\chi_{\alpha,\nu}^2} \quad \text{or} \quad z_{1-\alpha}^2 \widehat{Var}(\hat{\varsigma}) \approx \left(\frac{\nu\hat{\varsigma}}{\chi_{\alpha,\nu}^2} - \hat{\varsigma} \right)^2.$$

In the next step, let $\hat{\varsigma}$ be a linear combination of $a_q\hat{\varsigma}_q$, a_q constant, $q = 1, \ldots, Q$, i.e., $\hat{\varsigma} = \sum_{q=1}^{Q} a_q\hat{\varsigma}_q$, then an approximate upper confidence limit for $\varsigma = \sum_{q=1}^{Q} a_q\varsigma_q$ is

$$\hat{\varsigma} + \sqrt{\sum_{q=1}^{Q} z_{1-\alpha}^2 \widehat{Var}(a_q\hat{\varsigma}_q)}.$$

Let us for the moment assume that all a_q are greater than 0, then for each of the components of this approximate upper confidence limit we can exploit the above approximation which gives

$$\hat{\varsigma} + \sqrt{\sum_{q=1}^{Q} \left(\frac{\nu\, a_q\hat{\varsigma}_q}{\chi_{\alpha,\nu}^2} - a_q\hat{\varsigma}_q \right)^2}.$$

In the case where some a_q are smaller than 0, the corresponding limits have to be replaced by $\left(\nu\, a_q\hat{\varsigma}_q / \chi_{1-\alpha,\nu}^2 - a_q\hat{\varsigma}_q \right)^2$. This approach has been extended by Hyslop *et al.* (2000), by additionally allowing for a term not being a variance component, namely δ^2, the upper confidence limit of which can be calculated from a t-distribution with $n - 2$ degrees of freedom as

$$CI_{\delta,1-\alpha}^u = \left(\left| \hat{\delta} \right| + t_{1-\alpha,n-2}\sqrt{\frac{1}{4}\sum_{i=1}^{2}\frac{1}{n_i}\hat{\sigma}_i^2} \right)^2.$$

Let $CI^u_{\sigma^2_q,1-\alpha}$, $q = UT, UR, VT, VR$, denote the upper confidence limits for the above variance components,

$$\sigma^2_{UT},\; 0.5\,\sigma^2_{VT},\; -(1+\theta^{pop}_{mom})\sigma^2_{UR},\; -\frac{1+\theta^{pop}_{mom}}{2}\sigma^2_{VR},$$

with

$$CI^u_{\sigma^2_q,1-\alpha} = \begin{cases} \dfrac{(n-2)\,a_q\,\hat\sigma^2_q}{\chi^2_{1-\alpha,n-2}} & \text{if } a_q < 0 \\[3mm] \dfrac{(n-2)\,a_q\,\hat\sigma^2_q}{\chi^2_{\alpha,n-2}} & \text{if } a_q > 0. \end{cases}$$

This finally gives an approximate upper confidence limit for $\eta^{pop}_{mom,ref}$ as follows:

$$CI^u_{\eta^{pop}_{mom,\,ref},1-\alpha} = \hat\eta^{pop}_{mom,\,ref} + \left[\left(CI^u_{\delta,1-\alpha} - \hat\delta^2\right)^2 + \left(CI^u_{\sigma^2_{UT},1-\alpha} - \hat\sigma^2_{UT}\right)^2 + \left(CI^u_{\sigma^2_{VT},1-\alpha} - 0.5\hat\sigma^2_{VT}\right)^2 \right.$$

$$\left. + \left(CI^u_{\sigma^2_{UR},1-\alpha} + (1+\theta^{pop}_{mom})\hat\sigma^2_{UR}\right)^2 + \left(CI^u_{\sigma^2_{VR},1-\alpha} + \frac{1+\theta^{pop}_{mom}}{2}\hat\sigma^2_{VR}\right)^2 \right]^{1/2}$$

with e.g.,

$$CI^u_{\sigma^2_{VR},1-\alpha} = \frac{(n-2)\left(-\frac{1+\theta^{pop}_{mom}}{2}\right)\hat\sigma^2_{VR}}{\chi^2_{1-\alpha,n-2}}.$$

If $CI^u_{\eta^{pop}_{mom,ref},0.95} < 0$, population bioequivalence can be concluded. For the constant-scaled criterion this results in

$$CI^u_{\eta^{pop}_{mom,const},1-\alpha} = \hat\eta^{pop}_{mom,const} + \left[\left(CI^u_{\delta,1-\alpha} - \hat\delta^2\right)^2 + \left(CI^u_{\sigma^2_{UT},1-\alpha} - \hat\sigma^2_{UT}\right)^2 + \left(CI^u_{\sigma^2_{VT},1-\alpha} - 0.5\hat\sigma^2_{VT}\right)^2 \right.$$

$$\left. + \left(CI^u_{\sigma^2_{UR},1-\alpha} + \hat\sigma^2_{UR}\right)^2 + \left(CI^u_{\sigma^2_{VR},1-\alpha} + 0.5\,\hat\sigma^2_{VR}\right)^2 \right]^{1/2}$$

with

$$\hat\eta^{pop}_{mom,const} = \hat\delta^2 + \hat\sigma^2_{UT} + 0.5\,\hat\sigma^2_{VT} - \hat\sigma^2_{UR} - 0.5\,\hat\sigma^2_{VR} - \theta^{pop}_{mom}\,\sigma^2_0.$$

It should, however, be mentioned that the correct application of the above approach to construct a confidence interval for a linear function of variance components requires independence of the components. This assumption is not fulfilled. Hyslop (2001) therefore investigated the power of this approach by means of simulation results and observed that this parametric confidence interval for the moment-based criterion to assess population bioequivalence is strongly conservative.

9.4.2 Probability-based criteria

Probability-based criteria have not been recommended by the FDA. For the sake of completeness, they will be discussed in this section in some detail. We follow the approach by Schall and Luus (1993) who assumed a two-period crossover design for assessing PBE. As introduced in Section 9.3.4, population bioequivalence according to the probability-based criteria can be concluded if

$$\Theta^{pop}_{prob,d} = P^{pop}_{TR} - P^{pop}_{RR} > \theta^{pop}_{prob,d}$$

or analogously, if

$$\Theta^{pop}_{prob,r} = \frac{P^{pop}_{TR}}{P^{pop}_{RR}} > \theta^{pop}_{prob,r},$$

where $P^{pop}_{TR} = P_B(|Y_T - Y_R| \leq r)$ and $P^{pop}_{RR} = P_B(|Y_R - Y'_R| \leq r)$ here denote the probabilities for the between-subject deviations being smaller than a predefined value r. This value r is either a constant or $r = r_0 \sigma_{BR}$ with $r_0 = \gamma \sqrt{2}$ as suggested by Schall (1995a).

9.4.2.1 Statistical procedures

In the following we will focus on the ratio of the two probabilities since the discussion for the difference of P^{pop}_{TR} and P^{pop}_{RR} is exactly the same. The corresponding test problem of population bioequivalence is as follows:

$$H_0 : \Theta^{pop}_{prob,r} \leq \theta^{pop}_{prob,r} \text{ vs. } H_1 : \Theta^{pop}_{prob,r} > \theta^{pop}_{prob,r}.$$

This test problem will again be solved via a confidence interval where the null hypothesis is to be rejected at a 5 % significance level if the lower bound of the corresponding two-sided interval exceeds $\theta^{pop}_{prob,r}$.

9.4.2.1.1 A distribution-free approach

For solving this test problem Schall and Luus (1993) proposed a bootstrap confidence interval. Before presenting this approach (see Shao *et al.* 2000a), let us discuss how to estimate the above probabilities. For the sake of simplicity a standard crossover design *RT/TR* as in Schall and Luus (1993) and the additive model for the pharmacokinetic characteristic of interest as introduced in Section 3.4.1 are assumed,

$$Y_{ijk} = \mu + \tau_h + \pi_k + \lambda_f + s_{ij} + e_{ijk},$$

where μ is the overall mean; τ_h is the fixed effect under formulation h, where $h = R$, if $i = k$ and $h = T$ otherwise, and $\tau_R + \tau_T = 0$; μ_R and μ_T as introduced before are then given as $\mu + \tau_R$ and $\mu + \tau_T$, respectively; π_k is the fixed effect of the kth period with $\Sigma_k \pi_k = 0$; λ_f is the carryover effect of formulation R or T from period 1 to period 2, i.e., $f = R$ if $i = 1$, $k = 2$ and $f = T$ if $i = 2$, $k = 2$ with $\lambda_R + \lambda_T = 0$; s_{ij} is the random effect of the jth subject in the ith sequence.

For each subject j and each sequence i, taking the differences of two bioavailabilities under the reference formulation gives

$$Y_{1j1} - Y_{1j'1} = s_{1j} - s_{1j'} + e_{1j1} - e_{1j'1} \quad \text{(sequence 1)}$$

$$Y_{2j2} - Y_{2j'2} = s_{2j} - s_{2j'} + e_{2j2} - e_{2j'2} \quad \text{(sequence 2)}$$

$$Y_{1j1} - Y_{2j'2} = \varepsilon_{12} + s_{1j} - s_{2j'} + e_{1j1} - e_{2j'2} \quad \text{(sequences 1 and 2)},$$

where $\varepsilon_{12} = \pi_1 - \pi_2 - \lambda_T$ and $j < j'$ for subjects j, j' in the same sequence and $j \neq j'$ for subjects in different sequences. Note, that the distribution of $Y_{1j1} - Y_{2j'2}$ is not the same as that of $Y_R - Y'_R$ unless $\varepsilon_{12} = 0$, which is true when there is no period or carryover effect. Similarly, let us now consider the differences

$$Y_{1j2} - Y_{1j'1} = \tau_T - \tau_R + \varepsilon_{11} + s_{1j} - s_{1j'} + e_{1j2} - e_{1j'1} \quad \text{(sequence 1)}$$

$$Y_{1j2} - Y_{2j'2} = \tau_T - \tau_R + \varepsilon_{22} + s_{1j} - s_{2j'} + e_{1j2} - e_{2j'2} \quad \text{(sequences 1 and 2)}$$

$$Y_{2j1} - Y_{2j'2} = \tau_T - \tau_R + \varepsilon_{21} + s_{2j} + s_{2j'} + e_{2j1} - e_{2j'2} \quad \text{(sequence 2)}$$

$$Y_{2j1} - Y_{1j'1} = \tau_T - \tau_R + s_{2j} - s_{1j'} + e_{2j1} - e_{1j'1} \quad \text{(sequences 2 and 1)},$$

where $\varepsilon_{11} = \pi_2 - \pi_1 + \lambda_R$, $\varepsilon_{21} = \pi_1 - \pi_2 - \lambda_T$, and $\varepsilon_{22} = \lambda_R - \lambda_T$. Note, that the distribution of $Y_{1j2} - Y_{1j'1}$, $Y_{1j2} - Y_{2j'2}$ and $Y_{2j1} - Y_{2j'2}$ is not the same as that of $Y_T - Y_R$ unless $\varepsilon_{11} = \varepsilon_{21} = \varepsilon_{22} = 0$, which is true when there is no period and no carryover effect. Following Shao et al. (2000a) we first deal with the case where r is a constant. For simplicity, let $\boldsymbol{\varepsilon}$ denote the vector $(\varepsilon_{11}, \varepsilon_{12}, \varepsilon_{21}, \varepsilon_{22})$. If $\boldsymbol{\varepsilon}$ is known, unbiased estimators of the above probabilities can be easily obtained via the corresponding relative frequencies as follows:

$$\hat{P}_{RR}^{pop}(\boldsymbol{\varepsilon}) = \frac{2}{n(n-1)} \left\{ \sum_{j,j'=1, j<j'}^{n_1} I\left(\left|Y_{1j1} - Y_{1j'1}\right| \leq r\right) + \sum_{j=1}^{n_1}\sum_{j'=1}^{n_2} I\left(\left|Y_{1j1} - Y_{2j'2} - \varepsilon_{12}\right| \leq r\right) \right.$$

$$\left. + \sum_{j,j'=1, j<j'}^{n_2} I\left(\left|Y_{2j2} - Y_{2j'2}\right| \leq r\right) \right\}$$

$$\hat{P}_{TR}^{pop}(\boldsymbol{\varepsilon}) = \frac{1}{n(n-1)} \left\{ \sum_{j,j'=1, j\neq j'}^{n_1} I\left(\left|Y_{1j2} - Y_{1j'1} - \varepsilon_{11}\right| \leq r\right) + \sum_{j,j'=1, j\neq j'}^{n_2} I\left(\left|Y_{2j1} - Y_{2j'2} - \varepsilon_{21}\right| \leq r\right) \right.$$

$$\left. + \sum_{j=1}^{n_1}\sum_{j'=1}^{n_2} I\left(\left|Y_{1j2} - Y_{2j'2} - \varepsilon_{22}\right| \leq r\right) + \sum_{j'=1}^{n_1}\sum_{j=1}^{n_2} I\left(\left|Y_{2j1} - Y_{1j'1}\right| \leq r\right) \right\}$$

with $n = n_1 + n_2$ and $I(A)$ the indicator function of an event A. For a replicate crossover design the same idea, i.e., building pairs of different subjects within or between sequences, can be exploited for estimating the above probabilities, although it may result in some tedious calculations.

Since $\boldsymbol{\varepsilon}$ is usually unknown, Schall and Luus (1993) proposed a bootstrap procedure where $\boldsymbol{\varepsilon}$ is simultaneously estimated such that it can be replaced by its estimator based on the original dataset. The algorithm reads as follows:

Step 1: Let $Y_{ij} = (Y_{ij1}, Y_{ij2})'$ and $Y_i = (Y_{i1}, \ldots, Y_{in_i})'$. For each fixed sequence i, draw a simple random sample $Y_i^{*b} = (Y_{i1}^{*b}, \ldots, Y_{in_i}^{*b})'$ with replacement from Y_i. That is, the bootstrap samples are obtained using subjects as sampling units, stratified by sequence. Repeat this process for $b = 1, \ldots, B = 2000$ independently to obtain B bootstrap samples $Y_i^{*1}, \ldots, Y_i^{*B}$, $i = 1, 2$.

Step 2: Let $\hat{\varepsilon}$ be a REML or an ANOVA estimator of ε calculated from the original dataset. For each $b = 1, \ldots, B$, $\hat{P}_{TR}^{pop*b}(\varepsilon)$ and $\hat{P}_{RR}^{pop*b}(\varepsilon)$ are the same as $\hat{P}_{TR}^{pop}(\varepsilon)$ and $\hat{P}_{RR}^{pop}(\varepsilon)$ but calculated from the bootstrap data Y_{ijk}^{*b} instead of the original dataset. Then define $\tilde{\Theta}_{prob,r}^{pop*b}$ as

$$\tilde{\Theta}_{prob,r}^{pop*b} = \hat{P}_{TR}^{pop*b}(\hat{\varepsilon}) / \hat{P}_{RR}^{pop*b}(\hat{\varepsilon}).$$

Step 3: Let $\tilde{\Theta}_{prob,r,SL}^{pop}(5)$ denote the 5th percentile of $\tilde{\Theta}_{prob,r}^{pop*b}$, $b = 1, \ldots, B$. Then, population bioequivalence can be claimed if and only if $\tilde{\Theta}_{prob,r,SL}^{pop}(5) > \theta_{prob,r}^{pop}$.

It has been explicitly shown by Shao *et al.* (2000a) for the corresponding procedure to assess IBE that the above bootstrap procedure is inconsistent, which means for the procedure discussed here that

$$\lim P(\tilde{\Theta}_{prob,r,SL}^{pop}(5) < \theta_{prob,r}^{pop}) \neq 0.95 \text{ for } n \text{ tending to infinity.}$$

If ε is, however, estimated within each bootstrap sample, i.e., if we replace $\tilde{\Theta}_{prob,r}^{pop*b}$ by

$$\hat{\Theta}_{prob,r}^{pop*b} = \hat{P}_{TR}^{pop*b}(\hat{\varepsilon}^{*b}) / \hat{P}_{RR}^{pop*b}(\hat{\varepsilon}^{*b}),$$

then the bootstrap procedure presented above becomes the standard bootstrap percentile, which has been shown to be consistent (Shao *et al.* 2000a).

Until now it has been assumed that r is constant. Schall (1995a) suggested using $r = r_0 \sigma_{BR}$ instead of r in the definition of $\Theta_{prob,r}^{pop}$, i.e.,

$$\Theta_{prob,r}^{pop} = \frac{P_{TR}^{pop}}{P_{RR}^{pop}}$$

with $P_{TR}^{pop} = P_B(|Y_T - Y_R| \leq r_0 \sigma_{BR})$ and $P_{RR}^{pop} = P_B(|Y_R - Y_R'| \leq r_0 \sigma_{BR})$.

Defining estimators of P_{TR}^{pop} and P_{RR}^{pop}, we have therefore to account not only for the parameter ε but also for σ_{BR}, i.e.,

$$\hat{P}_{RR}^{pop}(\varepsilon, \sigma_{BR}) = \frac{2}{n(n-1)} \left\{ \sum_{j,j'=1, j<j'}^{n_1} I\left(|Y_{1j1} - Y_{1j'1}| \leq r_0 \sigma_{BR}\right) \right.$$

$$+ \sum_{j=1}^{n_1} \sum_{j'=1}^{n_2} I\left(|Y_{1j1} - Y_{2j'2} - \varepsilon_{12}| \leq r_0 \sigma_{BR}\right)$$

$$\left. + \sum_{j,j'=1, j<j'}^{n_2} I\left(|Y_{2j2} - Y_{2j'2}| \leq r_0 \sigma_{BR}\right) \right\}$$

$$\hat{P}_{TR}^{pop}(\varepsilon, \sigma_{BR}) = \frac{1}{n(n-1)} \left\{ \sum_{j,j'=1, j\neq j'}^{n_1} I\left(\left|Y_{1j2} - Y_{1j'1} - \varepsilon_{11}\right| \leq r_0 \sigma_{BR}\right) \right.$$

$$+ \sum_{j,j'=1, j\neq j'}^{n_2} I\left(\left|Y_{2j1} - Y_{2j'2} - \varepsilon_{21}\right| \leq r_0 \sigma_{BR}\right)$$

$$+ \sum_{j=1}^{n_1} \sum_{j'=1}^{n_2} I\left(\left|Y_{1j2} - Y_{2j'2} - \varepsilon_{22}\right| \leq r_0 \sigma_{BR}\right)$$

$$\left. + \sum_{j'=1}^{n_1} \sum_{j=1}^{n_2} I\left(\left|Y_{2j1} - Y_{1j'1}\right| \leq r_0 \sigma_{BR}\right) \right\}.$$

If ε and σ_{BR} are known then the above estimators are again unbiased for P_{TR}^{pop} and P_{RR}^{pop}. In the usual case of unknown ε and σ_{BR}, we can apply the bootstrap procedure presented above where for each bootstrap sample

$$\hat{\Theta}_{prob,r}^{pop*b} = \hat{P}_{TR}^{pop*b}(\hat{\varepsilon}^{*b}, \hat{\sigma}_{BR}^{*b})/\hat{P}_{RR}^{pop*b}(\hat{\varepsilon}^{*b}, \hat{\sigma}_{BR}^{*b})$$

has to be calculated with $\hat{P}_{TR}^{pop*b}$, $\hat{P}_{RR}^{pop*b}$, $\hat{\varepsilon}^{*b}$, and $\hat{\sigma}_{BR}^{*b}$ being the bootstrap analogues of $\hat{P}_{TR}^{pop}$, $\hat{P}_{RR}^{pop}$, $\hat{\varepsilon}$, and $\hat{\sigma}_{BR}$. Estimators of ε and σ_{BR} can again be obtained from an analysis of variance or using the restricted maximum likelihood estimator. Let us denote with $\hat{\Theta}_{prob,r,BP}^{pop}(5)$ the 5th percentile of $\hat{\Theta}_{prob,r}^{pop*b}$, $b = 1, \ldots, B$. Then, the standard bootstrap percentile rejects the hypothesis of population bioinequivalence if $\hat{\Theta}_{prob,r,BP}^{pop}(5) > \theta_{prob,r}^{pop}$ and population bioequivalance can be claimed. The same arguments as used in the proof for the bootstrap procedure above show that this bootstrap percentile test procedure is consistent, whereas analogously to the bootstrap procedure proposed by Schall and Luus (1993) the bootstrap test using the 5th percentile of

$$\tilde{\Theta}_{prob,r}^{pop*b} = \hat{P}_{TR}^{pop*b}(\hat{\varepsilon}, \hat{\sigma}_{BR})/\hat{P}_{RR}^{pop*b}(\hat{\varepsilon}, \hat{\sigma}_{BR}), \ b = 1, \ldots, B,$$

is inconsistent. To achieve consistency of the probability-based bootstrap procedure, it is therefore crucial that the unknown parameters ε and σ_{BR} are estimated from each bootstrap sample within the bootstrap algorithm and not only once based on the original dataset. It should be noted that this is in contrast to the moment-based approach investigated in Section 9.4.1.1.1, where consistency also holds if the decision about the reference-scaled or constant-scaled version is based on the original dataset.

9.4.2.1.2   A parametric approach

If we now assume a normal distribution for the transformed pharmacokinetic characteristic of interest, the above probabilities P_{TR}^{pop} and P_{RR}^{pop} can be calculated via the cumulative distribution function Φ of a standard normal variate as follows:

$$P_{TR}^{pop} = P_B(|Y_T - Y_R| \leq \gamma \cdot \sqrt{2} \cdot \sigma_{BR})$$

$$= P_B(-\gamma \cdot \sqrt{2} \cdot \sigma_{BR} \leq Y_T - Y_R \leq \gamma \cdot \sqrt{2} \cdot \sigma_{BR})$$

$$= P_B\left(-\gamma \cdot \sqrt{2} \cdot \sigma_{BR} - (\mu_T - \mu_R) \leq Y_T - Y_R - (\mu_T - \mu_R) \leq \gamma \cdot \sqrt{2} \cdot \sigma_{BR} - (\mu_T - \mu_R)\right)$$

$$= P_B\left(\frac{-\gamma \cdot \sqrt{2} \cdot \sigma_{BR} - (\mu_T - \mu_R)}{\sqrt{\sigma_{BT}^2 + \sigma_{BR}^2}} \leq \frac{Y_T - Y_R - (\mu_T - \mu_R)}{\sqrt{\sigma_{BT}^2 + \sigma_{BR}^2}} \leq \frac{\gamma \cdot \sqrt{2} \cdot \sigma_{BR} - (\mu_T - \mu_R)}{\sqrt{\sigma_{BT}^2 + \sigma_{BR}^2}}\right)$$

$$= \Phi\left(\frac{\gamma \cdot \sqrt{2} \cdot \sigma_{BR} - (\mu_T - \mu_R)}{\sqrt{\sigma_{BT}^2 + \sigma_{BR}^2}}\right) - \Phi\left(\frac{-\gamma \cdot \sqrt{2} \cdot \sigma_{BR} - (\mu_T - \mu_R)}{\sqrt{\sigma_{BT}^2 + \sigma_{BR}^2}}\right),$$

where $Var_B(Y_T - Y_R) = \sigma_{BT}^2 + \sigma_{BR}^2$. Analogously, since $Var_B(Y_R - Y_R') = 2\sigma_{BR}^2$ and $E_B(Y_R - Y_R') = 0$, we get

$$P_{RR}^{pop} = P_B(|Y_R - Y_R'| \leq \gamma \cdot \sqrt{2} \cdot \sigma_{BR})$$

$$= P_B\left(\frac{-\gamma \cdot \sqrt{2} \cdot \sigma_{BR}}{\sqrt{2\sigma_{BR}^2}} \leq \frac{Y_R - Y_R'}{\sqrt{2\sigma_{BR}^2}} \leq \frac{\gamma \cdot \sqrt{2} \cdot \sigma_{BR}}{\sqrt{2\sigma_{BR}^2}}\right)$$

$$= \Phi(\gamma) - \Phi(-\gamma),$$

which means that P_{RR}^{pop} is just a constant, e.g., equal to 0.68 if $\gamma = 1$. Thus, the probability-based criterion reduces to

$$P_{TR}^{pop} > MINP,$$

where the notation *MINP* is adopted from Schall (1995a) and Anderson and Hauck (1990) (see also Section 9.5.2.1.3 on TIER). *MINP* results from the above criteria as $MINP = P_{RR}^{pop} + \theta_{prob,d}^{pop}$ or $MINP = P_{RR}^{pop} \cdot \theta_{prob,r}^{pop}$ depending on whether the original criterion was the difference or the ratio of P_{TR}^{pop} and P_{RR}^{pop}. Schall (1995a) recommended a bias-corrected bootstrap (Efron and Tibshirani, 1993) to construct a confidence interval for P_{TR}^{pop}:

Step 1: Calculate $\hat{P}_{TR}^{pop}$ by estimating the parameters based on the original data, where the estimators $\hat{\mu}_T$, $\hat{\mu}_R$, $\hat{\sigma}_{BT}^2$, and $\hat{\sigma}_{BR}^2$ are obtained from an ANOVA or REML.

Step 2: Let $Y_{ij} = (Y_{ij1}, Y_{ij2}, Y_{ij3}, Y_{ij4})'$ and $Y_i = (Y_{i1}, \ldots, Y_{in_i})'$. For each fixed sequence i, draw a simple random sample $Y_i^{*b} = (Y_{i1}^{*b}, \ldots, Y_{in_i}^{*b})'$ with replacement from Y_i. That is, the bootstrap samples are obtained using subjects as sampling units, stratified by sequence. Repeat this process at least for $b = 1, \ldots, B = 1000$ to obtain B bootstrap samples $Y_i^{*1}, \ldots, Y_i^{*B}$, $i = 1, 2$.

Step 3: For each $b = 1, \ldots, B$, compute $\hat{\mu}_T^{*b}$, $\hat{\mu}_R^{*b}$, $\hat{\sigma}_{BT}^{*b}$, and $\hat{\sigma}_{BR}^{*b}$ by using the same methods as those in Step 1 but with the dataset (Y_1, Y_2) replaced by the bootstrap dataset (Y_1^{*b}, Y_2^{*b}) and obtain $\hat{P}_{TR}^{pop*b}$.

Step 4: Calculate $z_0 = \Phi^{-1}\left[(\textit{number of } \hat{P}^{pop*b}_{TR} < \hat{P}^{pop}_{TR})/B\right]$ and $z_{0.05}$ as the αth percentile of Φ. Let $\hat{\Theta}^{pop}_{prob, BC}(5)$ denote the $\Phi(z_{0.05} + 2z_0)$th percentile of $\hat{P}^{pop*b}_{TR}$, $b = 1, \ldots, B$, which gives the lower bound of the one-sided 95 % bias-corrected bootstrap interval for P^{pop}_{TR}. Then, population bioequivalence can be claimed if and only if this bound is greater than *MINP*.

9.5   Individual bioequivalence

9.5.1   Moment-based criteria

To derive the moment-based criterion for assessing IBE, the parameter Θ_{mom} introduced in Section 9.3.4 has to be calculated:

$$\Theta_{mom} = \frac{E(Y_R - Y_T)^2 - E(Y_R - Y'_R)^2}{\max\left\{\sigma_0^2, \sigma^2\right\}},$$

assuming a replicate crossover design and the additive model given in Section 9.3.3, where $\sigma^2 = E(Y_R - Y'_R)^2$ denotes the variance under the reference formulation. In contrast to Section 9.4.1, Y_T, Y_R and Y'_R can no longer be regarded as independent. Thus, the variance terms are somewhat more complicated. For convenience, let us recall that

$$\sigma_D^2 = \sigma_{BT}^2 + \sigma_{BR}^2 - 2\rho\sigma_{BR}\sigma_{BT}.$$

This yields

$$\begin{aligned}
E(Y_T - Y_R)^2 &= Var(Y_T - Y_R) + (E(Y_T - Y_R))^2 \\
&= Var(Y_T) + Var(Y_R) - 2Cov(Y_T, Y_R) + (\mu_T - \mu_R)^2 \\
&= (\mu_T - \mu_R)^2 + \sigma_{BT}^2 + \sigma_{WT}^2 + \sigma_{BR}^2 + \sigma_{WR}^2 - 2\rho\sigma_{BR}\sigma_{BT} \\
&= (\mu_T - \mu_R)^2 + \sigma_{WT}^2 + \sigma_{WR}^2 + \sigma_D^2
\end{aligned}$$

and $E(Y_R - Y'_R)^2 = 2\sigma_{WR}^2$.

Thus, a test and a reference formulation can be said to be individually bioequivalent if, in the case of the scaled criterion,

$$\Theta^{ind}_{mom} = \frac{(\mu_T - \mu_R)^2 + \sigma_D^2 + \sigma_{WT}^2 - \sigma_{WR}^2}{\max\left\{\sigma_{W0}^2, \sigma_{WR}^2\right\}} < \theta^{ind}_{mom},$$

where θ^{ind}_{mom} denotes the predetermined bound for the moment-based criterion assessing IBE. Here, the FDA (1997) specified 0.02 as the maximum difference for the within-variances under test and reference formulation, i.e., for $\sigma_{WT}^2 - \sigma_{WR}^2$; a maximum value of 0.03 for the interaction between subject and formulation, i.e., for σ_D^2; and 0.04 for σ_{W0}^2. Analogously to the scaled moment-based aggregate measure for assessing PBE, the value for σ_{W0}^2 is based on the individual difference ratio (*IDR*) and again on the corresponding criterion for average bioequivalence. As with the *PDR*, the *IDR* compares the expected squared difference of the bioavailabilities under test and reference formulation with the expected squared difference of the bioavailabilities under twice the reference formulation. Thus, this ratio results in

$$IDR = \sqrt{\frac{(\mu_T - \mu_R)^2 + \sigma_D^2 + \sigma_{WT}^2 + \sigma_{WR}^2}{2\sigma_{WR}^2}}.$$

The FDA also gives 1.25 as the largest tolerable value of the *IDR*, in analogy to the average bioequivalence criterion. As already observed for the *PDR*, the *IDR* is closely related to the reference-scaled version of the moment-based aggregate measure of IBE:

$$IDR = \sqrt{\Theta_{mom,ref}^{ind}/2 + 1} \quad with \quad \Theta_{mom,ref}^{ind} = \frac{(\mu_T - \mu_R)^2 + \sigma_D^2 + \sigma_{WT}^2 - \sigma_{WR}^2}{\sigma_{WR}^2}.$$

As for PBE, the reference-scaled measure $\Theta_{mom,ref}^{ind}$ is now replaced by $[\ln(1.25)]^2/\sigma_{W0}^2$ with $\ln(1.25)$ as the limit for $\mu_T - \mu_R$, again according to the criterion of average bioequivalence and assuming $\sigma_{WT}^2 = \sigma_{WR}^2$ as well as $\sigma_D^2 = 0$. Analogously to σ_0^2, solving the following inequality with respect to σ_{W0}^2,

$$IDR = \sqrt{\frac{[\ln(1.25)]^2}{2\sigma_{W0}^2} + 1} \leq 1.25$$

gives the same value for σ_{W0}^2 of about 0.04. Further assuming the 80/125 rule again, which means that the ratio of the expected bioavailability under test formulation and the expected bioavailability under reference formulation has to lie, with a certain probability, within a range from 80 % to 125 %, gives $\ln(1.25)$ as the upper bound for $\mu_T - \mu_R$. This results in the following value for θ_{mom}^{ind}:

$$\theta_{mom}^{ind} = \frac{[\ln(1.25)]^2 + 0.03 + 0.02}{0.04} \approx 2.49483.$$

The criticism against IBE, as for PBE, is that the criterion cannot be transferred to the original scale. For further analyses let us again consider the linearized version of the above criterion:

$$(\mu_T - \mu_R)^2 + \sigma_D^2 + \sigma_{WT}^2 - \sigma_{WR}^2 - \max\{\sigma_{W0}^2, \sigma_{WR}^2\} \, \theta_{mom}^{ind} < 0.$$

As for PBE, let us now assume that all variances are equal and that the correlation coefficient ρ equals 1, which implies that there is zero subject-by-formulation interaction:

$$\sigma_D^2 = \sigma_{BT}^2 + \sigma_{BR}^2 - 2\rho\sigma_{BR}\sigma_{BT} = 2\sigma_B^2 - 2\sigma_B\sigma_B = 0,$$

and which results in an upper bound θ_{mom}^{ind} of

$$\theta_{mom}^{ind} = \frac{[\ln(1.25)]^2}{0.04}.$$

Thus, we have for the above criterion

$$(\mu_T - \mu_R)^2 + \sigma_D^2 + \sigma_{WT}^2 - \sigma_{WR}^2 - \max\{\sigma_0^2, \sigma_{WR}^2\}\,\theta_{mom}^{ind} < 0$$

$$\Leftrightarrow (\mu_T - \mu_R)^2 + 0 + \sigma_W^2 - \sigma_W^2 - 0.04\frac{[\ln(1.25)]^2}{0.04} < 0$$

$$\Leftrightarrow (\mu_T - \mu_R)^2 < [\ln(1.25)]^2.$$

This means the above moment-based criterion for assessing IBE reduces to the usual criterion for average bioequivalence if the reasoning behind the concept of IBE, i.e., unequal variances and a non-zero subject-by-formulation interaction, does not hold.

9.5.1.1 Statistical procedures

For statistical assessment of IBE according to the moment-based criterion, Θ_{mom}^{ind} has to be estimated, where, analogously to Θ_{mom}^{pop}, the unknown parameters in the numerator and the denominator can be estimated using an analysis of variance (ANOVA) or the method of restricted maximum likelihood (REML) under mixed effects models. This can be done by using, for instance, the SAS® procedure PROC MIXED. Let us denote the resulting estimator as $\hat{\Theta}_{mom}^{ind}$.

The statistical test problem of individual bioequivalence now reads as follows:

$$H_0 : \Theta_{mom}^{ind} \geq \theta_{mom}^{ind} \text{ vs. } H_1 : \Theta_{mom}^{ind} < \theta_{mom}^{ind},$$

where IBE can be claimed if the null hypothesis is rejected at a significance level of 5 %. According to the FDA guidances (1997, 1999b) a two-sided 90 % confidence interval or a one-sided upper 95 % confidence interval for Θ_{mom}^{ind} should be calculated and the null hypothesis is to be rejected if the upper bound is smaller than θ_{mom}^{ind}. Since the estimator $\hat{\Theta}_{mom}^{ind}$ is even more complex than $\hat{\Theta}_{mom}^{pop}$, first the bootstrap approach will again be exploited to calculate a confidence interval for Θ_{mom}^{ind}.

9.5.1.1.1 The bootstrap procedure

The methods given above for assessing PBE can be used to construct a bootstrap confidence interval for IBE. The Monte Carlo algorithm for the bootstrap procedure proposed by the FDA (1997) reads as follows:

Step 1: The individual bioequivalence parameter Θ_{mom}^{ind} is estimated by

$$\hat{\Theta}_{mom}^{ind} = \frac{(\hat{\mu}_T - \hat{\mu}_R)^2 + \hat{\sigma}_D^2 + \hat{\sigma}_{WT}^2 - \hat{\sigma}_{WR}^2}{\max\{\sigma_{W0}^2, \hat{\sigma}_{WR}^2\}},$$

where $\hat{\sigma}_D^2 = \hat{\sigma}_{BT}^2 + \hat{\sigma}_{BR}^2 - 2\hat{\rho}\hat{\sigma}_{BR}\hat{\sigma}_{BT}$ and $\hat{\mu}_T, \hat{\mu}_R, \hat{\sigma}_{WT}^2, \hat{\sigma}_{WR}^2, \hat{\sigma}_{BT}^2, \hat{\sigma}_{BR}^2$ and $\hat{\rho}$ are obtained from ANOVA or REML.

Step 2: This step is the same as for population bioequivalence.

Step 3: For each $b = 1, \ldots, B$, compute $\hat{\mu}_T^{*b}, \hat{\mu}_R^{*b}, \hat{\sigma}_{WT}^{*b}, \hat{\sigma}_{WR}^{*b}, \hat{\sigma}_{BT}^{*b}, \hat{\sigma}_{BR}^{*b}$, and $\hat{\rho}^{*b}$ by using the same methods as those in Step 1 but with the dataset $(\mathbf{Y}_1, \mathbf{Y}_2)$ replaced by the bootstrap dataset $(\mathbf{Y}_1^{*b}, \mathbf{Y}_2^{*b})$ and let

$$
\tilde{\Theta}_{mom}^{ind*b} = \begin{cases} \dfrac{(\hat{\mu}_T^{*b} - \hat{\mu}_R^{*b})^2 + (\hat{\sigma}_D^{*b})^2 + (\hat{\sigma}_{WT}^{*b})^2 - (\hat{\sigma}_{WR}^{*b})^2}{(\hat{\sigma}_{WR}^{*b})^2} & if \quad \hat{\sigma}_{WR}^2 \geq \sigma_{W0}^2 \\[3ex] \dfrac{(\hat{\mu}_T^{*b} - \hat{\mu}_R^{*b})^2 + (\hat{\sigma}_D^{*b})^2 + (\hat{\sigma}_{WT}^{*b})^2 - (\hat{\sigma}_{WR}^{*b})^2}{\sigma_{W0}^2} & if \quad \hat{\sigma}_{WR}^2 < \sigma_{W0}^2. \end{cases}
$$

Step 4: Let $\tilde{\Theta}_{mom,FDA}^{ind}(95)$ denote the 95th percentile of $\tilde{\Theta}_{mom}^{ind*b}, b = 1, \ldots, B$. Then, individual bioequivalence can be claimed if and only if $\tilde{\Theta}_{mom,FDA}^{ind}(95) < \theta_{mom}^{ind}$. Again replacing $\tilde{\Theta}_{mom}^{ind*b}$ in Step 3 of the FDA bootstrap procedure by

$$
\hat{\Theta}_{mom}^{ind*b} = \begin{cases} \dfrac{(\hat{\mu}_T^{*b} - \hat{\mu}_R^{*b})^2 + (\hat{\sigma}_D^{*b})^2 + (\hat{\sigma}_{WT}^{*b})^2 - (\hat{\sigma}_{WR}^{*b})^2}{(\hat{\sigma}_{WR}^{*b})^2} & if \quad (\hat{\sigma}_{WR}^{*b})^2 \geq \sigma_{W0}^2 \\[3ex] \dfrac{(\hat{\mu}_T^{*b} - \hat{\mu}_R^{*b})^2 + (\hat{\sigma}_D^{*b})^2 + (\hat{\sigma}_{WT}^{*b})^2 - (\hat{\sigma}_{WR}^{*b})^2}{\sigma_{W0}^2} & if \quad (\hat{\sigma}_{WR}^{*b})^2 < \sigma_{W0}^2 \end{cases}
$$

yields the standard bootstrap percentile interval.

Shao *et al.* (2000a) showed that for $\sigma_{WR}^2 \neq \sigma_{W0}^2$ both procedures are consistent. Both procedures are, however, inconsistent for $\sigma_{WR}^2 = \sigma_{W0}^2$. Again the so-called *m*-out-of-*n* bootstrap procedure would lead to a consistent procedure regardless of whether $\sigma_{WR}^2 = \sigma_{W0}^2$ or not, with the disadvantage that the *m*-out-of-*n* bootstrap is not so efficient as the standard bootstrap if the latter is consistent.

Shao *et al.* (2000b) studied the size and power of different bootstrap procedures based on simulation studies and suggested a method for sample size determination. Their results will not be reviewed here. It should, however, be mentioned that they observed that $n = 24$ with the same number of subjects in both sequences is not enough to obtain a power of at least 70 % which is in contrast to the draft FDA guidance (1997).

9.5.1.1.2   *A parametric confidence interval*

As already mentioned above, the FDA (1999b) recommended a parametric approach in a revised draft guidance for assessing bioequivalence. This is based on a principle for constructing approximate confidence intervals for linear functions of variance components. For this purpose, Hyslop *et al.* (2000) assumed a normal distribution for the transformed pharmacokinetic characteristic of interest, e.g., the logarithm of *AUC*, and extended an idea of Graybill and Wang (1980) and Ting *et al.* (1990); see also the method by Howe (1974), which employs a Cornish–Fisher expansion. To exploit this approach, the linearized version of the moment-based criterion for assessing IBE has to be reparametrized such that the resulting estimator reads as a function of independent components for which exact confidence intervals can be computed. For simplicity, let us focus on the reference-scaled version, where the constant-scaled version can be treated analogously (see also Pigeot and Zierer, 2001).

The linearized version of the reference-scaled IBE criterion,

$$(\mu_T - \mu_R)^2 + \sigma_D^2 + \sigma_{WT}^2 - \sigma_{WR}^2 - \sigma_{WR}^2 \theta_{mom}^{ind} < 0$$

can be rewritten as follows:

$$\eta_{ref}^{ind} = \delta^2 + \sigma_I^2 + 0.5\,\sigma_{WT}^2 - (1.5 + \theta_{mom}^{ind})\sigma_{WR}^2 < 0$$

with $\delta = \mu_T - \mu_R$ and $\sigma_I^2 = \sigma_D^2 + 0.5\,\sigma_{WT}^2 + 0.5\,\sigma_{WR}^2$. An estimator, $\hat{\eta}_{ref}^{ind}$, of η_{ref}^{ind} can be obtained by replacing all unknown parameters with their REML estimators. Based on η_{ref}^{ind} the test problem of individual bioequivalence can be formulated as:

$$H_0 : \eta_{ref}^{ind} \geq 0 \text{ vs. } H_1 : \eta_{ref}^{ind} < 0.$$

This test problem will now be solved via a parametric confidence interval, which needs explicit calculation of the point estimators of the components of η_{ref}^{ind} and their distributions.

We start with the point estimator of δ. For each subject j in each sequence i let I_{ij} denote the difference of the mean bioavailabilities under test and reference formulation, i.e.,

$$I_{1j} = 0.5\,(Y_{1j1} + Y_{1j3}) - 0.5\,(Y_{1j2} + Y_{1j4}) \text{ and } I_{2j} = 0.5\,(Y_{2j2} + Y_{2j4}) - 0.5\,(Y_{2j1} + Y_{2j3}).$$

Using these reparametrizations, we get as estimator of δ

$$\hat{\delta} = \frac{1}{2} \sum_{i=1}^{2} \frac{1}{n_i} \sum_{j=1}^{n_i} I_{ij},$$

which is, due to the model assumptions above, normally distributed with

$$E(\hat{\delta}) = \delta \text{ and } Var(\hat{\delta}) = \frac{1}{4} \sum_{i=1}^{2} \frac{1}{n_i} \sigma_I^2.$$

An unbiased estimator of σ_I^2 can be obtained from results for the REML estimators of contrasts as:

$$\hat{\sigma}_I^2 = \frac{1}{n-2} \sum_{i=1}^{2} \sum_{j=1}^{n_i} (I_{ij} - \bar{I}_{i.})^2 \text{ with } n = n_1 + n_2, \bar{I}_{i.} = \frac{1}{n_i} \sum_{j=1}^{n_i} I_{ij},$$

which is then distributed as $(n-2)^{-1} \sigma_I^2 \chi_{n-2}^2$, where χ_{n-2}^2 denotes a χ^2-distribution with $n-2$ degrees of freedom.

Next, for each subject j in each sequence i let T_{ij} and R_{ij} denote the difference between the bioavailabilities under the test formulation and the reference formulation for the first and the second administration of the respective formulation, i.e.,

$$T_{1j} = Y_{1j1} - Y_{1j3}, \ T_{2j} = Y_{2j2} - Y_{2j4}, \ R_{1j} = Y_{1j2} - Y_{1j4}, \ R_{2j} = Y_{2j1} - Y_{2j3}$$

with $Var(T_{ij}) = 2\sigma^2_{WT}$ and $Var(R_{ij}) = 2\sigma^2_{WR}$ which can be understood as orthogonal contrasts of

$$Y_{1j} = (Y_{1j2}, Y_{1j4}, Y_{1j1}, Y_{1j3})', \quad Y_{2j} = (Y_{2j1}, Y_{2j3}, Y_{2j2}, Y_{2j4})'.$$

This implies that σ^2_{WT} and σ^2_{WR} can be estimated independently of $\hat{\delta}$ and $\hat{\sigma}^2_I$ (Patterson and Jones, 2002). Since the following applies for T_{ij} as well we only consider R_{ij} with

$$\frac{1}{\sqrt{2}} R_{ij} = \left(\frac{1}{\sqrt{2}}, -\frac{1}{\sqrt{2}}, 0, 0 \right) Y_{ij}.$$

Thus, an estimator of $Var(R_{ij}) = 2\sigma^2_{WR}$ can be calculated from the estimated covariance matrix of Y_{ij}, exploiting the representation of R_{ij} as a contrast. The REML estimator of σ^2_{WR} is

$$\hat{\sigma}^2_{WR} = \frac{1}{2} \frac{1}{n-2} \sum_{i=1}^{2} \sum_{j=1}^{n_i} (R_{ij} - \overline{R}_{i.})^2$$

with $\overline{R}_{i.} = \frac{1}{n_i} \sum_{j=1}^{n_i} R_{ij}$ and $\hat{\sigma}^2_{WR} \sim \frac{\sigma^2_{WR}}{n-2} \chi^2_{n-2}$. The REML estimator $\hat{\sigma}^2_{WT}$ can be derived analogously as

$$\hat{\sigma}^2_{WT} = \frac{1}{2} \frac{1}{n-2} \sum_{i=1}^{2} \sum_{j=1}^{n_i} (T_{ij} - \overline{T}_{i.})^2$$

with $\overline{T}_{i.} = \frac{1}{n_i} \sum_{j=1}^{n_i} T_{ij}$ and $\hat{\sigma}^2_{WT} \sim \frac{\sigma^2_{WT}}{n-2} \chi^2_{n-2}$.

Based on these preliminary steps, an upper confidence limit for η^{ind}_{ref} can be calculated following the approach outlined in Section 9.4.1.1.2. That is we have to combine the upper confidence limit of δ, i.e.,

$$CI^u_{\delta,1-\alpha} = \left(|\hat{\delta}| + t_{1-\alpha,n-2} \sqrt{\frac{1}{4} \sum_{i=1}^{2} \frac{1}{n_i} \hat{\sigma}^2_I} \right)^2$$

and the upper confidence limits for the above variance components σ^2_I, $0.5\,\sigma^2_{WT}$, $-(1.5 + \theta^{ind}_{mom})\sigma^2_{WR}$ denoted as $CI^u_{\sigma^2_q,1-\alpha}$, $q = WR, WT, I$, with

$$CI^u_{\sigma^2_q,1-\alpha} = \begin{cases} \dfrac{(n-2)\,a_q\hat{\sigma}^2_q}{\chi^2_{1-\alpha,n-2}} & \text{if } a_q < 0 \\[4mm] \dfrac{(n-2)\,a_q\hat{\sigma}^2_q}{\chi^2_{\alpha,n-2}} & \text{if } a_q > 0. \end{cases}$$

Finally, this gives an approximate upper confidence limit for η_{ref}^{ind} as follows:

$$CI_{\eta_{ref}^{ind},1-\alpha}^u = \hat{\eta}_{ref}^{ind} + \left[(CI_{\delta,1-\alpha}^u - \hat{\delta}^2)^2 + (CI_{\sigma_I^2,1-\alpha}^u - \hat{\sigma}_I^2)^2 + (CI_{\sigma_{WT}^2,1-\alpha}^u - 0.5\hat{\sigma}_{WT}^2)^2\right.$$

$$\left. + (CI_{\sigma_{WR}^2,1-\alpha}^u + (1.5 + \theta_{mom}^{ind})\hat{\sigma}_{WR}^2)^2\right]^{1/2}.$$

If $CI_{\eta_{mom,ref}^{ind},0.95}^u < 0$, individual bioequivalence can be concluded. For the constant-scaled criterion this results in

$$CI_{\eta_{const}^{ind},1-\alpha}^u = \hat{\eta}_{const}^{ind} + \left[(CI_{\delta,1-\alpha}^u - \hat{\delta}^2)^2 + (CI_{\sigma_I^2,1-\alpha}^u - \hat{\sigma}_I^2)^2 + (CI_{\sigma_{WT}^2,1-\alpha}^u - 0.5\hat{\sigma}_{WT}^2)^2\right.$$

$$\left. + (CI_{\sigma_{WR}^2,1-\alpha}^u + 1.5\hat{\sigma}_{WR}^2)^2\right]^{1/2}$$

with $\hat{\eta}_{const}^{ind} = \hat{\delta}^2 + \hat{\sigma}_I^2 + 0.5\,\hat{\sigma}_{WT}^2 - 1.5\,\hat{\sigma}_{WR}^2 - \theta_{mom}^{ind}\,\sigma_{W0}^2$.

9.5.2 Probability-based criteria

As already mentioned in Section 9.4.2, the probability-based criteria have not been recommended by the FDA. These criteria will be presented in this section for assessing IBE. We again follow the approach by Schall and Luus (1993) who assumed a three-period crossover design with one application of the test and two applications of the reference formulation. The proposed procedures, however, can be easily adapted to other designs e.g., the dual balanced design *TRT/RTR* presented in Table 9.3. Therefore, Shao *et al.* (2000a) followed the original design, which they specified as *TRR/RTR* in their theoretical investigations of the bootstrap approach for assessing individual bioequivalence although this design is inefficient compared to the above dual balanced design. As introduced in Section 9.3.4, individual bioequivalence according to the probability-based criteria can be stated if:

$$\Theta_{prob,d}^{ind} = P_{TR}^{ind} - P_{RR}^{ind} > \theta_{prob,d}^{ind}$$

or analogously, if

$$\Theta_{prob,r}^{ind} = \frac{P_{TR}^{ind}}{P_{RR}^{ind}} > \theta_{prob,r}^{ind},$$

where $P_{TR}^{ind} = P_W(|Y_T - Y_R| \le r)$ and $P_{RR}^{ind} = P_W(|Y_R - Y_R'| \le r)$ here denote the probabilities for the within-subject deviations being smaller than a predefined value r. This value r is either a constant or $r = r_0\sigma_{WR}$ with $r_0 = \gamma\sqrt{2}$ as suggested by Schall (1995a).

9.5.2.1 Statistical procedures

As in Section 9.4.2.1 we will consider the ratio of the two probabilities P_{TR}^{ind} and P_{RR}^{ind}. The corresponding test problem of individual bioequivalence then reads as follows:

$$H_0 : \Theta_{prob,r}^{ind} \le \theta_{prob,r}^{ind} \quad \text{vs.} \quad H_1 : \Theta_{prob,r}^{ind} > \theta_{prob,r}^{ind}.$$

This test problem will again be solved via a confidence interval where the null hypothesis is to be rejected at a 5 % significance level if the lower bound of the corresponding interval exceeds $\theta_{prob,r}^{ind}$.

9.5.2.1.1 A distribution-free approach

To solve this test problem Schall and Luus (1993) proposed the same bootstrap confidence interval as for assessing PBE. Before presenting the bootstrap (see Shao et al., 2000a) let us discuss how to estimate the above probabilities assuming the above replicate design *TRR/RTR* and in principle the additive model as summarized in Table 9.4 but with only three periods, i.e.,

$$Y_{ijk} = \mu + \tau_h + \pi_k + v_i + \gamma_{hik} + s_{ijh} + e_{ijk},$$

where all definitions remain unchanged besides the index for the formulation being administered: now we have $h = R$, if $(i, k) = (1, 2), (1, 3), (2, 1), (2, 3)$ and $h = T$ otherwise.

For each subject j and each sequence i, taking the differences of two bioavailabilities under the reference formulation gives

$$Y_{1j2} - Y_{1j3} = \varepsilon_{123} + e_{1j2} - e_{1j3} \quad (sequence\ 1)$$
$$Y_{2j1} - Y_{2j3} = \varepsilon_{213} + e_{2j1} - e_{2j3} \quad (sequence\ 2),$$

where $\varepsilon_{123} = \pi_2 - \pi_3 + \gamma_{R12} - \gamma_{R13}$ and $\varepsilon_{213} = \pi_1 - \pi_3 + \gamma_{R21} - \gamma_{R23}$. Analogously to the corresponding approach for PBE note that the distribution of $Y_{1j2} - Y_{1j3}$ or $Y_{2j1} - Y_{2j3}$ is not the same as that of $Y_R - Y_R'$ unless $\varepsilon_{123} = 0$ or $\varepsilon_{213} = 0$, which is true when there is no period or interaction effect. Similarly, let us now consider the differences

$$Y_{1j1} - Y_{1j2} = \tau_T - \tau_R + \varepsilon_{112} + s_{1jT} - s_{1jR} + e_{1j1} - e_{1j2} \quad (sequence\ 1)$$
$$Y_{1j1} - Y_{1j3} = \tau_T - \tau_R + \varepsilon_{113} + s_{1jT} - s_{1jR} + e_{1j1} - e_{1j3} \quad (sequence\ 1)$$
$$Y_{2j2} - Y_{2j1} = \tau_T - \tau_R + \varepsilon_{221} + s_{2jT} - s_{2jR} + e_{2j2} - e_{2j1} \quad (sequence\ 2)$$
$$Y_{2j2} - Y_{2j3} = \tau_T - \tau_R + \varepsilon_{223} + s_{2jT} - s_{2jR} + e_{2j2} - e_{2j3} \quad (sequence\ 2),$$

which do not have the same distribution as that of $Y_T - Y_R$ unless $\varepsilon_{112} = \varepsilon_{113} = \varepsilon_{221} = \varepsilon_{223} = 0$, where $\varepsilon_{112} = \pi_1 - \pi_2 + \gamma_{T11} - \gamma_{R12}$, $\varepsilon_{113} = \pi_1 - \pi_3 + \gamma_{T11} - \gamma_{R13}$, $\varepsilon_{221} = \pi_2 - \pi_1 + \gamma_{T22} - \gamma_{R21}$, and $\varepsilon_{223} = \pi_2 - \pi_3 + \gamma_{T22} - \gamma_{R23}$. As in Shao et al. (2000a) we first deal with the case that r is a constant. Let ε denote here the vector $(\varepsilon_{112}, \varepsilon_{113}, \varepsilon_{221}, \varepsilon_{223}, \varepsilon_{123}, \varepsilon_{213})$.

If ε is known, unbiased estimators of the above probabilities can easily be obtained via the corresponding relative frequencies as follows:

$$\hat{P}_{RR}^{ind}(\varepsilon) = \frac{1}{n}\left\{\sum_{j=1}^{n_1} I\left(\left|Y_{1j2} - Y_{1j3} - \varepsilon_{123}\right| \leq r\right) + \sum_{j=1}^{n_2} I\left(\left|Y_{2j1} - Y_{2j3} - \varepsilon_{213}\right| \leq r\right)\right\}$$

$$\hat{P}_{TR}^{ind}(\varepsilon) = \frac{1}{2n}\left\{\sum_{j=1}^{n_1}\left\{I\left(\left|Y_{1j1} - Y_{1j2} - \varepsilon_{112}\right| \leq r\right) + I\left(\left|Y_{1j1} - Y_{1j3} - \varepsilon_{113}\right| \leq r\right)\right\}\right.$$

$$\left. + \sum_{j=1}^{n_1}\left\{I\left(\left|Y_{2j2} - Y_{2j1} - \varepsilon_{221}\right| \leq r\right) + I\left(\left|Y_{2j2} - Y_{2j3} - \varepsilon_{223}\right| \leq r\right)\right\}\right\}$$

with $n = n_1 + n_2$ and $I(A)$ the indicator function of an event A.

Since ε is usually unknown, Schall and Luus (1993) proposed a bootstrap procedure where ε is simultaneously estimated such that it can be replaced by its estimator based on the original dataset. Analogously to the bootstrap procedure presented in Section 9.4.2.1.1 the algorithm is as follows:

Step 1: Let $Y_{ij} = (Y_{ij1}, Y_{ij2}, Y_{ij3})'$ and $Y_i = (Y_{i1}, \ldots, Y_{in_i})'$. For each fixed sequence i, draw a simple random sample $Y_i^{*b} = (Y_{i1}^{*b}, \ldots, Y_{in_i}^{*b})'$ with replacement from Y_i. That is, the bootstrap samples are obtained using subjects as sampling units, stratified by sequence. Repeat this process for $b = 1, \ldots, B = 2000$ independently to obtain B bootstrap samples $Y_i^{*1}, \ldots, Y_i^{*B}$, $i = 1, 2$.

Step 2: Let $\hat{\varepsilon}$ be a REML or an ANOVA estimator of ε calculated from the original dataset. For each $b = 1, \ldots, B$, $\hat{P}_{TR}^{ind*b}(\varepsilon)$ and $\hat{P}_{RR}^{ind*b}(\varepsilon)$ are the same as $\hat{P}_{TR}^{ind}(\varepsilon)$ and $\hat{P}_{RR}^{ind}(\varepsilon)$ but calculated from the bootstrap data Y_{ijk}^{*b} instead of the original dataset. Then define $\tilde{\Theta}_{prob,r}^{ind*b}$ as

$$\tilde{\Theta}_{prob,r}^{ind*b} = \hat{P}_{TR}^{ind*b}(\hat{\varepsilon})/\hat{P}_{RR}^{ind*b}(\hat{\varepsilon}).$$

Step 3: Let $\tilde{\Theta}_{prob,r,SL}^{ind}(5)$ denote the 5th percentile of $\tilde{\Theta}_{prob,r}^{ind*b}$, $b = 1, \ldots, B$. Then, individual bioequivalence can be claimed if and only if $\tilde{\Theta}_{prob,r,SL}^{ind}(5) > \theta_{prob,r}^{ind}$.

It has been shown by Shao et al. (2000a) that the above bootstrap procedure is inconsistent, which means that for n tending to infinity

$$\lim P(\tilde{\Theta}_{prob,r,SL}^{ind}(5) < \theta_{prob,r}^{ind}) \neq 0.95.$$

If, however, ε is estimated within each bootstrap sample, i.e., if we replace $\tilde{\Theta}_{prob,r}^{ind*b}$ by

$$\hat{\Theta}_{prob,r}^{ind*b} = \hat{P}_{TR}^{ind*b}(\hat{\varepsilon}^{*b})/\hat{P}_{RR}^{ind*b}(\hat{\varepsilon}^{*b}),$$

then the bootstrap procedure presented above becomes the standard bootstrap percentile, which has been shown to be consistent (Shao et al. 2000a).

Let us now consider the case of $r = r_0 \sigma_{WR}$ instead of constant r in the definition of $\Theta^{ind}_{prob,r}$, i.e.,

$$\Theta^{ind}_{prob,r} = \frac{P^{ind}_{TR}}{P^{ind}_{RR}}$$

with $P^{ind}_{TR} = P_W(|Y_T - Y_R| \leq r_0 \sigma_{WR})$ and $P^{ind}_{RR} = P_W(|Y_R - Y'_R| \leq r_0 \sigma_{WR})$.
Analogously to PBE, estimators of P^{ind}_{TR} and P^{ind}_{RR} have also to account for σ_{WR}, i.e.,

$$\hat{P}^{ind}_{RR}(\varepsilon, \sigma_{WR}) = \frac{1}{n} \left\{ \sum_{j=1}^{n_1} I\left(\left|Y_{1j2} - Y_{1j3} - \varepsilon_{123}\right| \leq r_0 \sigma_{WR}\right) + \sum_{j=1}^{n_2} I\left(\left|Y_{2j1} - Y_{2j3} - \varepsilon_{213}\right| \leq r_0 \sigma_{WR}\right) \right\}$$

$$\hat{P}^{ind}_{TR}(\varepsilon, \sigma_{WR}) = \frac{1}{2n} \left\{ \sum_{j=1}^{n_1} \left\{ I\left(\left|Y_{1j1} - Y_{1j2} - \varepsilon_{112}\right| \leq r_0 \sigma_{WR}\right) + I\left(\left|Y_{1j1} - Y_{1j3} - \varepsilon_{113}\right| \leq r_0 \sigma_{WR}\right) \right\} \right.$$

$$\left. + \sum_{j=1}^{n_1} \left\{ I\left(\left|Y_{2j2} - Y_{2j1} - \varepsilon_{221}\right| \leq r_0 \sigma_{WR}\right) + I\left(\left|Y_{2j2} - Y_{2j3} - \varepsilon_{223}\right| \leq r_0 \sigma_{WR}\right) \right\} \right\}.$$

If ε and σ_{WR} are known then the above estimators are again unbiased for P^{ind}_{TR} and P^{ind}_{RR}. If ε and σ_{WR} are unknown, we apply the bootstrap procedure presented above, where for each bootstrap sample

$$\hat{\Theta}^{ind*b}_{prob,r} = \hat{P}^{ind*b}_{TR}(\hat{\varepsilon}^{*b}, \hat{\sigma}^{*b}_{WR}) / \hat{P}^{ind*b}_{RR}(\hat{\varepsilon}^{*b}, \hat{\sigma}^{*b}_{WR})$$

has to be calculated with $\hat{P}^{ind*b}_{TR}$, $\hat{P}^{ind*b}_{RR}$, $\hat{\varepsilon}^{*b}$, and $\hat{\sigma}^{*b}_{WR}$ being the bootstrap analogues of $\hat{P}^{ind}_{TR}$, $\hat{P}^{ind}_{RR}$, $\hat{\varepsilon}$, and $\hat{\sigma}_{WR}$. Estimators of ε and σ_{WR} can again be obtained from an analysis of variance or using the restricted maximum likelihood estimator. Let us denote with $\hat{\Theta}^{ind}_{prob,r,BP}(5)$ the 5th percentile of $\hat{\Theta}^{ind}_{prob,r}$, $b = 1, \ldots, B$. Then, the standard bootstrap percentile rejects the hypothesis of individual bioinequivalence if $\hat{\Theta}^{ind}_{prob,r,BP}(5) > \theta^{ind}_{prob,r}$. The same arguments as for the proof of the bootstrap procedure above ensure that this bootstrap percentile test procedure is consistent, whereas analogously to the bootstrap procedure proposed by Schall and Luus (1993) the bootstrap test using the 5th percentile of

$$\tilde{\Theta}^{ind*b}_{prob,r} = \hat{P}^{ind*b}_{TR}(\hat{\varepsilon}, \hat{\sigma}_{WR}) / \hat{P}^{ind*b}_{RR}(\hat{\varepsilon}, \hat{\sigma}_{WR}), b = 1, \ldots, B,$$

is inconsistent.

9.5.2.1.2 A parametric approach

In analogy to PBE, let us now assume a normal distribution for the transformed pharmacokinetic characteristic of interest. Then the above probabilities P^{ind}_{TR} and P^{ind}_{RR} can be calculated via the cumulative density distribution Φ of a standard normal variate as follows:

$$
\begin{aligned}
P_{TR}^{ind} &= P_W(|Y_T - Y_R| \leq \gamma \cdot \sqrt{2} \cdot \sigma_{WR}) \\
&= P_W(-\gamma \cdot \sqrt{2} \cdot \sigma_{WR} \leq Y_T - Y_R \leq \gamma \cdot \sqrt{2} \cdot \sigma_{WR}) \\
&= P_W\left(-\gamma \cdot \sqrt{2} \cdot \sigma_{WR} - (\mu_T - \mu_R) \leq Y_T - Y_R - (\mu_T - \mu_R) \leq \gamma \cdot \sqrt{2} \cdot \sigma_{WR} - (\mu_T - \mu_R)\right) \\
&= P_W\left(\frac{-\gamma \cdot \sqrt{2} \cdot \sigma_{WR} - (\mu_T - \mu_R)}{\sqrt{\sigma_{WT}^2 + \sigma_{WR}^2 + \sigma_D^2}} \leq \frac{Y_T - Y_R - (\mu_T - \mu_R)}{\sqrt{\sigma_{WT}^2 + \sigma_{WR}^2 + \sigma_D^2}} \leq \frac{\gamma \cdot \sqrt{2} \cdot \sigma_{WR} - (\mu_T - \mu_R)}{\sqrt{\sigma_{WT}^2 + \sigma_{WR}^2 + \sigma_D^2}}\right) \\
&= \Phi\left(\frac{\gamma \cdot \sqrt{2} \cdot \sigma_{WR} - (\mu_T - \mu_R)}{\sqrt{\sigma_{WT}^2 + \sigma_{WR}^2 + \sigma_D^2}}\right) - \Phi\left(\frac{-\gamma \cdot \sqrt{2} \cdot \sigma_{WR} - (\mu_T - \mu_R)}{\sqrt{\sigma_{WT}^2 + \sigma_{WR}^2 + \sigma_D^2}}\right),
\end{aligned}
$$

where $Var_W(Y_T - Y_R) = \sigma_{WT}^2 + \sigma_{WR}^2 + \sigma_D^2$. Analogously, since $Var_W(Y_R - Y_R') = 2\sigma_{WR}^2$ and $E_W(Y_R - Y_R') = 0$, we get

$$
\begin{aligned}
P_{RR}^{ind} &= P_W(|Y_R - Y_R'| \leq \gamma \cdot \sqrt{2} \cdot \sigma_{WR}) \\
&= P_W\left(\frac{-\gamma \cdot \sqrt{2} \cdot \sigma_{WR}}{\sqrt{2} \cdot \sigma_{WR}} \leq \frac{Y_R - Y_R'}{\sqrt{2} \cdot \sigma_{WR}} \leq \frac{\gamma \cdot \sqrt{2} \cdot \sigma_{WR}}{\sqrt{2} \cdot \sigma_{WR}}\right) \\
&= \Phi(\gamma) - \Phi(-\gamma),
\end{aligned}
$$

which means that also for assessing IBE, P_{RR}^{ind} results in a constant and the probability-based criterion reduces to

$$
P_{TR}^{ind} > MINP.
$$

MINP can be obtained from the above criteria as $MINP = P_{RR}^{ind} + \theta_{prob,d}^{ind}$ or $MINP = P_{RR}^{ind} \cdot \theta_{prob,r}^{ind}$ depending on whether the original criterion was the difference or the ratio of P_{TR}^{ind} and P_{RR}^{ind}. According to Schall (1995a) we have the algorithm for a bias-corrected bootstrap confidence interval for P_{TR}^{ind}:

Step 1: Calculate $\hat{P}_{TR}^{ind}$ by estimating the required parameters based on the original data, where the estimators $\hat{\mu}_T$, $\hat{\mu}_R$, $\hat{\sigma}_{WT}^2$, $\hat{\sigma}_{WR}^2$, $\hat{\sigma}_{BT}^2$, $\hat{\sigma}_{BR}^2$, and $\hat{\rho}$ are obtained from ANOVA or REML and $\hat{\sigma}_D^2 = \hat{\sigma}_{BT}^2 + \hat{\sigma}_{BR}^2 - 2\hat{\rho}\hat{\sigma}_{BR}\hat{\sigma}_{BT}$.

Step 2: This step is the same as for PBE.

Step 3: For each $b = 1, \ldots, B$, compute $\hat{\mu}_T^{*b}$, $\hat{\mu}_R^{*b}$, $\hat{\sigma}_{WT}^{*b}$, $\hat{\sigma}_{WR}^{*b}$, $\hat{\sigma}_{BT}^{*b}$, $\hat{\sigma}_{BR}^{*b}$, and $\hat{\rho}^{*b}$ by using the same methods as those in Step 1 but with the dataset (Y_1, Y_2) replaced by the bootstrap dataset (Y_1^{*b}, Y_2^{*b}) and obtain $\hat{P}_{TR}^{ind*b}$.

Step 4: Calculate $z_{0.05}$ as the αth percentile of Φ and $z_0 = \Phi^{-1}(p)$, where p is the proportion of bootstrap replications $\hat{P}_{TR}^{ind\,b}$ smaller than $\hat{P}_{TR}^{ind}$. The lower bound $\hat{\Theta}_{prob,BC}^{ind}(5)$ of the one-sided 95 % bias-corrected bootstrap interval for P_{TR}^{ind} can be obtained as the

$\Phi(z_{0.05} + 2z_0)$th percentile of $\hat{P}_{TR}^{ind*b}$, $b = 1, \ldots, B$. Then, individual bioequivalence can be claimed if and only if this bound is greater than *MINP*.

Schall (1995a) also mentioned that under certain assumptions an exact parametric confidence interval for P_{TR}^{ind} can be constructed based on the non-central F-distribution. For details see Schall (1995a).

9.5.2.1.3   Test for individual equivalence ratio (TIER)

When Anderson and Hauck (1990) introduced the concept of individual bioequivalence they also proposed a criterion for assessing IBE as well as a statistical test procedure. Let X_T and X_R denote the pharmacokinetic response on the original scale, then average bioequivalence can be concluded if

$$\theta_1 \leq \frac{E(X_T)}{E(X_R)} \leq \theta_2 \text{ (cf. Section 4.3.2).}$$

Anderson and Hauck suggested replacing the expected pharmacokinetic responses under test and reference formulation by the subject-specific expected bioavailabilities, which yields the so-called individual equivalence ratio (*IER*)

$$1 - R_I \leq \frac{E(X_{jT})}{E(X_{jR})} \leq 1 + R_I.$$

The probability-based criterion based on *IER* reads then as

$$P_{TIER} = P_W \left(1 - R_I \leq \frac{E(X_{jT})}{E(X_{jR})} \leq 1 + R_I \right) > MINP,$$

where R_I and *MINP* have to be fixed by a regulatory agency. That is individual bioequivalence can be concluded if P_{TIER} is greater than the minimum proportion of the population *MINP*, in which the reference and the test formulation have to be bioequivalent. If R_I is chosen as 0.25 and *MINP* as 0.75 we get the well-known 75/75 rule. Anderson and Hauck, however, suggested the use of $R_I = 0.1$ and $MINP = 0.8$ which means that the test and reference formulation are regarded as individual bioequivalent if the ratio of the subject-specific expected bioavailabilities lies between 0.9 and 1.1 for more than 80 % of the population.

Assuming normality and equal variances under test and reference formulation (cf. Chapter 3), taking the logarithm of the pharmacokinetic responses yields the following equivalent criterion for adequately chosen values of R_I:

$$P_{TIER} = P_W \left(-r \leq E(Y_{jT}) - E(Y_{jR}) \leq r \right)$$
$$= P_W \left(-r \leq \mu_{jT} - \mu_{jR} \leq r \right) > MINP.$$

This reformulation is useful to investigate the relationship between P_{TIER} and the probability-based measures introduced by Schall and Luus (1993). Let us rewrite these probabilities by replacing Y_T, Y_R, Y_R' by their subject-specific expected values. This yields for P_{RR}^{ind},

$$P_{RR}^{ind} = P_W(|E(Y_{jR}) - E(Y_{jR}')| \leq r)$$
$$= P_W(|\mu_{jR} - \mu_{jR}| \leq r) = 1.$$

In addition, P_{TR}^{ind} results in

$$P_{TR}^{ind} = P_W(|E(Y_{jT}) - E(Y_{jR})| \leq r)$$
$$= P_W(|\mu_{jT} - \mu_{jR}| \leq r).$$

Thus, for the probability-based measure calculating the ratio of P_{TR}^{ind} and P_{RR}^{ind} we get

$$\Theta_{prob,r}^{ind} = \frac{P_{TR}^{ind}}{P_{RR}^{ind}}$$
$$= \frac{P_W(|\mu_{jT} - \mu_{jR}| \leq r)}{1} = P_{TIER}.$$

Analogously the probability-based measure calculating the difference of P_{TR}^{ind} and P_{RR}^{ind} can be expressed in terms of P_{TIER} as

$$\Theta_{prob,d}^{ind} = P_{TR}^{ind} - P_{RR}^{ind}$$
$$= P_W(|\mu_{jT} - \mu_{jR}| \leq r) - 1 = P_{TIER} - 1.$$

The test problem of individual bioequivalence based on the individual equivalence ratio reads as follows:

$$H_0 : P_{TIER} \leq MINP \text{ vs. } H_1 : P_{TIER} > MINP.$$

This test problem can be solved via a confidence interval where the null hypothesis is to be rejected at a 5 % significance level if the lower bound of the corresponding interval exceeds $MINP$ (Chow and Liu, 2000, p. 468f). Alternatively, we can proceed as follows: Since the probability P_{TIER} defines a Bernoulli experiment for each subject, the test procedure can be based on a binomial distribution. Let us therefore count the number of subjects N for which $Y_{jT} - Y_{jR}$ is within $-r$ and r, which is binomially distributed with $n = n_1 + n_2$ and success probability P_{TIER}, where the pharmacokinetic responses are obtained from a standard two-period, two-sequence crossover. Since for $0 \leq p \leq q \leq 1$,

$$P(N = J | P_{TIER} = p) \leq P(N = J | P_{TIER} = q),$$

individual bioequivalence can be concluded if

$$P(N \text{ or more subjects whose } Y_{jT} - Y_{jR} \text{ is within} - r \text{ and } r | P_{TIER} = MINP) \leq \alpha.$$

This test procedure has certain drawbacks as discussed by Ju (1997), who also proposed a modification to improve the *TIER* in certain respects. One crucial property of the *TIER* is that the decision on individual bioequivalence is based solely on whether a subject shows a bioequivalent reaction on the test and reference formulation, thus ignoring further information. In addition, the *TIER* can only be used with standard crossover designs. In the presence of period or carryover effects the *TIER* cannot be applied. Furthermore, the variabilities of the pharmacokinetic responses are not accounted for which may be a disadvantage for some formulations.

9.5.3 Relationships between aggregate bioequivalence criteria

Schall (1995b) gave a unified view of individual, population and average bioequivalence if their assessment is based on aggregate criteria. The main idea behind the criteria presented in the preceding sections is a comparison of measures of (expected) discrepancy (or similarity) between the pharmacokinetic characteristic of interest under test and reference formulation (Y_T and Y_R) and under twice the reference formulation (Y_R and Y_R'). Let $S(Y_T - Y_R)$ and $S(Y_R - Y_R')$ denote such measures. Then, bioequivalence criteria can be obtained by the difference or ratio of these measures. If we consider a measure of discrepancy then the test and reference formulation are said to be bioequivalent if the discrepancy between the test and the reference formulation is not much larger than the discrepancy between the reference and the reference formulation. A measure of discrepancy is e.g., the mean squared difference

$$S(Y_T - Y_R) = E(Y_T - Y_R)^2 \text{ and } S(Y_R - Y_R') = E(Y_R - Y_R')^2$$

which leads to the moment-based criterion (see Section 9.4.1 for PBE and Section 9.5.1 for IBE). If we consider a measure of similarity then the test and reference formulation are said to be bioequivalent if the similarity between the test and the reference formulation is not much less than the similarity between the reference and the reference formulation. A measure of similarity is e.g., the probability that the differences $Y_T - Y_R$ and $Y_R - Y_R'$ fall in a specified range, i.e.,

$$S(Y_T - Y_R) = P_{TR} = P\left(|Y_T - Y_R| \leq r\right) \text{ and } S(Y_R - Y_R') = P_{RR} = P\left(|Y_R - Y_R'| \leq r\right)$$

which leads to the probability-based criterion (see Section 9.4.2 for PBE and Section 9.5.2 for IBE).

The distinction between population and individual bioequivalence is made depending on whether the differences $Y_T - Y_R$ and $Y_R - Y_R'$ in the above measures represent between- or within-subject differences of bioavailabilities: If they represent between-subject differences, this will lead to criteria for assessing PBE; if they represent within-subject differences, we obtain criteria for the assessment of IBE.

Let us first focus on moment-based criteria for assessing IBE and especially on the unscaled criterion with some predefined bound Δ_d^2 which can be formulated as:

$$(\mu_T - \mu_R)^2 + \sigma_D^2 + \sigma_{WT}^2 - \sigma_{WR}^2 < \Delta_d^2.$$

Please note that we now use Δ as symbol for the bound to distinguish it from the specific ones to be fixed to assess PBE or IBE depending on the moment-based or probability-based approach. The lower index d or r will again indicate whether a difference or a ratio of measures is considered.

It can be easily seen, that if we have equal within-subject variances, i.e., $\sigma_W^2 = \sigma_{WT}^2 = \sigma_{WR}^2$, then the criterion reduces to

$$(\mu_T - \mu_R)^2 + \sigma_D^2 < \Delta_d^2.$$

If we now also assume that there is no subject-by-formulation interaction, i.e., $\sigma_D^2 = 0$, then the criterion further simplifies to

$$(\mu_T - \mu_R)^2 < \Delta_d^2 \text{ or equivalently} - \Delta_d < \mu_T - \mu_R < \Delta_d,$$

which is just the corresponding criterion of average bioequivalence.

In the case of the scaled criterion, i.e.,

$$\frac{(\mu_T - \mu_R)^2 + \sigma_D^2 + \sigma_{WT}^2 - \sigma_{WR}^2}{\sigma_{WR}^2} < \Delta_r^2,$$

the same assumptions finally lead to a scaled criterion of ABE, i.e.,

$$-\Delta_r < \frac{\mu_T - \mu_R}{\sigma_W} < \Delta_r.$$

It was pointed out by Schall (1995b) that – being monotonic functions of each other – the scaled criterion for assessing IBE is equivalent to the criterion *RIR* proposed by Sheiner (1992), which can be obtained from this scaled criterion by adding 1 to its left hand side, and also to the criteria proposed by Ekbohm and Melander (1989) and by Endrenyi (1994) as well as to the ratio of mean squared differences.

Let us now briefly look at the probability-based criteria, which we have already shown in Section 9.5.2.1.3 to be closely related to the criterion proposed by Anderson and Hauck (1990). In addition, using the scaled criterion with $r = r_0 \sigma_{WR}$ with $r_0 = \gamma \sqrt{2}$ as suggested by Schall (1995a) and assuming normality with $\sigma_W^2 = \sigma_{WT}^2 = \sigma_{WR}^2$ and $\sigma_D^2 = 0$, we get for the parametric criterion presented in Section 9.5.2.1.2 for assessing IBE,

$$
P_{TR}^{ind} = \Phi\left(\frac{\gamma \cdot \sqrt{2} \cdot \sigma_{WR} - (\mu_T - \mu_R)}{\sqrt{\sigma_{WT}^2 + \sigma_{WR}^2 + \sigma_D^2}}\right) - \Phi\left(\frac{-\gamma \cdot \sqrt{2} \cdot \sigma_{WR} - (\mu_T - \mu_R)}{\sqrt{\sigma_{WT}^2 + \sigma_{WR}^2 + \sigma_D^2}}\right)
$$

$$
= \Phi\left(\gamma + \frac{\mu_R - \mu_T}{\sqrt{2}\sigma_W}\right) - \Phi\left(-\gamma + \frac{\mu_R - \mu_T}{\sqrt{2}\sigma_W}\right) > MINP.
$$

Since P_{TR}^{ind} is a monotonic decreasing function of $|\mu_T - \mu_R|/\sigma_W$ this criterion is equivalent to the scaled criterion for assessing ABE.

Analogous relationships can be obtained for the corresponding criteria for assessing PBE where for instance the unscaled moment-based criterion (see Section 9.4.1) simplifies to the conventional criterion for assessing ABE if the total variances under test and reference formulation are the same, i.e., $\sigma^2 = \sigma_T^2 = \sigma_R^2$. For further details we refer the reader to Schall (1995b).

To summarize, if the variances of the pharmacokinetic response under test and reference formulation are the same and if there is no subject-by-formulation interaction there is no need for more complex bioequivalence criteria, i.e., average bioequivalence is sufficient. In addition, under these assumptions there is of course no distinction between individual and population bioequivalence.

9.5.4 Drawbacks of aggregate measures

Although at first glance appealing, aggregate measures have some major drawbacks as discussed e.g., in Hauschke and Steinijans (2000) and Steinijans (2001). The moment-based criteria for assessing population bioequivalence and individual bioequivalence are derived assuming an additive model for the pharmacokinetic response, which typically implies that the untransformed pharmacokinetic characteristic of interest has to be log transformed. In contrast to the criteria for assessing average bioequivalence (see Chapter 4), the test problems for PBE and IBE on the additive scale have no natural counterparts on the original scale if constructed using the moment-based measures since these are functions of both location and scale parameters and only defined on the logarithmic scale. It seems to be difficult or even impossible to relate these measures to the original scale, which makes the whole approach of limited practical application.

Another issue concerns the statistical methods for assessing PBE and ABE. First, no exact methods are available for calculating confidence intervals. Second, the estimators of the moment-based measures are not unbiased where the bias can be substantial in bioequivalence studies with small sample sizes and/or highly variable drugs. Third, further research would be necessary to study the finite-sample behavior of the proposed procedures and to investigate the impact of outliers and missing values. As a result of the lack of exact statistical methods, the sample size determination has to be performed on simulated data, where e.g., the simulation study by Shao et al. (2000b) has shown that 12 subjects in each sequence is not sufficient to obtain a power of at least 70 % which is in contrast to the draft FDA guidance (1997). In the guidance, sample sizes are provided under the assumption of no subject-by-formulation interaction and equal within-subject variances. Thus, it is not surprising that larger sample sizes seem to be required for assessing IBE where the main interest is in subject-by-formulation interaction and unequal within-subject variances.

The most important drawback is caused by the bias–variance trade-off being inherent in the moment-based measures, which means that a substantial difference between the population means can be compensated for by small variabilities. By this, the aggregate moment-biased criterion rewards a test formulation that has lower variability. This is an issue of major concern as has been illustrated e.g., by Midha et al. (1997) and by Hsuan (2000). Midha et al. (1997) demonstrated – by using the scaled individual bioequivalence criterion for a real dataset with no substantial subject-by-formulation interaction but an almost twofold difference in the within-subject variances – that the upper limit of the bootstrap confidence interval does not exceed the traditional average bioequivalence criterion of 1.25 until the ratio of geometric means exceeds 1.40. Moreover, the IBE criterion can be met without satisfying the ABE criterion. To summarize, these criteria do not necessarily imply the desirable hierarchy between average, population and individual bioequivalence, i.e., it might happen that individual bioequivalence is claimed without fulfilling the criterion of average bioequivalence.

Most of the above drawbacks can be overcome by a disaggregate approach. An example of such an approach will be presented in Section 9.6.

9.6   Disaggregate criteria

To achieve a testing procedure that maintains the hierarchy of the bioequivalence approaches a stepwise procedure should be considered, where a decision on population bioequivalence is only to be made if ABE has already been concluded and IBE is only to be claimed if PBE and ABE have already been shown. Vuorinen and Turunen (1996, 1997) proposed a three-step procedure where first ABE is tested at significance level α. If ABE cannot be approved the procedure stops. Otherwise, population bioequivalence will be assessed in the second step again using an appropriate statistical test at level α. If PBE cannot be approved the procedure stops with the conclusion that test and reference formulation are average bioequivalent. Otherwise, IBE will be assessed at level α in the third step. If IBE cannot be approved the procedure ends with the conclusion of population and average bioequivalence. Otherwise, the procedure terminates having approved ABE, PBE and IBE. Due to the stepwise character of the procedure no multiplicity adjustment is required to control for the multiple level α.

Vuorinen and Turunen (1996, 1997) assumed a standard two-period, two-sequence crossover bioequivalence trial (for an extension to higher-order crossover designs see Vuorinen, 1997). Preliminary to the stepwise procedure for assessing bioequivalence they recommended a test for unequal carryover and period effects. This problem is addressed in Chapter 4 and will therefore not be discussed further here. In the following, we will describe the stepwise procedure in more detail, where we have to distinguish whether the additive model can be assumed on the original scale or after logarithmic transformation. In addition, different statistical tests have to be conducted at each step depending on whether normality holds or not. We will focus on the parametric procedure while briefly mentioning the nonparametric alternative (see also Sections 3.4 and 4.3.3).

9.6.1   Stepwise procedure on the original scale

To be more precise let us assume the standard crossover design RT/TR and an additive model for the pharmacokinetic characteristic of interest on the original scale without carryover effects, but where we allow for a sequence effect, i.e.,

$$X_{ijk} = \mu + \tau_h + \pi_k + v_i + s_{ij} + e_{ijk},$$

where μ is the overall mean; τ_h is the fixed effect under formulation h, where $h = R$, if $i = k$ and $h = T$ otherwise, and $\tau_R + \tau_T = 0$; $\mu_R = \mu + \tau_R$ and $\mu_T = \mu + \tau_T$, respectively; π_k is the fixed effect of the kth period with $\Sigma_k \pi_k = 0$; v_i is the fixed effect of the ith sequence with $\Sigma_i \nu_i = 0$; s_{ij} is the random effect of the jth subject in the ith sequence. It is further assumed that s_{ij} are independent, $Var(s_{ij}) = \sigma_B^2$, i.e., independent of the formulation administered to the subjects, and e_{ijk} are independent random errors with expected mean 0 and variances σ_{WR}^2 and σ_{WT}^2, respectively. Furthermore, s_{ij} and e_{ijk} are assumed to be mutually independent. Under these assumptions, we have $Var(X_T) = \sigma_T^2 = \sigma_B^2 + \sigma_{WT}^2$, $Var(X_R) = \sigma_R^2 = \sigma_B^2 + \sigma_{WR}^2$, and $Cov(X_T, X_R) = \sigma_B^2$ where the latter can be easily derived. Let us e.g., consider the first sequence. Due to the independence of s_{ij} and e_{ijk} and because they have expected means 0 we obtain

$$
\begin{aligned}
Cov(X_{1jT}, X_{1jR}) &= Cov(s_{1j} + e_{1j2}, s_{1j} + e_{1j1}) \\
&= E\left[(s_{1j} + e_{1j2})(s_{1j} + e_{1j1})\right] - E(s_{1j} + e_{1j2})E(s_{1j} + e_{1j1}) \\
&= E(s_{1j}^2) + E(s_{1j}e_{1j2}) + E(s_{1j}e_{1j1}) + E(e_{1j2}e_{1j1}) - 0 \\
&= Var(s_{1j}) = \sigma_B^2.
\end{aligned}
$$

Hence, the within-subject correlation of two observations on the same subject, denoted by ρ is given as:

$$
\rho = \frac{Cov(X_T, X_R)}{\sqrt{Var(X_T)}\sqrt{Var(X_R)}} = \frac{\sigma_B^2}{\sigma_T \sigma_R}.
$$

Step 1: Average bioequivalence

For the assessment of ABE the following test problem has to be solved:

$$
H_0^1 : \frac{\mu_T}{\mu_R} \leq \theta_1 \text{ or } \frac{\mu_T}{\mu_R} \geq \theta_2 \quad \text{vs.} \quad H_1^1 : \theta_1 < \frac{\mu_T}{\mu_R} < \theta_2.
$$

From Chapter 4 we know that this test problem is equivalent to the following two one-sided test problems:

$$
H_{01}^1 : \frac{\mu_T}{\mu_R} \leq \theta_1 \quad \text{vs.} \quad H_{11}^1 : \frac{\mu_T}{\mu_R} > \theta_1
$$

and

$$
H_{02}^1 : \frac{\mu_T}{\mu_R} \geq \theta_2 \quad \text{vs.} \quad H_{12}^1 : \frac{\mu_T}{\mu_R} < \theta_2.
$$

This is equivalent to

$$
H_{01}^1 : \mu_T - \theta_1 \mu_R \leq 0 \quad \text{vs.} \quad H_{11}^1 : \mu_T - \theta_1 \mu_R > 0
$$

and

$$
H_{02}^1 : \mu_T - \theta_2 \mu_R \geq 0 \quad \text{vs.} \quad H_{12}^1 : \mu_T - \theta_2 \mu_R < 0.
$$

θ_1 and θ_2 give the equivalence range with, typically, $\theta_1 = 0.8$ and $\theta_2 = 1.25$. The null hypothesis of bioinequivalence, H_0, can be rejected at level α if both one-sided null hypotheses can be rejected at level α. Analogously to Chapter 3, let us consider the following differences

$$D_{ij\theta_1} = \begin{cases} \frac{1}{2}\left(X_{1j2} - \theta_1 X_{1j1}\right) & \text{if } i=1 \\ \frac{1}{2}\left(\theta_1 X_{2j2} - X_{2j1}\right) & \text{if } i=2 \end{cases} \quad \text{and} \quad D_{ij\theta_2} = \begin{cases} \frac{1}{2}\left(X_{1j2} - \theta_2 X_{1j1}\right) & \text{if } i=1 \\ \frac{1}{2}\left(\theta_2 X_{2j2} - X_{2j1}\right) & \text{if } i=2. \end{cases}$$

The expected values and variances can be calculated as

$$E(D_{ij\theta_1}) = \begin{cases} \frac{1}{2}\left[(\pi_2 - \theta_1 \pi_1) + (\mu_T - \theta_1 \mu_R)\right] & \text{if } i=1 \\ \frac{1}{2}\left[(\theta_1 \pi_2 - \pi_1) + (\theta_1 \mu_R - \mu_T)\right] & \text{if } i=2 \end{cases}$$

and

$$\sigma_{\theta_1}^2 = Var(D_{1j\theta_1}) = Var(D_{2j\theta_1}) = \frac{\sigma_T^2 + \theta_1^2 \sigma_R^2 - 2\theta_1 \sigma_B^2}{4}$$

and

$$E\left(D_{1j\theta_1} - D_{2j\theta_1}\right) = \mu_T - \theta_1 \mu_R,$$

where the latter results from the condition for reparametrization $\pi_1 + \pi_2 = 0$. Since under the above model assumptions $D_{1j\theta_1}, j = 1, \ldots, n_1$, and $D_{2j\theta_1}, j = 1, \ldots, n_2$, are independent normally distributed with the same variance $\sigma_{\theta_1}^2$, a two-sample t-test statistic can be used to test H_{01}^1, where H_{01}^1 can be rejected at level α if

$$T_{\theta_1} = \frac{\overline{D}_{1\theta_1} - \overline{D}_{2\theta_1}}{\hat{\sigma}_{\theta_1}\sqrt{\frac{1}{n_1} + \frac{1}{n_2}}} > t_{1-\alpha,n_1+n_2-2}$$

with

$$\overline{D}_{i\theta_1} = \frac{1}{n_i}\sum_{j=1}^{n_i} D_{ij\theta_1} \quad \text{and} \quad \hat{\sigma}_{\theta_1}^2 = \frac{1}{n_1+n_2-2}\sum_{i=1}^{2}\sum_{j=1}^{n_i}(D_{ij\theta_1} - \overline{D}_{i\theta_1})^2$$

denoting the sample means and the pooled sample variance. Analogously, we have that H_{01}^2 can be rejected at level α if

$$T_{\theta_2} = \frac{\overline{D}_{1\theta_2} - \overline{D}_{2\theta_2}}{\hat{\sigma}_{\theta_2}\sqrt{\frac{1}{n_1} + \frac{1}{n_2}}} < -t_{1-\alpha,n_1+n_2-2}.$$

Thus, average bioequivalence can be concluded at level α if $T_{\theta_1} > t_{1-\alpha,n_1+n_2-2}$ and $T_{\theta_2} < -t_{1-\alpha,n_1+n_2-2}$. The corresponding nonparametric test can be based on two one-sided Wilcoxon rank sum tests (cf. Section 4.3.3).

If average bioequivalence is approved, we can proceed with the next step.

Step 2: Population bioequivalence

Step 2 of the stepwise procedure for assessing bioequivalence is related to the assessment of population bioequivalence. For this purpose, the total variances under test and reference formulation can be compared, i.e., the following test problem can be considered:

$$H_0^2 : \frac{\sigma_T^2}{\sigma_R^2} \leq \eta_1^2 \quad \text{or} \quad \frac{\sigma_T^2}{\sigma_R^2} \geq \eta_2^2 \quad \text{vs.} \quad H_1^2 : \eta_1^2 < \frac{\sigma_T^2}{\sigma_R^2} < \eta_2^2.$$

Since the between-subject variances σ_{BT}^2 and σ_{BR}^2 are assumed to be identical, a possible difference between the variances under test and reference formulation is due to the difference in the within-subject variances σ_{WT}^2 and σ_{WR}^2. The corresponding test problem then reads as follows:

$$H_0^2 : \frac{\sigma_{WT}^2}{\sigma_{WR}^2} \leq \eta_{W1}^2 \quad \text{or} \quad \frac{\sigma_{WT}^2}{\sigma_{WR}^2} \geq \eta_{W2}^2 \quad \text{vs.} \quad H_1^2 : \eta_{W1}^2 < \frac{\sigma_{WT}^2}{\sigma_{WR}^2} < \eta_{W2}^2$$

which is equivalent to

$$H_{01}^2 : \sigma_{WT}^2 - \eta_{W1}^2 \sigma_{WR}^2 \leq 0 \quad \text{vs.} \quad H_{11}^2 : \sigma_{WT}^2 - \eta_{W1}^2 \sigma_{WR}^2 > 0$$

and

$$H_{02}^2 : \sigma_{WT}^2 - \eta_{W2}^2 \sigma_{WR}^2 \geq 0 \quad \text{vs.} \quad H_{12}^2 : \sigma_{WT}^2 - \eta_{W2}^2 \sigma_{WR}^2 < 0.$$

Liu and Chow (1992) proposed a testing procedure that may, however, show a poor behavior, since the ratio of the within-subject variances $\sigma_{WT}^2/\sigma_{WR}^2$ is a poor surrogate for σ_T^2/σ_R^2 whenever the magnitude of the between-subject variation is high compared to the within-subject variation, i.e., if there is a high within-subject correlation which is typical for bioequivalence studies (Vuorinen and Turunen, 1996, 1997). Vuorinen and Turunen therefore suggested modifying the test procedure by calculating bounds η_{W1}^2 and η_{W2}^2 that are related to η_1^2 and η_2^2, but keeping the test statistic as originally proposed. Their suggestion is to calculate

$$\eta_{W1}^2 = (\eta_1^2 - \eta_1 \rho)/(1 - \eta_1 \rho) \quad \text{and} \quad \eta_{W2}^2 = (\eta_2^2 - \eta_2 \rho)/(1 - \eta_2 \rho)$$

where e.g., $\eta_1 = 0.7$ and $\eta_2 = 1.43$ and ρ has to be estimated from the data (Vuorinen and Tuominen, 1994) which leads to approximate bounds.

To derive an adequate test statistic Vuorinen and Turunen (1997) proposed using not the original data, but residuals from sequence-by-period means, to account for period effects. According to Vuorinen and Turunen two types of residuals have to be calculated:

$$D_{ijn_W^2} = \begin{cases} \left(-X_{1j1} + \overline{X}_{1.1}\right) + \left(X_{1j2} - \overline{X}_{1.2}\right) & \text{if } i=1 \\ \left(X_{2j1} - \overline{X}_{2.1}\right) + \left(-X_{2j2} + \overline{X}_{2.2}\right) & \text{if } i=2 \end{cases}$$

and for the first test problem

$$D_{ij\eta_{W1}^2} = \begin{cases} \eta_{W1}^2 \left(X_{1j1} - \overline{X}_{1.1}\right) + \left(X_{1j2} - \overline{X}_{1.2}\right) & \text{if } i = 1 \\ \left(X_{2j1} - \overline{X}_{2.1}\right) + \eta_{W1}^2 \left(X_{2j2} - \overline{X}_{2.2}\right) & \text{if } i = 2 \end{cases}$$

as well as for the second test problem

$$D_{ij\eta_{W2}^2} = \begin{cases} \eta_{W2}^2 \left(X_{1j1} - \overline{X}_{1.1}\right) + \left(X_{1j2} - \overline{X}_{1.2}\right) & \text{if } i = 1 \\ \left(X_{2j1} - \overline{X}_{2.1}\right) + \eta_{W2}^2 \left(X_{2j2} - \overline{X}_{2.2}\right) & \text{if } i = 2 \end{cases}$$

with $\overline{X}_{i.k} = 1/n_i \sum_{j=1}^{n_i} X_{ijk}$.

Since the resulting test statistic is based on the empirical correlation coefficient of the above transformed variables, the variances and covariances of $D_{ij\eta_W^2}$, $D_{ij\eta_{W1}^2}$, and $D_{ij\eta_{W2}^2}$ have first to be calculated. We will give here only details for deriving $Var(D_{1j\eta_W^2})$. All other expressions can be obtained analogously. It holds that

$$Var(D_{1j\eta_W^2}) = Var\left(\left(-X_{1j1} + \overline{X}_{1.1}\right) + \left(X_{1j2} - \overline{X}_{1.2}\right)\right)$$

$$= Var\left(-X_{1j1} + \overline{X}_{1.1}\right) + Var\left(X_{1j2} - \overline{X}_{1.2}\right) + 2Cov\left(-X_{1j1} + \overline{X}_{1.1}, X_{1j2} - \overline{X}_{1.2}\right),$$

where

$$Var\left(-X_{1j1} + \overline{X}_{1.1}\right) = Var\left(-X_{1j1}\left(1 - \frac{1}{n_1}\right) + \frac{1}{n_1} \sum_{j'=1, j' \neq j}^{n_1} X_{1j'1}\right)$$

$$= \left(1 - \frac{1}{n_1}\right)^2 \sigma_R^2 + \frac{1}{n_1^2}(n_1 - 1)\sigma_R^2 = \frac{n_1 - 1}{n_1}\sigma_R^2,$$

$$Var\left(X_{1j2} - \overline{X}_{1.2}\right) = \frac{n_1 - 1}{n_1}\sigma_T^2,$$

and

$$Cov\left(-X_{1j1} + \overline{X}_{1.1}, X_{1j2} - \overline{X}_{1.2}\right) = Cov\left(-X_{1j1}\left(1 - \frac{1}{n_1}\right) + \frac{1}{n_1} \sum_{j'=1, j' \neq j}^{n_1} X_{1j'1},\right.$$

$$\left. X_{1j2}\left(1 - \frac{1}{n_1}\right) - \frac{1}{n_1} \sum_{j'=1, j' \neq j}^{n_1} X_{1j'2}\right)$$

$$= Cov\left(-X_{1j1}(1 - \frac{1}{n_1}), X_{1j2}(1 - \frac{1}{n_1})\right)$$

$$+ Cov\left(\frac{1}{n_1} \sum_{j'=1, j' \neq j}^{n_1} X_{1j'1}, -\frac{1}{n_1} \sum_{j'=1, j' \neq j}^{n_1} X_{1j'2}\right)$$

$$= -\left(\frac{n_1 - 1}{n_1}\right)^2 Cov\left(X_{1j1}, X_{1j2}\right)$$

$$-\frac{1}{n_1^2} \sum_{j'=1,j'\neq j}^{n_1} Cov\left(X_{1j'1}, X_{1j'2}\right)$$

$$= -\left(\frac{n_1-1}{n_1}\right)^2 Cov\left(X_{1j1}, X_{1j2}\right)$$

$$-\frac{n_1-1}{n_1^2} Cov\left(X_{1j'1}, X_{1j'2}\right) = -\frac{n_1-1}{n_1}\sigma_B^2$$

which in total gives

$$Var(D_{1j\eta_W^2}) = \frac{n_1-1}{n_1}\sigma_R^2 + \frac{n_1-1}{n_1}\sigma_T^2 - 2\frac{n_1-1}{n_1}\sigma_B^2$$

$$= \frac{n_1-1}{n_1}\left(\sigma_B^2 + \sigma_{WR}^2 + \sigma_B^2 + \sigma_{WT}^2 - 2\sigma_B^2\right) = \frac{n_1-1}{n_1}\left(\sigma_{WR}^2 + \sigma_{WT}^2\right).$$

Thus, the variances and covariances of $D_{ij\eta_W^2}$, $D_{ij\eta_{W1}^2}$ and $D_{ij\eta_{W2}^2}$ are as follows:

$$Var(D_{ij\eta_W^2}) = \frac{n_i-1}{n_i}\left(\sigma_{WR}^2 + \sigma_{WT}^2\right),$$

$$Var(D_{ij\eta_{W1}^2}) = \frac{n_i-1}{n_i}\left(\sigma_{WT}^2 + \left(\eta_{W1}^2\right)^2\sigma_{WR}^2 + \left(1+\eta_{W1}^2\right)^2\sigma_B^2\right),$$

$$Var(D_{ij\eta_{W2}^2}) = \frac{n_i-1}{n_i}\left(\sigma_{WT}^2 + \left(\eta_{W2}^2\right)^2\sigma_{WR}^2 + \left(1+\eta_{W2}^2\right)^2\sigma_B^2\right),$$

$$Cov\left(D_{ij\eta_W^2}, D_{ij\eta_{W1}^2}\right) = \frac{n_i-1}{n_i}\left(\sigma_{WT}^2 - \eta_{W1}^2\sigma_{WR}^2\right),$$

$$Cov\left(D_{ij\eta_W^2}, D_{Ij\eta_{W2}^2}\right) = \frac{n_i-1}{n_i}\left(\sigma_{WT}^2 - \eta_{W2}^2\sigma_{WR}^2\right).$$

Let ρ denote the Bravais–Pearson correlation coefficient, then $\rho_{\eta_{W1}^2}$ is defined as follows:

$$\rho_{\eta_{W1}^2} = \frac{Cov\left(D_{ij\eta_W^2}, D_{ij\eta_{W1}^2}\right)}{\sqrt{Var(D_{ij\eta_W^2})}\sqrt{Var(D_{ij\eta_{W1}^2})}}$$

with $\rho_{\eta_{W2}^2}$ being defined analogously. $\rho_{\eta_{W1}^2}$ now has to be estimated by replacing all unknown quantities with e.g., their REML estimators obtained from the mixed-effect model introduced above or just by calculating the corresponding sample correlation coefficient, $\hat{\rho}_{\eta_{W1}^2}$. This gives the following t-test statistic

$$T_{\eta_{W1}^2} = \frac{\hat{\rho}_{\eta_{W1}^2}}{\sqrt{\dfrac{1-\hat{\rho}_{\eta_{W1}^2}^2}{n_1+n_2-3}}}$$

(see Chow and Liu, 2000, p. 196ff), i.e., H_{01}^2 can be rejected at level α if $T_{\eta_{W1}^2} > t_{1-\alpha, n_1+n_2-3}$. Analogously, H_{02}^2 can be rejected at level α if

$$T_{\eta_{W2}^2} = \frac{\hat{\rho}_{\eta_{W2}^2}}{\sqrt{\dfrac{1 - \hat{\rho}_{\eta_{W2}^2}^2}{n_1 + n_2 - 3}}} < -t_{1-\alpha, n_1+n_2-3}.$$

Population bioequivalence can be concluded at level α if H_{01}^2 and H_{02}^2 are both rejected at level α. Vuorinen and Turunen (1997) noted that the resulting test is a two one-sided Pitman–Morgan's test procedure given in terms of the correlation between crossover differences and subject totals. The corresponding nonparametric test can be based on the sample Spearman rank correlation coefficient.

If population bioequivalence is approved, we can proceed with the last step.

Step 3: Individual bioequivalence

For the last step, i.e., assessing individual bioequivalence, Vuorinen and Turunen (1996, 1997) suggested solving the following test problem:

$$H_0^3 : \rho \leq \varsigma \quad \text{vs.} \quad H_1^3 : \rho > \varsigma.$$

Here, ρ again denotes the within-subject correlation coefficient and ς is a positive bound to be chosen e.g., as 0.5. As for the second step, residuals from sequence-by-period means have to be calculated:

$$D_{ijs}^R = \begin{cases} (X_{1j1} - \overline{X}_{1.1}) & \text{if } i = 1 \\ (X_{2j2} - \overline{X}_{2.2}) & \text{if } i = 2 \end{cases} \quad \text{and} \quad D_{ijs}^T = \begin{cases} (X_{1j2} - \overline{X}_{1.2}) & \text{if } i = 1 \\ (X_{2j1} - \overline{X}_{2.1}) & \text{if } i = 2. \end{cases}$$

Analogous to the variance and covariance calculations in Step 2 we get

$$Var(D_{ijs}^R) = \frac{n_i - 1}{n_i} \sigma_R^2, \ Var(D_{ijs}^T) = \frac{n_i - 1}{n_i} \sigma_T^2 \quad \text{and} \quad Cov(D_{ijs}^R, D_{ijs}^T) = \frac{n_i - 1}{n_i} \sigma_B^2$$

and thus

$$\rho = \frac{Cov(D_{ijs}^R, D_{ijs}^T)}{\sqrt{Var(D_{ijs}^R)} \sqrt{Var(D_{ijs}^T)}} = \frac{\sigma_B^2}{\sigma_R \sigma_T}.$$

The corresponding sample Bravais–Pearson correlation coefficient calculated from the observed D_{ijs}^R and D_{ijs}^T and Fisher's z-transformation can be used for assessing IBE, i.e., H_0^3 can be rejected at level α if

$$Z_\varsigma = \frac{1}{2} \sqrt{n_1 + n_2 - 3} \left\{ \ln\left(\frac{1 - \hat{\rho}}{1 + \hat{\rho}}\right) - \ln\left(\frac{1 - \varsigma}{1 + \varsigma}\right) \right\} > z_{1-\alpha},$$

where $z_{1-\alpha}$ denotes the $(1-\alpha)$ quantile of the standard normal distribution. The corresponding nonparametric test can again be carried out based on the sample Spearman rank correlation coefficient.

If finally H_0^3 is rejected, individual, population and average bioequivalence can be concluded.

9.6.2 Stepwise procedure on the logarithmic scale

Let us now assume that the additive model introduced in Section 9.6.1 holds for the pharmacokinetic characteristic after its logarithmic transformation, i.e.,

$$Y_{ijk} = \ln X_{ijk} = \mu + \tau_h + \pi_k + \nu_i + s_{ij} + e_{ijk}$$

(cf. Section 4.2.1). To perform the stepwise procedure outlined above on the logarithmic scale such that it can still be interpreted on the original scale, the first step of the procedure has to be formulated via the ratio of medians. As pointed out by Vuorinen and Turunen (1997), the remaining steps need not be modified since it can be easily shown via the delta method that the standard deviations of the logarithmically transformed variables approximately coincide with the respective coefficients of variation on the original scale. Assuming further that average bioequivalence is fulfilled, so that the expected means 'cancel out' in the ratio of coefficients of variation on the original scale, the ratio of the variances of the logarithmically transformed variables approximately coincide with the respective ratio of variances on the original scale.

Let us therefore focus on the first step, which deals with the assessment of average bioequivalence. Now, it has to be shown that

$$\theta_1 < \frac{M(X_T)}{M(X_R)} < \theta_2$$

with $M(X)$ denoting the median of a random variable X (see Section 4.2.1). Since $M(X_h) = \exp(\mu_h)$, $h = R, T$, the test problem of ABE can be formulated as:

$$H_0^1 : \frac{\exp(\mu_T)}{\exp(\mu_R)} \leq \theta_1 \quad \text{or} \quad \frac{\exp(\mu_T)}{\exp(\mu_R)} \geq \theta_2 \quad \text{vs.} \quad H_1^1 : \theta_1 < \frac{\exp(\mu_T)}{\exp(\mu_R)} < \theta_2.$$

After logarithmic transformation this becomes:

$$H_0^1 : \mu_T - \mu_R \leq \ln \theta_1 \quad \text{or} \quad \mu_T - \mu_R \geq \ln \theta_2 \quad \text{vs.} \quad H_1^1 : \ln \theta_1 < \mu_T - \mu_R < \ln \theta_2,$$

which is equivalent to the following two one-sided test problems:

$$H_{01}^1 : \mu_T - \mu_R - \ln \theta_1 \leq 0 \quad \text{vs.} \quad H_{11}^1 : \mu_T - \mu_R - \ln \theta_1 > 0$$

and

$$H_{02}^1 : \mu_T - \mu_R - \ln \theta_2 \geq 0 \quad \text{vs.} \quad H_{12}^1 : \mu_T - \mu_R - \ln \theta_2 < 0$$

(see Section 4.3.2). This test problem can be solved as described in Section 4.3.2. According to Vuorinen and Turunen, the following modified period differences have to be defined:

$$D_{ij\ln\theta_1} = \begin{cases} \frac{1}{2}\left(Y_{1j2} - Y_{1j1}\right) - \ln\theta_1 & \text{if } i=1 \\ \frac{1}{2}\left(Y_{2j2} - Y_{2j1}\right) & \text{if } i=2 \end{cases} \quad \text{and } D_{ij\ln\theta_2} = \begin{cases} \frac{1}{2}\left(Y_{1j2} - Y_{1j1}\right) - \ln\theta_2 & \text{if } i=1 \\ \frac{1}{2}\left(Y_{2j2} - Y_{2j1}\right) & \text{if } i=2. \end{cases}$$

The expected values and variances can be calculated as

$$E(D_{ij\ln\theta_1}) = \begin{cases} \frac{1}{2}\left[(\pi_2 - \pi_1) + (\mu_T - \mu_R)\right] - \ln\theta_1 & \text{if } i=1 \\ \frac{1}{2}\left[(\pi_2 - \pi_1) + (\mu_R - \mu_T)\right] & \text{if } i=2 \end{cases}$$

and

$$\sigma_{\theta_1}^2 = Var(D_{1j\ln\theta_1}) = Var(D_{2j\ln\theta_1}) = \frac{\sigma_{WT}^2 + \sigma_{WR}^2}{4}$$

and

$$E\left(D_{1j\ln\theta_1} - D_{2j\ln\theta_1}\right) = \mu_T - \mu_R - \ln\theta_1.$$

Thus, a two-sample t-test statistic can be used to test H_{01}^1, where H_{01}^1 can be rejected at level α if

$$T_{\ln\theta_1} = \frac{\overline{D}_{1\ln\theta_1} - \overline{D}_{2\ln\theta_1}}{\hat{\sigma}_{\ln\theta_1}\sqrt{\frac{1}{n_1} + \frac{1}{n_2}}} > t_{1-\alpha,n_1+n_2-2}$$

with

$$\overline{D}_{i\ln\theta_1} = \frac{1}{n_i}\sum_{j=1}^{n_i} D_{ij\ln\theta_1} \quad \text{and} \quad \hat{\sigma}_{\ln\theta_1}^2 = \frac{1}{n_1+n_2-2}\sum_{i=1}^{2}\sum_{j=1}^{n_i}(D_{ij\ln\theta_1} - \overline{D}_{i\ln\theta_1})^2$$

denoting the sample means and the pooled sample variance. In analogy, we have that H_{02}^1 can be rejected at level α if

$$T_{\ln\theta_2} = \frac{\overline{D}_{1\ln\theta_2} - \overline{D}_{2\ln\theta_2}}{\hat{\sigma}_{\ln\theta_2}\sqrt{\frac{1}{n_1} + \frac{1}{n_2}}} < -t_{1-\alpha,n_1+n_2-2}.$$

Thus, average bioequivalence can be concluded at level α if $T_{\ln\theta_1} > t_{1-\alpha,n_1+n_2-2}$ and $T_{\ln\theta_2} < -t_{1-\alpha,n_1+n_2-2}$. The corresponding nonparametric test can be based on two one-sided Wilcoxon rank sum tests (cf. Section 9.4.3.3).

9.7   Other approaches

Further proposals for assessing PBE and IBE can be found in the literature, which will not be reviewed here. Instead, we would like to present some non-standard methods to indicate the variety of the approaches for assessing population or individual bioequivalence.

The above aggregate measures are based on calculating discrepancies between the pharmacokinetic responses under test and reference formulation, where ABE only compares their population means, thus ignoring other distributional characteristics. Therefore, the idea was born to compare the entire distributions of the bioavailabilities under test and reference to assess bioequivalence. However, most of the measures are constructed such that they compare, besides the means, the variabilities and the subject-by-formulation interaction under test and reference, depending on whether PBE or IBE is to be assessed. If it is justified to assume that the bioavailabilities under test and reference are normally or lognormally distributed, a comparison of their distributions can in fact be reduced to a comparison of their means and variances, due to the unique characterization of a (log)normal distribution by its first two moments. If the assumption of a (log)normal distribution is, however, not justified it might instead be reasonable to not only compare moments but also the entire distributions.

9.7.1   Trimmed Mallows distance

This approach was exploited by Freitag *et al.* (2005) who proposed a completely nonparametric test for assessing the marginals F and G of a bivariate distribution $H = (F, G)$, where F represents the distribution of the pharmacokinetic response under test and G under reference, respectively. For this purpose they considered the β-trimmed version of Mallows distance $(0 \le \beta < 0.5)$ which is defined for continuous cumulative distribution functions with finite second moments as:

$$\Gamma_\beta(F, G) = \sqrt{\frac{1}{1 - 2\beta} \int_\beta^{1-\beta} [F^{-1}(t) - G^{-1}(t)]^2 \, dt},$$

where F^{-1} and G^{-1} denote the corresponding quantile functions, i.e.,

$$F^{-1}(t) = \inf \{u; F(u) \ge t\}.$$

In contrast to other nonparametric tests, Freitag *et al.* argued that the trimmed Mallows distance combines various advantages such that (i) it achieves a certain degree of robustness against outliers due to trimming; (ii) it shows a reasonable behavior in the sense that in the case of a location-scale family the Mallows distance reduces to an aggregate measure combining the means and variances and in the case of a pure location family it leads to a classical measure of ABE, thus, giving a criterion for PBE that contains ABE as a special case; and (iii) that it can be calculated without any transformation of the pharmacokinetic response of interest, i.e., based on the original scale.

The authors assumed a standard two-period, two-sequence crossover design for deriving a PBE criterion based on Mallows distance. Let F_1 (G_1) denote the cumulative distribution function under test (reference), first (second) period, first sequence and G_2 (F_2) the respective cumulative distribution function under reference (test), first (second) period, second sequence. Then PBE can be concluded if

$$\Gamma_{\beta,pop}^2 = \frac{1}{2} \left\{ \Gamma_\beta(F_1, G_2)^2 + \Gamma_\beta(F_2, G_1)^2 \right\} \leq \Delta_0^2$$

for a fixed bound Δ_0^2. In the case of no period effects, it can be assumed that $F_1 = F_2 = F$ and $G_1 = G_2 = G$ which leads to the following simplified criterion:

$$\Gamma_{\beta,pop} = \Gamma_\beta(F, G) \leq \Delta_0.$$

In an example, Freitag et al. determined the bound Δ_0 by assuming an additive model and normal distributions with homogenous variances, which gives $\Gamma_{\beta,pop} = \Gamma_\beta(F, G) = \mu_T - \mu_R$ and $\Delta_0 = \ln(1.25)$. This implies a rather conservative criterion because in contrast to the criteria in Section 9.4.1 no additional tolerance limits for the variances are allowed.

To perform the statistical test procedure, the bootstrap percentile or the bias-corrected and accelerated bootstrap confidence interval can be used (Efron and Tibshirani, 1993), where the latter was shown by means of simulation results to perform better than the simple bootstrap percentile. For more details on the asymptotic behavior we refer the reader to Freitag et al. (2005).

9.7.2 Kullback–Leibler divergence

A second approach that is based on calculating a distance measure of the entire distributions uses the Kullback–Leibler divergence. We assume an additive model, where a standard two-period, two-sequence crossover design suffices. Let us further assume that densities f_T and f_R of the pharmacokinetic response of interest under test, Y_T, and reference, Y_R, exist with respect to a dominant measure ν. Then, the Kullback–Leibler divergence,

$$d(f_T, f_R) = \int [f_T(x) - f_R(x)] [\ln f_T(x) - \ln f_R(x)] d\nu$$

can be used to obtain a bioequivalence measure, which again guarantees that not only the first two moments are accounted for when calculating a similarity measure, but also other distributional characteristics. Depending on whether the two densities refer to metrics based on differences for the same or different individuals, we obtain measures for IBE (in the first case) and for PBE (in the latter case).

Bioequivalence can be concluded if

$$d(f_T, f_R) \leq d_0$$

for a predefined d_0. To calculate the Kullback–Leibler divergence further assumptions regarding the underlying distributions have to be made. For instance, Dragalin et al. (2003) assumed a normal distribution. In this case they were able to show that the resulting criterion implies hierarchy of the three bioequivalence concepts IBE, PBE and ABE, i.e., if IBE is shown then also PBE and ABE follow. For more details, we refer the reader to Dragalin et al. (2003).

9.7.3   Structural equation model

The above two approaches represent aggregate measures. Finally, we present a disaggregate criterion based on a structural equation model (SEM) where we assume the additive model introduced in Section 9.3.3 and a linear relationship between μ_T and μ_R, i.e., there exist α and β such that

$$\mu_T = \alpha + \beta\mu_R.$$

This linear relationship implies

$$\sigma_{BT}^2 = \beta^2 \sigma_{BR}^2,$$

$$\rho = 1,$$

$$\sigma_D^2 = \sigma_{BT}^2 + \sigma_{BR}^2 - 2\rho\sigma_{BT}\sigma_{BR} = \beta^2\sigma_{BR}^2 + \sigma_{BR}^2 - 2\beta\sigma_{BR}^2 = (\beta-1)^2\sigma_{BR}^2,$$

$$\delta = \mu_T - \mu_R = \alpha + (\beta-1)\mu_R.$$

Individual bioequivalence can now be concluded, if it holds for predefined $\theta_s, s = 1, \ldots, 5$, that:

$$\theta_1 \le \beta \le \theta_2$$

$$\theta_3 \le \delta \le \theta_4$$

$$\frac{\sigma_{WT}^2}{\sigma_{WR}^2} \le \theta_5.$$

Carrasco and Jover (2003) suggested the use of:

$$\theta_1 = \theta_5 = 1.5 = \frac{1}{\theta_2}$$

$$\theta_3 = -\ln(1.25) = -\theta_4,$$

where the authors tried to adapt suggestions by the FDA to SEM components. These bounds can of course be further modified depending on the user's requirements, e.g., in the case of a reference formulation with a large variance.

The parameters are estimated via a partial likelihood approach. The test problem of individual bioequivalence is formulated via 5 test problems with:

$$H_{01} : \beta \le \theta_1 \quad \text{vs} \quad H_{11} : \beta > \theta_1$$

$$H_{02} : \beta \ge \theta_2 \quad \text{vs} \quad H_{12} : \beta < \theta_2$$

$$H_{03} : \delta \le \theta_3 \quad \text{vs} \quad H_{13} : \delta > \theta_3$$

$$H_{04} : \delta \ge \theta_4 \quad \text{vs} \quad H_{14} : \delta < \theta_4$$

$$H_{05} : \frac{\sigma_{WT}^2}{\sigma_{WR}^2} \ge \theta_5 \quad \text{vs} \quad H_{15} : \frac{\sigma_{WT}^2}{\sigma_{WR}^2} < \theta_5.$$

The overall test problem of individual bioequivalence can then be expressed as:

$$H_0 = H_{01} \cup H_{02} \cup H_{03} \cup H_{04} \cup H_{05} \quad \text{vs.} \quad H_1 = H_{11} \cap H_{12} \cap H_{13} \cap H_{14} \cap H_{15}.$$

Based on Berger's intersection-union principle the above overall null hypothesis is rejected at significance level α if all hypotheses are rejected at level α. For test statistics to investigate the individual test problems and for the power of the resulting procedure see Carrasco and Jover (2003).

9.8 Average bioequivalence in replicate designs

We will close this section with a discussion of methods to assess ABE in replicate designs. In Section 9.3.2 we introduced replicate crossover designs that are in general required for assessing IBE, although we have seen that under certain conditions IBE may also be investigated in two-period, two-sequence crossover trails. It also became obvious that PBE can be assessed in standard crossover trials as well as in replicate designs. Techniques for assessing ABE have been demonstrated in preceding chapters always assuming a standard two-period, two-sequence crossover trial. However, it is of course possible to assess ABE in a crossover study with more than two periods. For the sake of completeness, therefore, we present a parametric approach for the assessment of ABE in a four-period, two-sequence crossover study *TRTR/RTRT* (see Table 9.1).

Let us again assume that the additive model holds for the pharmacokinetic characteristic on the logarithmic scale. In addition, we assume normality after transformation. Average bioequivalence can then be tested via the medians of the bioavailability under test and reference, i.e.,

$$\theta_1 < \frac{M(X_T)}{M(X_R)} < \theta_2$$

with $M(X)$ denoting the median of a random variable X (see Sections 4.2.1, 9.6.2). As discussed in Section 4.3.2 (cf. Section 9.6.2) the test problem of ABE can be formulated as the following two one-sided test problems:

$$H_{01} : \mu_T - \mu_R \leq \ln \theta_1 \quad \text{vs.} \quad H_{11} : \mu_T - \mu_R > \ln \theta_1$$

and

$$H_{02} : \mu_T - \mu_R \geq \ln \theta_2 \quad \text{vs.} \quad H_{12} : \mu_T - \mu_R < \ln \theta_2$$

with $\ln M(X_h) = \mu_h$, $h = R, T$. Typically θ_1 is chosen as 0.8 and θ_2 as 1.25. Thus, with $\theta = \ln(1.25)$ we get the following simplified test problems:

$$H_{01} : \mu_T - \mu_R \leq -\theta \quad \text{vs.} \quad H_{11} : \mu_T - \mu_R > -\theta$$

and

$$H_{02} : \mu_T - \mu_R \geq \theta \quad \text{vs.} \quad H_{12} : \mu_T - \mu_R < \theta.$$

Let us now define random variables I_{ij}, $i = 1, 2$, $j = 1, \ldots, n_i$, with

$$I_{1j} = 0.5\left(Y_{1j1} + Y_{1j3}\right) - 0.5\left(Y_{1j2} + Y_{1j4}\right) \text{ and } I_{2j} = 0.5\left(Y_{2j2} + Y_{2j4}\right) - 0.5\left(Y_{2j1} + Y_{2j3}\right)$$

(cf. the parametric approach in Section 9.4.1.1.2). Obviously, it holds that

$$E(I_{ij}) = \mu_T - \mu_R \text{ and } Var(I_{ij}) = \sigma_I^2 = \sigma_D^2 + \frac{1}{2}\sigma_{WT}^2 + \frac{1}{2}\sigma_{WR}^2.$$

As already discussed in Section 9.4.1.1.2, unbiased estimators of $\delta = \mu_T - \mu_R$ and of σ_I^2 can be obtained as:

$$\hat{\delta} = \frac{1}{2}\sum_{i=1}^{2}\frac{1}{n_i}\sum_{j=1}^{n_i} I_{ij} \text{ and } \hat{\sigma}_I^2 = \frac{1}{n-2}\sum_{i=1}^{2}\sum_{j=1}^{n_i}(I_{ij} - \bar{I}_{i.})^2 \text{ with } n = n_1 + n_2,$$

$$\bar{I}_{i.} = \frac{1}{n_i}\sum_{j=1}^{n_i} I_{ij},$$

where $\hat{\delta}$ is normally distributed with

$$E(\hat{\delta}) = \delta \text{ and } Var(\hat{\delta}) = \frac{1}{4}\sum_{i=1}^{2}\frac{1}{n_i}\sigma_I^2$$

and $\hat{\sigma}_I^2$ is distributed as $(n-2)^{-1}\sigma_I^2 \chi_{n-2}^2$ (see Chinchilli and Esinhart, 1996).

Thus, we get the following test procedure: ABE can be concluded at level α if both, H_{01} and H_{02} are rejected at level α, i.e., if

$$\frac{\hat{\delta} + \theta}{\hat{\sigma}_I\sqrt{\frac{1}{4}\left(\frac{1}{n_1} + \frac{1}{n_2}\right)}} > t_{1-\alpha, n-2} \text{ and } \frac{\hat{\delta} - \theta}{\hat{\sigma}_I\sqrt{\frac{1}{4}\left(\frac{1}{n_1} + \frac{1}{n_2}\right)}} < -t_{1-\alpha, n-2}.$$

The advantage of assessing ABE in a four-period, two-sequence crossover trial is the reduction in variance which of course leads to a reduction in sample size to achieve the same power compared to a two-period, two-sequence crossover trial. This advantage might, however, be counterbalanced by the longer duration of a crossover trial with more than two periods and the presumably higher number of dropouts. For more details see Patterson and Jones (2002).

9.9 Example: The antihypertensive patch dataset

The antihypertensive patch dataset (see Section 9.3.5) will now be used to illustrate the application of the linearized moment-based criteria that have been recommended by the FDA (FDA Guidance, 2001) for assessing PBE and IBE. In addition to PBE and IBE we also investigate whether the data fulfill the criterion for ABE in a replicate design as given in Section 9.8. Here, the FDA (FDA Guidance, 2001) recommends not using an unrestricted variance-covariance structure. Thus, we followed the recommendation in the guidance and constrained the covariance matrix to be non negative-definite. Two different variance-covariance structures that may be applied are mentioned by the FDA (FDA Guidance, 2001; see also SAS, 2000): *CSH*, which specifies the heterogeneous compound symmetry structure so that the covariance matrix is constrained to the following structure:

$$\Sigma = \begin{pmatrix} \sigma_{11}^2 & \rho\sigma_{12}\sigma_{21} \\ \rho\sigma_{12}\sigma_{21} & \sigma_{22}^2 \end{pmatrix},$$

and *FA0(2)*, which stands for 'no diagonal factor analytic of grade 2' which means that the covariance matrix has the following structure

$$\Sigma = \begin{pmatrix} \lambda_{11}^2 & \lambda_{11}\lambda_{21} \\ \lambda_{11}\lambda_{21} & \lambda_{21}^2 + \lambda_{22}^2 \end{pmatrix}.$$

Although the three variance-covariance structures (the unrestricted, *CSH*, and *FA0(2)*) should result in the same estimated covariance matrix, the individual parameter estimates can differ due to the different parameterizations and due to the internal calculations of SAS® (cf. Patterson and Jones, 2002, p. 23).

To assess PBE and IBE we apply the SAS® code provided in Table 9.7 for the logarithmically transformed *AUC* data; the C_{max} data can be dealt with analogously. To assess ABE we follow the FDA recommendation preferring the use of *FA0(2)* (we also performed the analysis using CSH but obtained comparable results not shown here).

Table 9.8 summarizes the results obtained for assessing ABE, PBE, and IBE where the given values are already retransformed using the exponential function. Thus, ABE can be concluded if the upper limit is below 1.25 and the lower limit exceeds 0.8. Please note that for PBE and IBE only the upper limits are shown since PBE and IBE can be concluded according to the linearized criteria if the corresponding upper limits are below 0.

As can be seen from the above results ABE can be concluded based on the values obtained for *AUC*, but the C_{max} data fail the criterion since the lower limit of the 90 % confidence interval is slightly below 0.8.

PBE can be concluded in either case, i.e., based on the *AUC* and on the C_{max} data, since for both datasets the upper confidence limit is below 0. For this dataset we obviously face the situation that the desired hierarchy of ABE, PBE, and IBE is not fulfilled for the C_{max} data where ABE could not be concluded but PBE was.

Finally, IBE has to be investigated. Here, the upper limits both exceed 0 and IBE cannot be concluded in either case. This may be due to a high subject-by-formulation interaction that seems to be present in this dataset, as pointed out by the FDA at the corresponding webpage (http://www.fda.gov/cder/bioequivdata/index.htm).

Table 9.7 SAS® procedure for calculating confidence intervals for assessing PBE and IBE according to the linearized criterion presented in Sections 9.4.1.1.2 and 9.5.1.1.2 for the example introduced in Section 9.3.5.

```
data data;
  infile datalines delimiter=',';
  input ID sequence $ period treatment $ AUC;
  cards;
1,RTTR,1,R,1020.65
1,RTTR,2,T,1321.23
1,RTTR,3,T,900.42
1,RTTR,4,R,1173.61
2,TRRT,1,T,950.59
2,TRRT,2,R,1637.71
2,TRRT,3,R,2076.75
2,TRRT,4,T,1485.93
3,RTTR,1,R,1188.82
3,RTTR,2,T,1440.99
3,RTTR,3,T,1501.2
3,RTTR,4,R,1481.27
4,TRRT,1,T,774.44
4,TRRT,2,R,585.89
4,TRRT,3,R,801.26
4,TRRT,4,T,773.51
5,TRRT,1,T,1563.08
5,TRRT,2,R,1571.75
5,TRRT,3,R,1917.37
5,TRRT,4,T,1886.05
6,RTTR,1,R,1119.22
6,RTTR,2,T,781.2
6,RTTR,3,T,800.85
6,RTTR,4,R,942.5
7,RTTR,1,R,1876.81
7,RTTR,2,T,1726.01
7,RTTR,3,T,1653.7
7,RTTR,4,R,1111.1
8,TRRT,1,T,2549.54
8,TRRT,2,R,3738.21
8,TRRT,3,R,3800.33
8,TRRT,4,T,5408.38
9,TRRT,1,T,2291.93
9,TRRT,2,R,1223.74
9,TRRT,3,R,1949.1
9,TRRT,4,T,3184.15
```

Table 9.7 Continued.

```
10,RTTR,1,R,1392.92
10,RTTR,2,T,826.36
10,RTTR,3,T,1220
10,RTTR,4,R,1607.52
11,RTTR,1,R,5239.22
11,RTTR,2,T,8894.11
11,RTTR,3,T,7726.47
11,RTTR,4,R,7451.66
12,TRRT,1,T,1044.18
12,TRRT,2,R,1023
12,TRRT,3,R,1178.2
12,TRRT,4,T,1155.25
13,TRRT,1,T,744.57
13,TRRT,2,R,985.58
13,TRRT,3,R,1721.01
13,TRRT,4,T,4217.64
14,RTTR,1,R,1629.67
14,RTTR,2,T,2081.88
14,RTTR,3,T,1302.65
14,RTTR,4,R,2805.07
15,RTTR,1,R,3054.97
15,RTTR,2,T,3370.78
15,RTTR,3,T,2644.44
15,RTTR,4,R,5941.36
16,TRRT,1,T,3469
16,TRRT,2,R,1712.59
16,TRRT,3,R,1680.07
16,TRRT,4,T,3285.23
17,TRRT,1,T,3006.95
17,TRRT,2,R,3063.28
17,TRRT,3,R,1764.34
17,TRRT,4,T,2055.51
18,RTTR,1,R,2323.41
18,RTTR,2,T,1063.45
18,RTTR,3,T,960.1
18,RTTR,4,R,2629.35
19,TRRT,1,T,4989.43
19,TRRT,2,R,6439.82
19,TRRT,3,R,4945.42
19,TRRT,4,T,2321.03
20,RTTR,1,R,2673.38
20,RTTR,2,T,1686.63
20,RTTR,3,T,2260.34
```

```
20,RTTR,4,R,4632.96
21,TRRT,1,T,2081.19
21,TRRT,2,R,1028.75
21,TRRT,3,R,758.83
21,TRRT,4,T,1168.12
22,RTTR,1,R,10843.61
22,RTTR,2,T,13162.65
22,RTTR,3,T,13505.79
22,RTTR,4,R,13575.9
23,TRRT,1,T,736.5
23,TRRT,2,R,947.58
23,TRRT,3,R,1426.96
23,TRRT,4,T,681.66
24,RTTR,1,R,2747.09
24,RTTR,2,T,3651.63
24,RTTR,3,T,2543.63
24,RTTR,4,R,1056.48
25,TRRT,1,T,2064.25
25,TRRT,2,R,2251.24
25,TRRT,3,R,2228.06
25,TRRT,4,T,2633.27
26,TRRT,1,T,1092.48
26,TRRT,2,R,1141.68
26,TRRT,3,R,1550.98
26,TRRT,4,T,996.55
27,RTTR,1,R,2011.28
27,RTTR,2,T,2109.67
27,RTTR,3,T,2902.35
27,RTTR,4,R,2283.6
28,RTTR,1,R,3793.47
28,RTTR,2,T,4165.73
28,RTTR,3,T,4666.95
28,RTTR,4,R,3274.41
29,RTTR,1,R,1427.53
29,RTTR,2,T,1591.38
29,RTTR,3,T,1909.97
29,RTTR,4,R,1911.43
30,TRRT,1,T,2333.74
30,TRRT,2,R,2878.94
30,TRRT,3,R,1698.3
30,TRRT,4,T,1142.33
31,RTTR,1,R,1932.8
31,RTTR,2,T,1620.69
31,RTTR,3,T,2279.44
```

Table 9.7   Continued.

```
31,RTTR,4,R,3251.14
32,TRRT,1,T,1835.61
32,TRRT,2,R,2760.92
32,TRRT,3,R,3188.04
32,TRRT,4,T,2480.39
33,TRRT,1,T,8330.61
33,TRRT,2,R,6064.54
33,TRRT,3,R,8737.6
33,TRRT,4,T,8353.62
34,RTTR,1,R,3612.64
34,RTTR,2,T,2494.45
34,RTTR,3,T,3153.79
34,RTTR,4,R,6386.19
35,RTTR,1,R,1061.92
35,RTTR,2,T,987.86
35,RTTR,3,T,1422.71
35,RTTR,4,R,1220.58
36,TRRT,1,T,2212.39
36,TRRT,2,R,1438.48
36,TRRT,3,R,1984.76
36,TRRT,4,T,2640.43
37,RTTR,1,R,2252.76
37,RTTR,2,T,2262.88
37,RTTR,3,T,1957.66
37,RTTR,4,R,3084.05
;
run;

* outputfile;
filename file "Result_BE.lis" ;

%GLOBAL thetaP thetaI sigma02 alpha
        model design scale log
        BAC
        treatmentR treatstring
        ntreatments nperiods nsequences;


%macro initial;
    /* model specifications, here multiplicative */
    %let model=multiplicative;

    /* kind of scale in the population or individual BE
       criterion, here: mixed */
    %let scale=mixed;
```

```
    %let thetaP = 1.74482611;   /* ((log(1.25)**2+0.02)/0.04) */
    %let thetaI = 2.49482611;   /* ((log(1.25)**2+0.05)/0.04) */
    %let sigma02 = 0.04;
    %let alpha = 0.05;

    %let BAC = AUC;             /* parameter */
%mend initial;

%macro manage_dataderivations;
    %LOCAL nseq nper ntreat;

    /* extract level of periods, sequence, treatment */
    proc glm data=data;
        class sequence ID period treatment;
        model &BAC = ID;
        ods output classlevels=cldata;
    run;

    /* set macro variables nsequences for number of sequences,
       nperiods for number of periods, ntreatments for number of
treatments */
    data _null_;
        set cldata;
        select (Class);
            when ("sequence") call symput('nseq',Levels);
            when ("period") call symput('nper',Levels);
            when ("treatment") call symput('ntreat',Levels);
            otherwise;
        end;
    run;

    %let nsequences = %scan(&nseq,1,' ');
    %let nperiods = %scan(&nper,1,' ');
    %let ntreatments = %scan(&ntreat,1,' ');

    /* get the study design */
    data _null_;
        set cldata;
        if Class = "sequence" then call symput("design",Values);
    run;

    /* identify sequence with sequence number */
    %do inds=1 %to &nsequences;
        %local designseq&inds;
        %let designseq&inds = %scan(&design,&inds,' ');
    %end;
```

Table 9.7 Continued.

```
      /* add seqno to dataset */
      data datacomp;
         set data;
         select (sequence);
         %do inds=1 %to &nsequences;
             when ("&&designseq&inds") seqno=&inds;
         %end;
         otherwise;
       end;
run;

      /* derivation of variable model */
      %if &model=multiplicative %then %let log=log; ;
%mend manage_dataderivations;

%macro manage_extractn;
      /* sort data, then calculate means to get number of subjects
        per sequence */
      proc sort data=datacomp;
         by seqno period;
      run;
      proc means data=datacomp;
         by seqno period;
         var &BAC;
         output out=nsequence;
      run;

      /* keep only necessary data */
      data nsequence;
         modify nsequence;
         if (period~=1 or _STAT_~="N") then remove;
      run;

      /* extract data and move it into separate data sets */
      data %do ind=1 %to &nsequences;
                  N&ind(rename=(&BAC=N&ind))
           %end; ;
         set nsequence;
         %do ind=1 %to &nsequences;
             if seqno=&ind then do;
                 keep &BAC;
                 output N&ind;
             end;
        %end;
      run;
```

```
      /* combine data and add total number of subjects */
      data nsequencetotal;
            merge %do ind=1 %to &nsequences;
                        N&ind
                  %end; ;
            N= 0 %do ind=1 %to &nsequences;
                              + N&ind
                  %end; ;
      run;
%mend manage_extractn;

%macro manage_logtransform;
      %if &model=multiplicative %then %do;
            data logdatacomp;
            set datacomp;
            log&BAC=log(&BAC);
            drop &BAC;
      run;
      %end;
%mend manage_logtransform;

%macro manage_dataperiod;
      /* divide data into data of each period */
      %do indp = 1 %to &nperiods;
            data period&indp;
            set datacomp(rename=(treatment=treatment&indp
      &BAC=&BAC&indp));
            run;
          data period&indp;

          modify period&indp;
          if period ~= &indp then remove;
          run;

          proc sort data=period&indp;
             by ID ;
          run;
      %end;

      /* combine the divided data into one data set*/
      data dataperiod;
          merge %do indp = 1 %to &nperiods;
          period&indp
          %end; ;
          by ID ;
          drop period;
```

Table 9.7   Continued.

```
    run;
    /* if necessary: same with log-data*/
    %if &model = multiplicative %then %do;
    %do indp = 1 %to &nperiods;
        data logperiod&indp;
        set logdatacomp(rename=(treatment=treatment&indp
                      log&BAC=log&BAC&indp));
        run;
        data logperiod&indp;
        modify logperiod&indp;
        if period ~= &indp then remove;
        run;
        proc sort data=logperiod&indp;
        by ID ;
        run;
    %end;

    data logdataperiod;
        merge %do indp = 1 %to &nperiods;
                logperiod&indp
            %end; ;
        by ID ;
          drop period;
    run;
    %end;
%mend manage_dataperiod;

%macro manage_extractorder;
    %local treatstring;

    /* put information about treatments into string */
    data _null_;
    set cldata;
    if Class = "treatment" then do;
        call symput('treatstring', Values);
    end;
    run;

    /* identify which treatment is reference */
    %do indt=1 %to &ntreatments;
     %global treatno&indt;
     %let treatno&indt = %scan(&treatstring, &indt, ' ');
     %if &&treatno&indt = R %then %let treatmentR = &indt; ;
     %end;
```

```
    data test;
        design=tranwrd(trim("&design")," " ,"-");
        %do indt=1 %to &ntreatments;
            design=tranwrd(design,   "&&treatno&indt",
   "&&treatno&indt*");
    %end;
    call symput('design',design);
run;

    /* define macro variable (L)s(S)ind and (L)r(R)s(S);
                            (L) is treatment, (S) sequence,
                            (R) is the (R)th replicate of
(L) in sequence (S) */
    %do indt=1 %to &ntreatments;
        %do inds=1 %to &nsequences;
            %global &&treatno&indt..s&inds.ind;
            %do indp=1 %to &nperiods;
                %global &&treatno&indt..r&indp.s&inds;
            %end;
        %end;
    %end;

    /* set the macro variables*/
    %do indt=1 %to &ntreatments;
        %do inds=1 %to &nsequences;
            %let &&treatno&indt..s&inds.ind = 1;
            %do indp=1 %to &nperiods;
                %if (%scan(%scan(&&design,&inds,-),&&indp,*)=
   &&treatno&indt) %then
                %do;
                  %let
&&treatno&indt..r&&&&&&treatno&indt..s&inds.ind.s&inds = &indp;
                %let    &&treatno&indt..s&inds.ind    =
%eval(&&&&&&treatno&indt..s&inds.ind + 1);
                %end;
            %end;
        %end;
    %end;

    /* undone last incrimination of (L)s(S)ind */
    %do indt=1 %to &ntreatments;
    %do inds=1 %to &nsequences;
        %let &&treatno&indt..s&inds.ind =
```

Table 9.7   Continued.

```
%eval(&&&&&&treatno&indt..s&inds.ind - 1);
        %end;
     %end;
%mend manage_extractorder;


%macro manage_studyP_fdamethod;


    /* do analysis for BAC (AUC) */
            data dataI_P;
            set &log.dataperiod;
            %do inds=1 %to &nsequences;
              if seqno=&inds then do;
              I = 0.5*(&log&BAC&&Tr1s&inds+&log&BAC&&Tr2s&inds)
                  -
0.5*(&log&BAC&&Rr1s&inds+&log&BAC&&Rr2s&inds);
                UT                                                 =
(0.5)*(&log&BAC&&Tr1s&inds+&log&BAC&&Tr2s&inds);
                UR                                                 =
(0.5)*(&log&BAC&&Rr1s&inds+&log&BAC&&Rr2s&inds);
                VT      =       sqrt(0.5)*(&log&BAC&&Tr1s&inds-
&log&BAC&&Tr2s&inds);
                VR      =       sqrt(0.5)*(&log&BAC&&Rr1s&inds-
&log&BAC&&Rr2s&inds);
                  end;
            %end;
             drop treatment1 treatment2 treatment3 treatment4;
      run;
            /* calculation of delta */
      proc means data=dataI_P;
        var I;
          output out=meanI_P;
      run;

      data resultP_delta(rename=(I=delta));
          set meanI_P;
            if _STAT_="MEAN" then do;
          keep I;
            output resultP_delta;
          end;
      run;
```

```
      /* calculation of M_I */
    PROC GLM data=dataI_P outstat=resultP_MI noprint;
        CLASS seqno ID;
        MODEL I = seqno;
      run;


    data resultP_MI;
        modify resultP_MI;
        if _TYPE_ ~= "ERROR" then remove;
      run;

    data resultP_MI;
     set resultP_MI;
        MI=SS/DF;
        keep MI;
      run;


      /* calculation of MU_T, MU_R, MV_T, MV_R */
  %manage_calc_MUVTR(UV=U, TR=T)
     %manage_calc_MUVTR(UV=U, TR=R)
     %manage_calc_MUVTR(UV=V, TR=T)
     %manage_calc_MUVTR(UV=V, TR=R)


      /* combine data and point estimate*/
      %if &scale=mixed %then %do;
       data resultsP_&log&BAC;
           merge resultP_delta resultP_MI resultP_MUT
                 resultP_MUR    resultP_MVT    resultP_MVR
nsequencetotal;
        theta = delta**2 + MUT + 0.5*MVT - (MUR+0.5*MVR) -
&thetaP * max((MUR+0.5*MVR),&sigma02);
          run;
         %end;


/* calculation of upper CI-limit */
      %if &scale=mixed %then
   %do;
      data CI_limit_P_&log&BAC;
          merge resultsP_&log&BAC;
          HD = (abs(delta)+tinv(%sysevalf(1 - &alpha),
N-&nsequences)
                   *          sqrt(MI*(&nsequences**(-2))
*(1/N1+1/N2)))**2;
```

Table 9.7   Continued.

```
        H1 = ((N-&nsequences)*MUT )/cinv(&alpha,
(N-&nsequences));
        H2 = ((N-&nsequences)*0.5*MVT)/cinv(&alpha,
(N-&nsequences));
        UD=(HD-delta)**2;
          U1=(H1-MUT)**2;
            U2=(H2-0.5*MVT)**2;


        MR=MUR+0.5*MVR;
        if MR<&sigma02 then do;
           H3cs = ((N-&nsequences)*-1*MUR )
              / cinv(%sysevalf(1 - &alpha),(N- &nsequences));
           H4cs = ((N-&nsequences)*-0.5*MVR )
                 / cinv(%sysevalf(1  -  &alpha),(N-
&nsequences));
           U3cs = (H3cs+MUR)**2;
             U4cs = (H4cs+0.5*MVR)**2;
             thetauplimit = theta + sqrt(UD+U1+U2+U3cs+U4cs)
- &thetaP*&sigma02;
        end;
        else
        do;
           H3rs   =   ((N-&nsequences)*-(1+&thetaP)*MUR )
                 /  cinv(%sysevalf(1   -   &alpha),(N-
&nsequences));
           H4rs = ((N-&nsequences)*-(1+&thetaP)*0.5*MVR )
                 /  cinv(%sysevalf(1 - &alpha),
(N-&nsequences));
           U3rs = (H3rs+(1+&thetaP)*MUR)**2;
             U4rs = (H4rs+(1+&thetaP)*0.5*MVR)**2;
             thetauplimit = theta + sqrt(UD+U1+U2+U3rs+U4rs);
        end;
        keep theta thetauplimit;
           run;
        %end;


    data CI_limit_P_&log&BAC;
        set CI_limit_P_&log&BAC;
        length character $ 4;
        character = "&BAC";
        study ="PBE";
    run;
```

```
           data CI_limit_P;
                  set CI_limit_P_&log.&BAC;
           run;


%mend manage_studyP_fdamethod;


%macro manage_studyI_fdamethod;
       /* do analysis for BAC (AUC) */

           /* construction of I_ij,T_ij, R_ij*/
       data dataI_I;
     set &log.dataperiod;
     %do inds=1 %to &nsequences;
         if seqno=&inds then do;
         I = 0.5*(&log&BAC&&Tr1s&inds+&log&BAC&&Tr2s&inds)

-0.5*(&log&BAC&&Rr1s&inds+&log&BAC&&Rr2s&inds);
         Tdiff = &log&BAC&&Tr1s&inds-&log&BAC&&Tr2s&inds;
               Rdiff    =    &log&BAC&&Rr1s&inds-
&log&BAC&&Rr2s&inds;
           end;
             %end;
     drop treatment1 treatment2 treatment3 treatment4;
     run;


       /* calculation of delta */
       proc means data=dataI_I ;
       var I;
           output out=meanI_I;
       run;
       data resultI_delta(rename=(I=delta));
           set meanI_I;
              if _STAT_="MEAN" then do;
            keep I;
            output resultI_delta;
           end;
     run;


        /* calculation of M_I */
        PROC GLM data=dataI_I outstat=resultI_MI noprint;
        CLASS seqno ID;
        MODEL I = seqno;
        run;
```

Table 9.7   Continued.

```
data resultI_MI;
modify resultI_MI;
       if _TYPE_ ~= "ERROR" then remove;
run;

data resultI_MI;
    set resultI_MI;
  MI=SS/DF;
  keep MI;
run;

/* calculation of M_T */
PROC GLM data=dataI_I outstat=resultI_MT noprint;
   CLASS seqno ID;
   MODEL Tdiff = seqno;
run;

data resultI_MT;
 modify resultI_MT;
 if _TYPE_ ~= "ERROR" then remove;
run;

data resultI_MT;
 set resultI_MT;
 MT=SS/(2*DF);
 keep MT;
run;
/* calculation of M_R */
PROC GLM data=dataI_I outstat=resultI_MR noprint;
       CLASS seqno ID;
        MODEL Rdiff = seqno;
 run;

data resultI_MR;
modify resultI_MR;
if _TYPE_ ~= "ERROR" then remove;
run;

data resultI_MR;
 set resultI_MR;
MR=SS/(2*DF);
 keep MR;
 run;
```

```
      /* combine data and point estimate*/
      %if &scale=mixed %then %do;
          data resultsI_&log&BAC;
            merge resultI_delta resultI_MI
                resultI_MT resultI_MR nsequencetotal;
            theta = delta**2 + MI+ 0.5*MT - 1.5*MR - &thetaI *
max(MR,&sigma02);
            run;
      %end;


      /* calculation of upper CI-limit */
       %if &scale=mixed %then %do;
       data CI_limit_I_&log&BAC;
            set resultsI_&log&BAC;
       HD  =  (abs(delta)+tinv(%sysevalf(1   -   &alpha),N-
&nsequences)
             *    sqrt(MI*(&nsequences**(-
2))*(1/N1+1/N2)))**2;
       HI  =  ((N-&nsequences)*MI   )/cinv(&alpha,(N-
&nsequences));
       HT = ((N-&nsequences)*0.5*MT )/cinv(&alpha,(N-
&nsequences));
      if MR<&sigma02 then do;
            HR   =   ((N-&nsequences)*(-1.5)*MT)/cinv(&alpha,
            (N-&nsequences));
            UD = (HD-delta)**2;
            UI = (HI-MI)**2;
            UT = (HT-0.5*MT)**2;
            UR = (HR+1.5*MR)**2;
                  thetauplimit=theta+sqrt(UD+UI+UT+UR)-
&thetaI*&sigma02;
      end;
      else do;
            HR = ((N-&nsequences)*(-1.5-&thetaI)*MT )
               / cinv(&alpha,(N-&nsequences));
            UD = (HD-delta)**2;
            UI = (HI-MI)**2;
            UT = (HT-0.5*MT)**2;
            UR = (HR+(1.5+&thetaI)*MR)**2;
            thetauplimit=theta+sqrt(UD+UI+UT+UR);
      end;
            keep theta thetauplimit;
            run;
      %end;
```

Table 9.7 Continued.

```
      data CI_limit_I_&log&BAC;
          set CI_limit_I_&log&BAC;
          length character $ 4;
          character = "&BAC";
          study ="IBE";
      run;

data CI_limit_I;
      set CI_limit_I_&log.&BAC;
run;

%mend manage_studyI_fdamethod;

%macro manage_calc_MUVTR(UV=, TR=);
      PROC GLM data=dataI_P outstat=resultP_M&UV&TR noprint;
          CLASS seqno ID;
          MODEL &UV&TR = seqno;
run;

data resultP_M&UV&TR;
      modify resultP_M&UV&TR;
      if _TYPE_ ~= "ERROR" then remove;
run;
data resultP_M&UV&TR;
      set resultP_M&UV&TR;
      M&UV&TR=SS/DF;
      keep M&UV&TR;
run;
 %mend manage_calc_MUVTR;

%macro report;
/* general reportings - input data */

options nodate pageno=1 linesize=80 pagesize=60;

data CI_limits;
      merge CI_limit_P CI_limit_I;
      by descending study;
      if thetauplimit < 0 then
          decision = "Yes";
      else decision = "NO!";
run;
```

```
proc report data=CI_limits headskip box nowd;
     title "Bioavailability study - results";
     title2 "&model model, PBE and IBE";
     column study character theta thetauplimit decision;
     define study / descending group format= $3. "";
     define character / display format= $8. "BE-char.";
     define theta / display format= 15.10 "point estimate of
theta";
     define thetauplimit / display format= 15.10
             "upper     %sysevalf(100*(1-&alpha))%
confidence limit";
     define decision / display format = $5. "BE concluded?";
run;
%mend report;

%macro control;

/* setting global macro variables*/
%initial

/* derive of further SAS datasets */
%manage_dataderivations
/* extract number of subjects in sequences and total */
%manage_extractn

/* logarithmic transformation, if necessary */
%manage_logtransform

/* combination of data for each subject */
%manage_dataperiod

/* extract order of given formulas*/
%manage_extractorder

%manage_studyP_fdamethod
%manage_studyI_fdamethod

proc printto Print=file new;
run;

%report

proc printto;
run;

%mend control;

%control
```

Table 9.8 Point estimate and 90% confidence interval for $\exp(\mu_T)/\exp(\mu_R)$ for assessing ABE; Point estimates and upper confidence limits for $\eta^{pop}_{mom,\ ref}$ and $\eta^{ind}_{mom,\ ref}$ for assessing PBE and IBE, respectively.

Bioequivalence concept	Pharmacokinetic characteristic	Point estimate	Confidence limits	
			Lower	Upper
ABE	AUC	0.959	0.867	1.061
	C_{max}	0.900	0.796	1.017
PBE	AUC	−0.687		−0.271
	C_{max}	−0.997		−0.434
IBE	AUC	−0.085		0.271
	C_{max}	−0.199		0.407

9.10 Conclusions

Let us finally reappraise whether the above criteria for assessing individual and population bioequivalence really capture the concepts of population and individual bioequivalence, i.e., whether they meet the requirements formulated by Anderson and Hauck (1990) with respect to prescribability and switchability. Let us first consider the criteria that have been recommended by the FDA.

Hauck and Anderson (1994) introduced the concept of population bioequivalence to ensure that drug-naïve patients can be safely prescribed either formulation, reference or test. This requires that the distributions of the pharmacokinetic characteristic under reference and test formulation are essentially the same. The constant-scaled moment-based criterion for the assessment of PBE,

$$\frac{(\mu_T - \mu_R)^2 + \sigma_T^2 - \sigma_R^2}{\sigma_0^2} < \theta^{pop}_{mom}$$

is fulfilled e.g., if the difference of expected means is small and if the variance under the test formulation is not much larger than that under the reference formulation. Since the FDA recommended this measure under the assumption of normality, where the normal distribution is uniquely characterized by its first two moments, this criterion meets the requirements of Hauck and Anderson fairly well. The only problem might be caused by the potential trade-off between the difference in means and the variance.

The concept of individual bioequivalence was introduced to ensure that a patient who gets the reference drug can be safely switched to the test drug. In this respect, Hsuan (2000) showed that for a highly variable drug with a within-subject CV reaching 40%, the allowable limits for the ratio of formulation means could reach 55–180% in an IBE investigation, as compared with the usual allowable limit of 80–125% in an ABE investigation. He raised doubts as to whether the implied standard of the new IBE criteria would adequately ensure switchability in highly variable drugs. In addition, switchability formally requires that the marginal distributions under test and reference formulation do not differ too much in the majority of patients. The FDA constant-scaled moment-based criterion for the assessment of IBE, which is given as

$$\frac{(\mu_T - \mu_R)^2 + \sigma_D^2 + \sigma_{WT}^2 - \sigma_{WR}^2}{\sigma_{W0}^2} < \theta_{mom}^{ind}$$

is fulfilled e.g., if the difference of expected means and the subject-by-formulation interaction are small and if the within-subject variance under the test formulation is not much larger than the within-subject variance under the reference formulation. Let us for the moment assume that s_{ijh} in the model introduced in Section 9.3.3 is fixed for a single subject. Then, again the similarity of the two marginal distributions is assessed by a comparison of their expected means and their within-subject variabilities. It was hoped that the subject-by-formulation variance component would capture the variation in results from subject to subject. The latter, however, has been criticized by Endrenyi et al. (2000). They showed that the estimated variance component for the subject-by-formulation interaction (σ_D^2) increases with the within-subject variability of the reference formulation (σ_{WR}^2). Thus, a fixed, set level of σ_D^2 (such as $\sigma_D = 0.15$ as suggested by the FDA) may not be regarded as a basis to demonstrate substantial interactions (see also Chow and Liu, 2000, p. 27). Since the prevalence of subject-by-formulation interaction in the replicate studies published by the FDA was based on this fixed criterion, the possibility cannot be excluded that this prevalence was too high. In line with this, Endrenyi and Tothfalusi (1999) were able to show that the FDA datasets are compatible with the hypothesis $\sigma_D = 0$. Meaning that these studies do not demonstrate the prevalence of a subject-by-formulation interaction, which had been put forward as a major motivation for IBE. In summary, this criterion is not very convincing.

In contrast to the aggregate criteria, the disaggregate criterion has the advantage that the different steps are closely related to the corresponding concepts of bioequivalence. The first step compares the expected means, which implies the classical criterion of ABE. The second step compares the variabilities under test and reference formulation, which together with Step 1 gives similarity of the first two moments. Assuming normality, this is sufficient to conclude similarity of the entire distributions and thus to conclude PBE. Furthermore, in contrast to the aggregate criterion, the criterion for PBE cannot be fulfilled by compensating for a large difference in means by a low variance for the pharmacokinetic response under the test formulation. The last step then tries to capture individual bioequivalence by investigating whether the within-subject correlation is sufficiently large. Since the similarity of the two distributions has already been proved by the first two steps, a positive within-correlation indicates that the bioavailabilities under test and reference should be sufficiently similar within a patient. In addition, since it can be assumed that the bioavailability under reference is sufficiently high, it can be concluded that – due to a high positive within-subject correlation – it should also be sufficiently high under the test formulation if a patient is switched from reference to test. It remains, however, questionable as to whether this disaggregate criterion meets the requirement by Anderson and Hauck (1990) that bioequivalence should be fulfilled in the majority of patients.

References

Anderson, S. and Hauck, W.W. (1990) Consideration of individual bioequivalence. *Journal of Pharmacokinetics and Biopharmaceutics* **18**, 259–73.

Barrett, J.S., Batra, V., Chow, A., Cook, J., Gould, A.L., Heller, A.H., Lo, M-W., Patterson, S.D., Smith, B.P., Stritar, J.A., Vega, J.M. and Zariffa, N. (2000a) PhRMA perspective on population and individual bioequivalence. *Journal of Clinical Pharmacology* **40**, 561–70.

Barrett, J.S., Batra, V., Chow, A., Cook, J., Gould, A.L., Heller, A.H., Lo, M-W., Patterson, S.D., Smith, B.P., Stritar, J.A., Vega, J.M. and Zariffa, N. (2000b) Update to the PhRMA perspective on population and individual bioequivalence. *Journal of Clinical Pharmacology* **40**, 571–2.

Carrasco, J-L. and Jover, L. (2003) Assessing individual bioequivalence using the structural equation model. *Statistics in Medicine* **22**, 901–12.

Chen, M-L. (1997) Individual bioequivalence – a regulatory update. *Journal of Biopharmaceutical Statistics* **7**, 5–11.

Chinchilli, V.M. (1996) The assessment of individual and population bioequivalence. *Journal of Biopharmaceutical Statistics* **6**, 1–14.

Chinchilli, V.M. and Esinhart, J.D. (1996) Design and analysis of intra-subject variability in cross-over experiments. *Statistics in Medicine* **15**, 1619–34.

Chow, S-C. and Liu, J-P. (1995) Current issues in bioequivalence trials. *Drug Information Journal* **29**, 795–804.

Chow, S-C. and Liu, J-P. (2000) *Design and analysis of bioavailability and bioequivalence studies.* Marcel Dekker, New York.

Dragalin, V., Fedorov, V., Patterson, S. and Jones, B. (2003) Kullback–Leibler divergence for evaluating bioequivalence. *Statistics in Medicine* **22**, 913–20.

Efron, B. and Tibshirani, R.J. (1993) *An introduction to the bootstrap.* Chapman & Hall, New York.

Elze, M. and Blume, H.H. (1999) Bioequivalence trials – status and perspectives. *Informatik, Biometrie und Epidemiologie in Medizin und Biologie* **30**, 87–95.

Ekbohm, G. and Melander, H. (1989) The subject-by-formulation interaction as a criterion of interchangeability of drugs. *Biometrics* **45**, 1249–54.

Endrenyi, L. (1994) A method for evaluation of individual bioequivalence. *International Journal of Clinical Pharmacology and Therapeutics* **32**, 497–508.

Endrenyi, L. and Tothfalusi, L. (1999) Subject-by-formulation interaction in determinations of individual bioequivalence: Bias and prevalence. *Pharmaceutical Research* **16**, 186–190.

Endrenyi, L., Amidon, G.L., Midha, K.K. and Skelly, J.P. (1998) Individual bioequivalence: attractive in principle, difficult in practice. *Pharmaceutical Research* **15**, 1321–5.

Endrenyi, L., Taback, N. and Tothfalusi, L. (2000) Properties of the estimated variance component for subject-by-formulation interaction in studies of individual bioequivalence. *Statistics in Medicine* **19**, 2867–78.

Esinhart, J.D. and Chinchilli, V.M. (1994) Extension to the use of tolerance intervals for the assessment of individual bioequivalence. *Journal of Biopharmaceutical Statistics* **4**, 39–52.

Food and Drug Administration (1997) *In vivo bioequivalence studies based on population and individual bioequivalence approaches. Guidance for Industry.* Center for Drug Evaluation and Research, Rockville, MD.

Food and Drug Administration (1999a) *BA and BE studies for orally administered drug products: General considerations.* Center for Drug Evaluation and Research, Rockville, MD.

Food and Drug Administration (1999b) *Average, population and individual approaches to establishing bioequivalence.* Center for Drug Evaluation and Research, Rockville, MD.

Food and Drug Administration (2000) *Bioavailability and bioequivalence studies for orally admin-istered drug products: General considerations.* Center for Drug Evaluation and Research, Rockville, MD.

Food and Drug Administration (2001) *Statistical approaches to establishing bioequivalence.* Center for Drug Evaluation and Research, Rockville, MD.

Food and Drug Administration (2003) *Bioavailability and bioequivalence studies for orally admin-istered drug products: General considerations.* Center for Drug Evaluation and Research, Rockville, MD.

Freitag, G., Czado, C. and Munk, A. (2005) A nonparametric test for similarity of marginals – with application to the assessment of population bioequivalence. *Journal of Statistical Planning and Inference* (to appear).

Graybill, F.A. and Wang, C.M. (1980) Confidence intervals on nonnegative linear combinations of variances. *Journal of the American Statistical Association* **75**, 869–73.

Hauck, W.W. and Anderson, S. (1992) Types of bioequivalence and related statistical considera-tions. *International Journal of Clinical Pharmacology, Therapy, and Toxicology* **30**, 181–7.

Hauck, W.W. and Anderson, S. (1994) Measuring switchability and prescribability: when is average bioequivalence sufficient? *Journal of Pharmacokinetics and Biopharmaceutics* **22**, 551–64.

Hauschke, D. and Steinijans, V.W. (2000) The US draft guidance regarding population and indi-vidual bioequivalence approaches: comments by a research-based pharmaceutical company. *Statistics in Medicine* **19**, 2769–74.

Holder, D.J. and Hsuan, F. (1993) Moment-based criteria for determining bioequivalence. *Biometrika* **80**, 835–46.

Howe, W.G. (1974) Approximate confidence limits on the mean of $X + Y$ where X and Y are two tabled independent random variables, *Journal of the American Statistical Association* **69**, 789–94.

Hsuan, F.C. (2000) Some statistical considerations on the FDA draft guidance for individual bioequivalence. *Statistics in Medicine* **19**, 2879–84.

Hwang, J.T.G. and Wang, W. (1997) The validity of the test of individual equivalence ratios. *Biometrika* **84**, 893–900.

Hyslop, T. (2001) *Assessment of individual and population bioequivalence in crossover and parallel designs.* Ph.D. Thesis, Temple University.

Hyslop, T., Hsuan, F. and Holder, D.J. (2000) A small sample confidence interval approach to assess individual bioequivalence. *Statistics in Medicine* **19**, 2885–97.

Ju, H.L. (1997) On TIER method for assessment of individual bioequivalence. *Journal of Biophar-maceutical Statistics* **7**, 63–85.

Liu, J-P. and Chow, S-C. (1992) On the assessment of variability in bioavailability/bioequivalence studies. *Communications in Statistics – Theory and Methods* **21**, 2591–2607.

Midha, K.K., Rawson, M.J. and Hubbard, J.W. (1997) Individual and average bioequivalence of highly variable drugs and drug products. *Journal of Pharmaceutical Sciences* **86**, 1193–7.

Patnaik, R.N., Lesko, L.J., Chen, M.L. and Williams, R.L. (1997) Individual bioequivalence. New concepts in the statistical assessment of bioequivalence metrics. *Clinical Pharmacokinetics* **33**, 1–6.

Patterson, S. (2001) A review of the development of biostatistical design and analysis techniques for assessing in vivo bioequivalence: Part two. *Indian Journal of Pharmaceutical Sciences* **63**, 169–86.

Patterson, S. and Jones, B. (2002) Replicate designs and average, individual, and population bioequivalence – I. estimation, inference, and retrospective assessment of performance on novel procedures and the proposed FDA methods for bioequivalence assessment. *Technical Report*, GlaxoSmithKline BDS.

Pigeot, I. and Zierer, A. (2001) Issues of bioequivalence. In: Kunert, J. and Trenkler, G. (eds) *Festschrift in Honour of Siegfried Schach: Mathematical Statistics with Applications in Biometry*, 81–96. Eul-Verlag, Lohmar, Köln.

SAS Institute Inc. (2000) *SAS/STAT user's guide, version 8*. SAS Institute Inc., Cary, NC.

Schall, R. (1995a) Assessment of individual and population bioequivalence using the probability that bioavailabilities are similar. *Biometrics* **51**, 615–26.

Schall, R. (1995b) A unified view of individual, population and average bioequivalence. In: Blume, H.H. and Midha, K.K. (eds) *Bio-International 2: Bioavailability, bioequivalence and pharmacokinetic studies*, 91–106. Medpharm Scientific Publishers, Stuttgart.

Schall, R. and Luus, H.G. (1993). On population and individual bioequivalence. *Statistics in Medicine* **12**, 1109–24.

Schall, R. and Williams, R.L. (1996). Towards a practical strategy for assessing individual bioequivalence. *Journal of Pharmacokinetics and Biopharmaceutics* **24**, 133–49.

Senn, S. (2001). Statistical issues in bioequivalence. *Statistics in Medicine* **20**, 2785–99.

Shao, J. and Tu, D. (1995) *The jackknife and the bootstrap*. Springer-Verlag, New York.

Shao, J., Kübler, J. and Pigeot, I. (2000a) Consistency of the bootstrap procedure in individual bioequivalence. *Biometrika* **87**, 573–85.

Shao, J., Chow, S-C. and Wang, B. (2000b) The bootstrap procedure in individual bioequivalence. *Statistics in Medicine* **19**, 2741–54.

Sheiner, L.B. (1992) Bioequivalence revisited. *Statistics in Medicine* **11**, 1777–88.

Steinijans, V.W. (2001) Some conceptual issues in the evaluation of average, population, and individual bioequivalence. *Drug Information Journal* **35**, 893–9.

Ting, N., Burdick, R.K., Graybill, F.A., Jeyaratnam, S. and Lu, T.-F.C (1990) Confidence intervals on linear combinations of variance components that are unrestricted in sign. *Journal of Statistical Computation and Simulation* **35**, 135–43.

Vuorinen, J. (1997) A practical approach for the assessment of bioequivalence under selected higher-order cross-over designs. *Statistics in Medicine* **16**, 2229–43.

Vuorinen, J. and Tuominen, J. (1994) Fieller's confidence intervals for the ratio of two means in the assessment of average bioequivalence from crossover data. *Statistics in Medicine* **13**, 2531–45.

Vuorinen, J. and Turunen, J. (1996) A three-step procedure for assessing bioequivalence in the general mixed model framework. *Statistics in Medicine* **15**, 2635–55.

Vuorinen, J. and Turunen, J. (1997) A simple three-step procedure for parametric and nonparametric assessment of bioequivalence. *Drug Information Journal* **31**, 167–80.

Wellek, S. (1993) Basing the analysis of comparative bioavailability trials on an individualized statistical definition of equivalence. *Biometrical Journal* **35**, 47–55.

10

Equivalence assessment for clinical endpoints

10.1 Introduction

Many clinical trials have the objective of showing equivalence between two treatments, usually a test drug under development and an existing reference drug for treatment of the same disease. In such studies the aim is no longer to detect a difference between the treatments but to demonstrate that the two active treatments are equivalent within a priori stipulated acceptance limits. If the endpoints follow a lognormal distribution as for example the concentration-related pharmacokinetic characteristics in bioequivalence trials, there is international consensus (CPMP, 2001; FDA, 2001) that the statistical assessment of equivalence should be based on the logarithmic scale, i.e., after logarithmic transformation of the original variables (see Chapter 4).

However, for bioequivalence assessment, there are situations in which the assumption of normality is acceptable for the original data without a logarithmic transformation, as it is in the case, for instance, for the pharmacokinetic characteristic AUC for topical dermatologic corticosteroids (FDA, 1995). Moreover, there are other situations in clinical trials for which the normality assumption for the untransformed clinical outcome may be justified, e.g., as for the assessment of therapeutic equivalence for two inhalers applied for the relief of asthma attacks using the morning peak expiratory flow rate as a measure of airflow obstruction (Jones *et al.*, 1996).

The following example refers to a respiratory clinical trial where the clinical outcome follows a normal distribution. In this multicenter randomized, double-blind, double-dummy, two-period and two-sequence crossover study, the aim was to demonstrate the equivalence of salbutamol administration in a new dry powder inhaler (Test: MAGhaler®) using no chlorofluorocarbon (CFC) propellants and a conventional CFC-containing

Bioequivalence Studies in Drug Development: Methods and Applications   D. Hauschke, V. Steinijans and I. Pigeot
© 2007 John Wiley & Sons, Ltd

metered-dose inhaler (Reference: MDI) (Kieser and Hauschke, 2000). On each of the two study days, which were separated by an appropriate washout period, the patients inhaled $200\,\mu g$ salbutamol from the MAGhaler® or the MDI. Forced expiratory volume in one second (FEV_1) was measured 10 minutes, 20 minutes, 30 minutes, 45 minutes, 1 hour, 2 hours, 4 hours, and 6 hours after inhalation. Primary efficacy variables were the area under the FEV_1 versus time curve during the first six hours after inhalation, $AUC(0-6)$, and the maximum value of FEV_1. An equivalence range of (0.80, 1.25) for the ratio of the expected means for test and reference was defined in the study protocol.

For illustrative purposes only the results for $AUC(0-6)$ are presented in the following. Fifty patients completed the study, $n_1 = 26$ for the sequence: MDI – MAGhaler® (RT) and $n_2 = 24$ for the sequence MAGhaler® – MDI (TR). The FEV_1 time profiles after inhalation were almost identical for both devices with arithmetic mean (median, lower quartile–upper quartile) for $AUC(0-6)$ of 1001 (956, 788–1250) and 993 (978, 787–1199) $(L \cdot min)$ for the MAGhaler® and the MDI, respectively. This leads to the quite narrow two-sided 95 % confidence interval $(0.99, 1.02) \subset (0.80, 1.25)$ proving the equivalence of salbutamol inhalation with the MAGhaler® and the MDI with regard to FEV_1.

The rather narrow 95 % confidence interval for the ratio of FEV_1 is not surprising as $AUC(0-6)$ of this lung function variable is dominated by the AUC below the FEV_1 baseline, denoted as baseline-AUC, which can easily account for more than 80 % of the total AUC. As this baseline-AUC does not reflect the drug-induced changes, the total AUC will favor the conclusion of equivalence. In recognition of this, Steinijans et al. (1996) proposed using the excess-AUC above the baseline, which has a greater discriminatory power than the total AUC = baseline-AUC + excess-AUC. This recommendation applies generally to pharmacodynamic endpoints that either have a physiological or endogenous baseline. The example given by Steinijans et al. (1996) referred to the excess-$AUC(0-168)$ of the prothrombin time as pharmacodynamic endpoint in a pantoprazole–warfarin drug–drug interaction study.

The purpose of this chapter is to provide a test procedure for the equivalence problem assuming that the untransformed variable is normally distributed with unknown variance. Furthermore, the corresponding power is derived and appropriate sample sizes are determined. In the case of the parallel group and of the crossover design, the calculation is based on the exact power of the corresponding two one-sided tests procedure. Additionally, approximate formulas for sample size calculation are given. These methods according to Hauschke et al. (1999) have been implemented in the software package nQuery Advisor® (Elashoff, 2005) and the application is illustrated at the end of this chapter.

The equivalence ranges (0.80, 1.25) and (0.75, 1/0.75) have been chosen for presentation of the appropriate sample sizes and the attained power. This was motivated by the fact that the test problem and the decision for intervals of the form $(\theta_1, \theta_2) = (\theta_1, 1/\theta_1)$ are invariant with respect to taking the reciprocal of the ratio of expected means μ_T/μ_R. Additionally, it can be shown that, only for equivalence limits so defined, the maximum power stabilizes at the point of equality, i.e., $\mu_T/\mu_R = 1$, as the sample size increases (Hauschke et al., 1999).

10.2 Design and testing procedure

10.2.1 Parallel group design

Let Y_T and Y_R designate the primary clinical outcome of interest for the test and reference treatment, respectively. A two-sample situation is considered where it is assumed that the outcomes are mutually independent and normally distributed with unknown but common variance σ^2,

$$Y_{Tj} \sim N(\mu_T, \sigma^2), j = 1, \ldots, n_1, \text{ and } Y_{Rj} \sim N(\mu_R, \sigma^2), j = 1, \ldots, n_2.$$

For equivalence testing it is reasonable to assume that the signs of the corresponding population means μ_T and μ_R are the same and, without loss of generality, positive. Let the interval (δ_1, δ_2), $\delta_1 < 0 < \delta_2$, denote the prespecified equivalence range, so that the corresponding test problem can be formulated as follows:

$$H_0 : \mu_T - \mu_R \leq \delta_1 \text{ or } \mu_T - \mu_R \geq \delta_2$$

vs.

$$H_1 : \delta_1 < \mu_T - \mu_R < \delta_2.$$

By assuming that the acceptance limits δ_1 and δ_2 are known numbers, expressed in the same units as the primary variable, H_0 can be rejected at level α in favor of H_1 (equivalence) if the classical $(1 - 2\alpha)100\,\%$ confidence interval for the difference of expected means $\mu_T - \mu_R$ is entirely included in the equivalence range (δ_1, δ_2). This procedure is equivalent to the two one-sided tests procedure using two-sample t-tests (Schuirmann, 1987).

In clinical practice the equivalence limits δ_1 and δ_2 are often expressed as fractions of the unknown reference mean $\mu_R \neq 0$, i.e., $\delta_1 = f_1\mu_R$ and $\delta_2 = f_2\mu_R$, $-1 < f_1 < 0 < f_2$. For example $f_1 = -f_2 = -0.2$ corresponds to the common $\pm 20\,\%$ criterion. The test problem for equivalence can then be formulated as:

$$H_0 : \frac{\mu_T}{\mu_R} \leq \theta_1 \text{ or } \frac{\mu_T}{\mu_R} \geq \theta_2$$

vs.

$$H_1 : \theta_1 < \frac{\mu_T}{\mu_R} < \theta_2,$$

where (θ_1, θ_2), $\theta_1 = 1 + f_1$, $\theta_2 = 1 + f_2$, $0 < \theta_1 < 1 < \theta_2$, is the corresponding equivalence range for the ratio of the expected means μ_T and μ_R. As shown in Section 3.3.3.1, the null hypothesis can be rejected in favor of equivalence, if

$$T_{\theta_1} = \frac{\overline{Y}_T - \theta_1 \overline{Y}_R}{\hat{\sigma}\sqrt{\frac{1}{n_1} + \frac{\theta_1^2}{n_2}}} > t_{1-\alpha, n_1+n_2-2}$$

and

$$T_{\theta_2} = \frac{\overline{Y}_T - \theta_2 \overline{Y}_R}{\hat{\sigma}\sqrt{\frac{1}{n_1} + \frac{\theta_2^2}{n_2}}} < -t_{1-\alpha, n_1+n_2-2},$$

where $\overline{Y}_T$ and $\overline{Y}_R$ denote the corresponding sample means and

$$\hat{\sigma}^2 = \frac{1}{n_1 + n_2 - 2}\left(\sum_{j=1}^{n_1}(Y_{Tj} - \overline{Y}_T)^2 + \sum_{j=1}^{n_2}(Y_{Rj} - \overline{Y}_R)^2\right).$$

Hauschke *et al.* (1999) have shown that rejection of H_0 by the two tests T_{θ_1} and T_{θ_2} each at level α is equivalent to inclusion of the $(1 - 2\alpha)100\,\%$ confidence interval for μ_T/μ_R, given by Fieller (1954), in the equivalence range (θ_1, θ_2), with

$$[\theta_l, \theta_u] \subset (\theta_1, \theta_2) \text{ and } \overline{Y}_R^2 > a_R,$$

where

$$\theta_l = \frac{\overline{Y}_T\overline{Y}_R - \sqrt{a_R\overline{Y}_T^2 + a_T\overline{Y}_R^2 - a_T a_R}}{\overline{Y}_R^2 - a_R}, \quad \theta_u = \frac{\overline{Y}_T\overline{Y}_R + \sqrt{a_R\overline{Y}_T^2 + a_T\overline{Y}_R^2 - a_T a_R}}{\overline{Y}_R^2 - a_R},$$

$$a_T = \frac{\hat{\sigma}^2}{n_1}t_{1-\alpha, n_1+n_2-2}^2, \quad a_R = \frac{\hat{\sigma}^2}{n_2}t_{1-\alpha, n_1+n_2-2}^2.$$

Note that the condition $\overline{Y}_R^2 > a_R$ implies that $\mu_R \neq 0$

$$\overline{Y}_R^2 > \frac{\hat{\sigma}^2}{n_2}t_{1-\alpha, n_1+n_2-2}^2 \Leftrightarrow \frac{|\overline{Y}_R|}{\hat{\sigma}\sqrt{\frac{1}{n_2}}} > t_{1-\alpha, n_1+n_2-2}.$$

Hence, the following two procedures for the equivalence assessment in parallel group trials lead to the same decision: Conclude equivalence if H_0 is rejected by the tests T_{θ_1} and T_{θ_2} each at level α, or conclude equivalence if $\overline{Y}_R^2 > a_R$ and Fieller's $(1 - 2\alpha)100\,\%$ confidence interval for μ_T/μ_R is included in the equivalence range (θ_1, θ_2).

It should be noted that in clinical trials, a significance level of $\alpha = 0.025$ is required for equivalence testing and this refers to the calculation of two-sided 95 % confidence intervals (CPMP, 2000). Hence, equivalence can be concluded at level $\alpha = 0.025$ if the corresponding two one-sided test problems (see Section 3.3.3.1) can be rejected each at level $\alpha = 0.025$. Only in the special case of bioequivalence have two-sided 90 % confidence intervals been established (CPMP, 2001) and this refers to a significance level of $\alpha = 0.05$.

10.2.2 Crossover design

The two-period, two-sequence crossover design is used in clinical trials where a difference in carryover effects can be excluded with reasonable assurance (Senn, 1993). Let sequences and periods be indexed by i and k, respectively, and suppose that n_i subjects are randomized to sequence i. If Y_{ijk} denotes the primary clinical endpoint variable of the jth subject in the ith sequence during period k, the following model is considered:

$$Y_{ijk} = \mu_h + s_{ij} + \pi_k + v_i + e_{ijk},$$

where μ_h is the effect of treatment h, with $h = R$ if $i = k$ and $h = T$ if $i \neq k$, π_k is the effect of the kth period with $\pi_1 + \pi_2 = 0$, and v_i is the sequence effect with $v_1 + v_2 = 0$, $i, k = 1, 2$, $j = 1, \ldots, n_i$. The subject terms s_{ij} are independent normally distributed with expected mean 0 and between-subject variance σ_B^2. The random errors e_{ijk} are independent and normally distributed with expected mean 0 and within-subject variances σ_{WT}^2 and σ_{WR}^2 for the test and reference treatment, respectively. Furthermore, s_{ij} and e_{ijk} are assumed to be mutually independent. The treatment variances are given by $\sigma_T^2 = \sigma_B^2 + \sigma_{WT}^2$ and $\sigma_R^2 = \sigma_B^2 + \sigma_{WR}^2$ for test and reference, respectively. The intraindividual outcomes within a sequence are correlated and the corresponding covariance is $\sigma_{TR} = \sigma_B^2$.

In analogy to the parallel group design, it can be demonstrated that in the case of a crossover design the test problem for equivalence,

$$H_0 : \frac{\mu_T}{\mu_R} \leq \theta_1 \text{ or } \frac{\mu_T}{\mu_R} \geq \theta_2$$

vs.

$$H_1 : \theta_1 < \frac{\mu_T}{\mu_R} < \theta_2$$

can be rejected, if

$$T_{\theta_1}^* = \frac{\overline{Y}_T - \theta_1 \overline{Y}_R}{\hat{\sigma}_1 \sqrt{\frac{1}{4}\left(\frac{1}{n_1} + \frac{1}{n_2}\right)}} > t_{1-\alpha, n_1 + n_2 - 2}$$

and

$$T_{\theta_2}^* = \frac{\overline{Y}_T - \theta_2 \overline{Y}_R}{\hat{\sigma}_2 \sqrt{\frac{1}{4}\left(\frac{1}{n_1} + \frac{1}{n_2}\right)}} < -t_{1-\alpha, n_1 + n_2 - 2}.$$

Where $\overline{Y}_T$ and $\overline{Y}_R$ denote the corresponding treatment least square means, and

$$\hat{\sigma}_1^2 = \hat{\sigma}_T^2 + \theta_1^2 \hat{\sigma}_R^2 - 2\theta_1 \hat{\sigma}_B^2 \quad \text{and} \quad \hat{\sigma}_2^2 = \hat{\sigma}_T^2 + \theta_2^2 \hat{\sigma}_R^2 - 2\theta_2 \hat{\sigma}_B^2$$

the unbiased estimators of

$$\sigma_1^2 = \sigma_T^2 + \theta_1^2 \sigma_R^2 - 2\theta_1 \sigma_B^2 \text{ and } \sigma_2^2 = \sigma_T^2 + \theta_2^2 \sigma_R^2 - 2\theta_2 \sigma_B^2,$$

respectively. These estimators are obtained by pooling sums of squares and sums of products from the two samples defined by the sequences (see Table 3.8), i.e.,

$$\hat{\sigma}_T^2 = \frac{1}{n_1 + n_2 - 2} \left(\sum_{j=1}^{n_1} (Y_{1j2} - \overline{Y}_{1T2})^2 + \sum_{j=1}^{n_2} (Y_{2j1} - \overline{Y}_{2T1})^2 \right)$$

$$\hat{\sigma}_R^2 = \frac{1}{n_1 + n_2 - 2} \left(\sum_{j=1}^{n_1} (Y_{1j1} - \overline{Y}_{1R1})^2 + \sum_{j=1}^{n_2} (Y_{2j2} - \overline{Y}_{2R2})^2 \right)$$

$$\hat{\sigma}_{TR} = \hat{\sigma}_B^2 = \frac{1}{n_1 + n_2 - 2} \left(\sum_{j=1}^{n_1} (Y_{1j2} - \overline{Y}_{1T2})(Y_{1j1} - \overline{Y}_{1R1}) + \sum_{j=1}^{n_2} (Y_{2j1} - \overline{Y}_{2T1})(Y_{2j2} - \overline{Y}_{2R2}) \right).$$

The same arguments as in the previous section lead to the conclusion that for the crossover design the rejection of H_0 at level α is equivalent to the condition

$$[\theta_l^*, \theta_u^*] \subset (\theta_1, \theta_2) \quad \text{and} \quad \overline{Y}_R^2 > a_R^*,$$

where

$$\theta_l^* = \frac{(\overline{Y}_T \overline{Y}_R - a_{TR}^*) - \sqrt{(\overline{Y}_T \overline{Y}_R - a_{TR}^*)^2 - (\overline{Y}_T^2 - a_T^*)(\overline{Y}_R^2 - a_R^*)}}{\overline{Y}_R^2 - a_R^*}$$

$$\theta_u^* = \frac{(\overline{Y}_T \overline{Y}_R - a_{TR}^*) + \sqrt{(\overline{Y}_T \overline{Y}_R - a_{TR}^*)^2 - (\overline{Y}_T^2 - a_T^*)(\overline{Y}_R^2 - a_R^*)}}{\overline{Y}_R^2 - a_R^*},$$

$$a_T^* = \frac{1}{4} \left(\frac{1}{n_1} + \frac{1}{n_2} \right) \hat{\sigma}_T^2 \, t_{1-\alpha, n_1+n_2-2}^2, \quad a_R^* = \frac{1}{4} \left(\frac{1}{n_1} + \frac{1}{n_2} \right) \hat{\sigma}_R^2 \, t_{1-\alpha, n_1+n_2-2}^2,$$

$$a_{TR}^* = \frac{1}{4} \left(\frac{1}{n_1} + \frac{1}{n_2} \right) \hat{\sigma}_{TR} \, t_{1-\alpha, n_1+n_2-2}^2.$$

The assumption that the within-subject variances are independent of the treatment, that is $\sigma_{WT}^2 = \sigma_{WR}^2 = \sigma_W^2$, results in $\sigma_T^2 = \sigma_R^2 = \sigma_B^2 + \sigma_W^2$, and hence

$$\sigma_1^2 = \sigma_T^2 + \theta_1^2 \sigma_R^2 - 2\theta_1 \sigma_B^2$$
$$= \sigma_B^2 + \sigma_W^2 + \theta_1^2 (\sigma_B^2 + \sigma_W^2) - 2\theta_1 \sigma_B^2 = \sigma_W^2 + \theta_1^2 \sigma_W^2 + \sigma_B^2 + \theta_1^2 \sigma_B^2 - 2\theta_1 \sigma_B^2$$
$$= \sigma_W^2 (1 + \theta_1^2) + \sigma_B^2 (1 - \theta_1)^2$$

and

$$\sigma_2^2 = \sigma_T^2 + \theta_2^2 \sigma_R^2 - 2\theta_2 \sigma_B = \sigma_W^2 (1 + \theta_2^2) + \sigma_B^2 (1 - \theta_2)^2.$$

The test statistics can be reformulated as

$$T^*_{\theta_1} = \frac{\overline{Y}_T - \theta_1 \overline{Y}_R}{\sqrt{\hat{\sigma}^2_W(1+\theta^2_1) + \hat{\sigma}^2_B(1-\theta_1)^2}\sqrt{\frac{1}{4}\left(\frac{1}{n_1}+\frac{1}{n_2}\right)}}$$

and

$$T^*_{\theta_2} = \frac{\overline{Y}_T - \theta_2 \overline{Y}_R}{\sqrt{\hat{\sigma}^2_W(1+\theta^2_2) + \hat{\sigma}^2_B(1-\theta_2)^2}\sqrt{\frac{1}{4}\left(\frac{1}{n_1}+\frac{1}{n_2}\right)}}.$$

The estimators $\hat{\sigma}^2_W$ and $\hat{\sigma}^2_B$ can be derived from the analysis of variance for the two-period, two-sequence crossover (see Chapter 4). It should be noted that this approach results in a conservative testing procedure and is a reasonable approach for practical use (Vuorinen and Tuominen, 1994).

As above, the following two procedures for the equivalence assessment for the crossover design lead to the same decisions: Conclude equivalence if H_0 is rejected by $T^*_{\theta_1}$ and $T^*_{\theta_2}$ each at nominal level α, or conclude equivalence if $\overline{Y}^2_R > a^*_R$ and Fieller's $(1-2\alpha)100$ % confidence interval for μ_T/μ_R is included in the equivalence range (θ_1, θ_2).

10.3 Power and sample size calculation

10.3.1 Parallel group design

For power and sample size determination it is assumed that $n_1 = n_2 = n/2$. In case of a parallel group design the probability of correctly accepting H_1 is given by

$$P(T_{\theta_1} > t_{1-\alpha,n-2} \quad \text{and} \quad T_{\theta_2} < -t_{1-\alpha,n-2} \,|\, \theta_1 < \mu_T/\mu_R < \theta_2 \,, \sigma).$$

The random vector $(T_{\theta_1}, T_{\theta_2})$ has a bivariate noncentral t-distribution with $n-2$ degrees of freedom and noncentrality parameters

$$\Theta_1 = \frac{\mu_T - \theta_1 \mu_R}{\sigma\sqrt{\frac{2(1+\theta^2_1)}{n}}} = \frac{\frac{\mu_T}{\mu_R} - \theta_1}{CV_R\sqrt{\frac{2(1+\theta^2_1)}{n}}}$$

and

$$\Theta_2 = \frac{\mu_T - \theta_2 \mu_R}{\sigma\sqrt{\frac{2(1+\theta^2_2)}{n}}} = \frac{\frac{\mu_T}{\mu_R} - \theta_2}{CV_R\sqrt{\frac{2(1+\theta^2_2)}{n}}},$$

where the standard deviation σ is expressed as a percentage of the reference mean, i.e., $\sigma = CV_R \mu_R$. The method of Owen (1965) for power calculation can only be applied if the correlation between the test statistics equals 1, i.e., $Corr(T_{\theta_1}, T_{\theta_2}) = 1$. However, Hauschke *et al.* (1999) have shown that

$$Corr(T_{\theta_1}, T_{\theta_2}) = \frac{1 + \theta_1 \theta_2}{\sqrt{(1 + \theta_1^2)(1 + \theta_2^2)}},$$

because

$$Var(\overline{Y}_T - \theta_1 \overline{Y}_R) = Var(\overline{Y}_T) + \theta_1^2 \, Var(\overline{Y}_R) = \frac{\sigma^2}{n_1} + \frac{\theta_1^2 \sigma^2}{n_2} = \frac{2\sigma^2(1 + \theta_1^2)}{n}$$

$$Var(\overline{Y}_T - \theta_2 \overline{Y}_R) = \frac{2\sigma^2(1 + \theta_2^2)}{n}$$

$$Cov(\overline{Y}_T - \theta_1 \overline{Y}_R, \overline{Y}_T - \theta_2 \overline{Y}_R) = Var(\overline{Y}_T) + \theta_1 \theta_2 Var(\overline{Y}_R) = \frac{2\sigma^2(1 + \theta_1 \theta_2)}{n},$$

and hence

$$Corr(\overline{Y}_T - \theta_1\overline{Y}_R, \overline{Y}_T - \theta_2\overline{Y}_R) = \frac{Cov(\overline{Y}_T - \theta_1 \overline{Y}_R, \overline{Y}_T - \theta_2 \overline{Y}_R)}{\sqrt{Var(\overline{Y}_T - \theta_1 \overline{Y}_R)Var(\overline{Y}_T - \theta_2 \overline{Y}_R)}}$$

$$= \frac{\dfrac{2\sigma^2(1 + \theta_1\theta_2)}{n}}{\sqrt{\dfrac{2\sigma^2(1 + \theta_1^2)}{n} \dfrac{2\sigma^2(1 + \theta_2^2)}{n}}} = \frac{\dfrac{2\sigma^2(1 + \theta_1\theta_2)}{n}}{\dfrac{2\sigma^2}{n}\sqrt{(1 + \theta_1^2)(1 + \theta_2^2)}} = \frac{1 + \theta_1\theta_2}{\sqrt{(1 + \theta_1^2)(1 + \theta_2^2)}}.$$

For an equivalence acceptance range of the type $(\theta_1, \theta_2) = (\theta_1, 1/\theta_1)$ the correlation reduces to

$$Corr(T_{\theta_1}, T_{\theta_2}) = \frac{1 + \theta_1 \theta_2}{\sqrt{(1 + \theta_1^2)(1 + \theta_2^2)}}$$

$$= \frac{2}{\sqrt{(1 + \theta_1^2)\left(1 + \frac{1}{\theta_1^2}\right)}}.$$

The method of Genz and Bretz (2002) for the computation of multivariate t-probabilities under more general correlation structures is used to create the figures and tables that follow (see Appendix at end of the chapter).

In Figures 10.1 and 10.2, the power curves are shown for two coefficients of variation CV_R of 30 % and 25 %, selected values of μ_T/μ_R from the alternative as a function of the sample size and for classical equivalence ranges of $(\theta_1, \theta_2) = (0.80, 1.25)$ and $(\theta_1, \theta_2) = (0.75, 1/0.75)$, respectively.

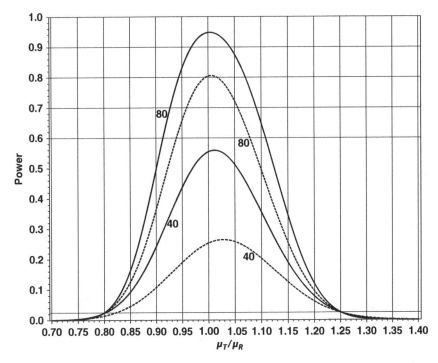

Figure 10.1 Parallel group design: Power curves refer to the equivalence range $(\theta_1, 1/\theta_1) = (0.80, 1.25)$, total sample sizes of $n = 40, 80$, $\alpha = 0.025$, $CV_R = 30\%$ (dotted line) and $CV_R = 25\%$ (solid line).

Figure 10.1 indicates that the proposed two one-sided test procedure is biased. For small sample sizes the actual level is smaller than the nominal significance level for $\mu_T/\mu_R = 0.80$. The method converges to an unbiased test of level α as the sample size increases (Hauschke *et al.*, 1999). This result had already been obtained by Schuirmann (1989).

The corresponding sample sizes necessary to attain a power of at least 0.80 and 0.90 are given for these acceptance ranges in Tables 10.1 and 10.2 for a significance level $\alpha = 0.025$, certain ratios μ_T/μ_R from the alternative and various coefficients of variation. The tables give an idea of the increase in sample size needed to attain a given power when the ratio approaches the limits of the equivalence range. However, from the investigations of Pigeot *et al.* (2003) it becomes evident that in equivalence trials with regard to the ratio of expected means for normally distributed outcomes, an unbalanced allocation of the total sample size implies a reduction in the required number of patients to achieve a certain power. For determination of the optimal allocation of the sample size we refer the reader to the publication by Pigeot *et al.* (2003).

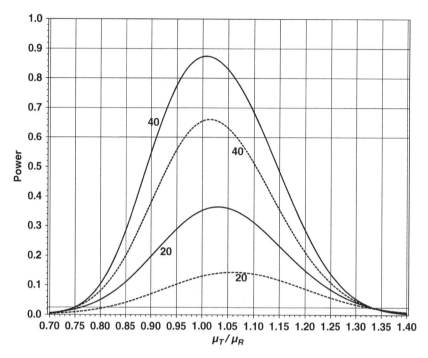

Figure 10.2 Parallel group design: Power curves refer to the equivalence range $(\theta_1, 1/\theta_1) = (0.75, 1.3333)$, total sample sizes of $n = 20, 40$, $\alpha = 0.025$, $CV_R = 30\%$ (dotted line) and $CV_R = 25\%$ (solid line).

10.3.2 Crossover design

Assuming a balanced two-period, two-sequence crossover design, i.e., $n_1 = n_2 = n/2$, the power is given by

$$P(T^*_{\theta_1} > t_{1-\alpha, n-2} \text{ and } T^*_{\theta_2} < -t_{1-\alpha, n-2} \mid \theta_1 < \mu_T/\mu_R < \theta_2, \sigma_1, \sigma_2).$$

The random vector $(T^*_{\theta_1}, T^*_{\theta_2})$ has a bivariate noncentral t-distribution with $n-2$ degrees of freedom and noncentrality parameters

$$\Theta^*_1 = \frac{\mu_T - \theta_1 \mu_R}{\sigma_1 \sqrt{\dfrac{1}{n}}} \text{ and } \Theta^*_2 = \frac{\mu_T - \theta_2 \mu_R}{\sigma_2 \sqrt{\dfrac{1}{n}}},$$

where

$$\sigma_1^2 = \sigma_T^2 + \theta_1^2 \sigma_R^2 - 2\theta_1 \sigma_B^2 \text{ and } \sigma_2^2 = \sigma_T^2 + \theta_2^2 \sigma_R^2 - 2\theta_2 \sigma_B^2.$$

Table 10.1 Parallel group design: Total sample sizes n needed to attain a power of 0.80 and 0.90 in the case of an equivalence range $(\theta_1, 1/\theta_1) = (0.80, 1.25)$, $\alpha = 0.025$ and CV_R ranging from 10 % to 40 %.

Power	CV_R (%)	μ_T/μ_R							
		0.85	0.90	0.95	1.00	1.05	1.10	1.15	1.20
0.80	10.0	106	28	14	12	14	20	44	164
	12.5	164	44	22	16	20	30	66	254
	15.0	234	60	30	22	26	44	94	364
	17.5	318	82	38	30	34	58	126	496
	20.0	414	106	50	38	44	74	164	646
	22.5	524	134	62	46	54	94	206	818
	25.0	646	164	76	56	66	114	254	1008
	27.5	782	198	90	68	80	138	308	1220
	30.0	930	234	108	80	96	164	364	1452
	32.5	1090	274	126	94	112	192	428	1702
	35.0	1264	318	146	108	128	222	496	1974
	37.5	1452	364	166	124	146	254	568	2266
	40.0	1650	414	188	140	166	288	646	2578
0.90	10.0	140	38	18	14	16	28	56	218
	12.5	218	56	28	20	24	40	88	340
	15.0	314	80	38	28	34	56	124	488
	17.5	426	108	50	36	44	76	168	662
	20.0	554	140	64	46	58	98	218	864
	22.5	700	178	80	56	72	124	276	1094
	25.0	864	218	98	70	88	152	340	1350
	27.5	1046	264	120	84	106	184	410	1632
	30.0	1244	314	142	98	124	218	488	1942
	32.5	1460	366	166	116	146	256	572	2278
	35.0	1692	426	190	134	168	296	662	2642
	37.5	1942	488	218	152	192	340	760	3032
	40.0	2208	554	248	174	220	386	864	3450

Assuming that the within-subject variances are independent of the treatment, that is $\sigma^2_{WT} = \sigma^2_{WR} = \sigma^2_W$, gives $\sigma^2_T = \sigma^2_R = \sigma^2_B + \sigma^2_W$ and hence

$$\sigma^2_1 = \sigma^2_W(1 + \theta^2_1) + \sigma^2_B(1 - \theta_1)^2, \quad \sigma^2_2 = \sigma^2_W(1 + \theta^2_2) + \sigma^2_B(1 - \theta_2)^2.$$

Table 10.2 Parallel group design: Total sample sizes n needed to attain a power of 0.80 and 0.90 in the case of an equivalence range $(\theta_1, 1/\theta_1) = (0.75, 1.3333)$, $\alpha = 0.025$ and CV_R ranging from 15 % to 50 %.

Power	CV_R %	\multicolumn{10}{c}{μ_T/μ_R}
		0.80	0.85	0.90	0.95	1.00	1.05	1.10	1.15	1.20	1.25
0.80	15.0	224	58	28	18	16	16	22	32	58	144
	17.5	304	78	36	22	20	20	28	42	78	196
	20.0	396	102	46	28	24	26	36	54	102	254
	22.5	500	128	58	36	30	32	44	68	128	322
	25.0	616	156	72	42	36	38	54	84	156	396
	27.5	744	188	86	52	42	46	64	102	188	478
	30.0	886	224	102	60	50	54	76	120	224	568
	32.5	1040	262	118	70	58	64	88	140	262	666
	35.0	1204	304	136	82	68	72	102	162	304	772
	37.5	1382	348	156	92	76	84	116	186	348	886
	40.0	1572	396	178	106	88	94	132	210	396	1008
	42.5	1776	446	200	118	98	106	148	238	446	1138
	45.0	1990	500	224	132	110	118	166	266	500	1276
	47.5	2216	556	248	148	122	132	184	296	556	1420
	50.0	2456	616	276	162	134	146	204	328	616	1574
0.90	15.0	298	76	36	22	18	20	28	42	76	192
	17.5	406	104	48	28	24	26	36	56	104	260
	20.0	528	134	62	36	30	32	46	72	134	340
	22.5	668	170	76	46	36	40	58	90	170	428
	25.0	824	208	94	54	44	50	70	112	208	528
	27.5	996	252	114	66	52	58	84	134	252	640
	30.0	1186	298	134	78	62	70	100	160	298	760
	32.5	1390	350	158	90	72	80	116	186	350	892
	35.0	1612	406	182	104	82	94	134	216	406	1034
	37.5	1850	464	208	120	94	106	154	248	464	1186
	40.0	2104	528	236	136	106	122	174	280	528	1348
	42.5	2376	596	266	152	120	136	196	316	596	1522
	45.0	2662	668	298	172	134	152	220	354	668	1706
	47.5	2966	744	332	190	150	170	244	394	744	1900
	50.0	3286	824	368	210	166	188	272	438	824	2106

Again, expressing σ_W and σ_B relative to the reference mean, i.e., $\sigma_W = CV_W \mu_R$ and $\sigma_B = CV_B \mu_R$, the noncentrality parameters read as

$$\Theta_1^* = \frac{\dfrac{\mu_T}{\mu_R} - \theta_1}{\sqrt{\dfrac{CV_W^2(1+\theta_1^2) + CV_B^2(1-\theta_1)^2}{n}}}$$

and

$$\Theta_2^* = \frac{\dfrac{\mu_T}{\mu_R} - \theta_2}{\sqrt{\dfrac{CV_W^2(1 + \theta_2^2) + CV_B^2(1 - \theta_2)^2}{n}}}.$$

The correlation between the test statistics $T_{\theta_1}^*$ and $T_{\theta_2}^*$ depends on the equivalence limits and on the within- and between-subject coefficients of variation. As with the parallel group design, the corresponding variance and covariance can be calculated for the crossover design as follows:

$$Var(\overline{Y}_T - \theta_1 \overline{Y}_R) = Var(\overline{Y}_T) + \theta_1^2 Var(\overline{Y}_R) - 2\theta_1 Cov(\overline{Y}_T, \overline{Y}_R)$$

$$= \frac{\sigma_B^2 + \sigma_W^2}{n} + \frac{\theta_1^2(\sigma_B^2 + \sigma_W^2)}{n} - \frac{2\theta_1\sigma_B^2}{n} = \frac{1}{n}(\sigma_W^2(1 + \theta_1^2) + \sigma_B^2(1 - \theta_1)^2).$$

Using $\sigma_W = CV_W \mu_R$ and $\sigma_B = CV_B \mu_R$ results in

$$Var(\overline{Y}_T - \theta_1 \overline{Y}_R) = \frac{\mu_R^2}{n}(CV_W^2(1 + \theta_1^2) + CV_B^2(1 - \theta_1)^2)$$

$$Var(\overline{Y}_T - \theta_2 \overline{Y}_R) = \frac{\mu_R^2}{n}(CV_W^2(1 + \theta_2^2) + CV_B^2(1 - \theta_2)^2).$$

The covariance can be derived as

$$Cov(\overline{Y}_T - \theta_1 \overline{Y}_R, \overline{Y}_T - \theta_2 \overline{Y}_R) = Var(\overline{Y}_T) + Var(\overline{Y}_R)\theta_1\theta_2 - Cov(\overline{Y}_T, \overline{Y}_R)(\theta_1 + \theta_2)$$

$$= \frac{1}{n}(\sigma_W^2 + \sigma_B^2 + (\sigma_B^2 + \sigma_W^2)\theta_1\theta_2 - \sigma_W^2(\theta_1 + \theta_2))$$

$$= \frac{1}{n}(\sigma_W^2(1 + \theta_1\theta_2) + \sigma_B^2(1 + \theta_1\theta_2 - \theta_1 - \theta_2))$$

$$= \frac{\mu_R^2}{n}(CV_W^2(1 + \theta_1\theta_2) + CV_B^2(1 + \theta_1\theta_2 - \theta_1 - \theta_2)),$$

and hence

$$Corr(\overline{Y}_T - \theta_1 \overline{Y}_R, \overline{Y}_T - \theta_2 \overline{Y}_R) = \frac{Cov(\overline{Y}_T - \theta_1 \overline{Y}_R, \overline{Y}_T - \theta_2 \overline{Y}_R)}{\sqrt{Var(\overline{Y}_T - \theta_1 \overline{Y}_R) Var(\overline{Y}_T - \theta_2 \overline{Y}_R)}}$$

$$= \frac{\frac{\mu_R^2}{n}(CV_W^2(1 + \theta_1\theta_2) + CV_B^2(1 + \theta_1\theta_2 - \theta_1 - \theta_2))}{\sqrt{\frac{\mu_R^2}{n}(CV_W^2(1 + \theta_1^2) + CV_B^2(1 - \theta_1)^2)\frac{\mu_R^2}{n}(CV_W^2(1 + \theta_2^2) + CV_B^2(1 - \theta_2)^2)}}$$

$$= \frac{CV_W^2(1 + \theta_1\theta_2) + CV_B^2(1 + \theta_1\theta_2 - \theta_1 - \theta_2)}{\sqrt{(CV_W^2(1 + \theta_1^2) + CV_B^2(1 - \theta_1)^2)(CV_W^2(1 + \theta_2^2) + CV_B^2(1 - \theta_2)^2)}}.$$

For an equivalence of the form $(\theta_1, \theta_2) = (\theta_1, 1/\theta_1)$ the correlation reduces to

$$Corr(T^*_{\theta_1}, T^*_{\theta_2}) = \frac{2CV_W^2 + CV_B^2\left(2 - \theta_1 - \frac{1}{\theta_1}\right)}{\sqrt{\left(CV_W^2(1+\theta_1^2) + CV_B^2(1-\theta_1)^2\right)\left(CV_W^2\left(1 + \frac{1}{\theta_1^2}\right) + CV_B^2\left(1 - \frac{1}{\theta_1}\right)^2\right)}}.$$

The computation of the corresponding integrals for the power calculation is analogous to that for the parallel group design (see Appendix at end of the chapter).

In Figures 10.3 and 10.4 the power curves are shown for equivalence ranges of $(\theta_1, \theta_2) = (0.80, 1.25)$ and $(\theta_1, \theta_2) = (0.75, 1/0.75)$, coefficients of variation $CV_W = 15\%, 20\%$ and $CV_B = 60\%$, selected values μ_T/μ_R and various sample sizes.

The figures show that as the within-subject coefficient of variation CV_W increases, the power decreases and larger sample sizes are needed to achieve a given power.

The minor influence of the between-subject coefficient of variation CV_W is demonstrated in Tables 10.3a and 10.3b, where the sample sizes necessary to attain a power of at least 0.80 and 0.90 are given in the case of an equivalence range of $(0.80, 1.25)$.

Tables 10.4a and 10.4b give the sample sizes to attain a power of at least 0.80 and 0.90 for the equivalence range $(0.75, 1/0.75)$. As already shown in the tables above,

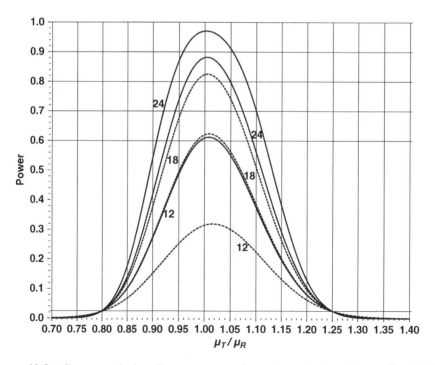

Figure 10.3 Crossover design: Power curves refer to the equivalence range $(\theta_1, 1/\theta_1) = (0.80, 1.25)$, total sample sizes of $n = 12, 18, 24$, $\alpha = 0.025$, $CV_W = 15\%$ (solid line) and $CV_W = 20\%$ (dotted line) and $CV_B = 60\%$.

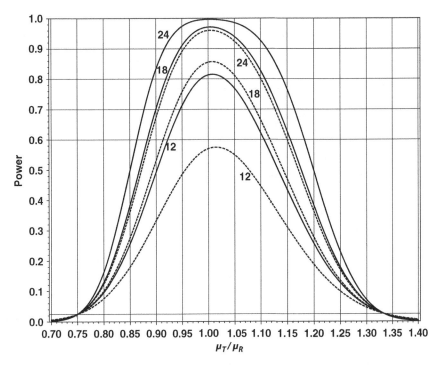

Figure 10.4   Crossover design: Power curves refer to the equivalence range $(\theta_1, 1/\theta_1) =$ (0.75, 1.3333), total sample sizes of $n = 12, 18, 24$, $\alpha = 0.025$, $CV_W = 15\%$ (solid line) and $CV_W = 20\%$ (dotted line) and $CV_B = 60\%$.

sample sizes are practicable for a clinical trial only for values from the alternative not far away from 1 and moderate within-subject coefficients of variation.

10.3.3   Approximate formulas for sample size calculation

The following formulas give a simple approach to sample size calculation for the proof of equivalence for hypotheses formulated in terms of the ratio of expected means assuming a normal distribution for the underlying characteristic of interest (Kieser and Hauschke, 1999, 2000).

In analogy to the sample size determination for bioequivalence (see Section 5.4), Kieser and Hauschke (1999) derived the approximate total sample size n needed to achieve a power of $1 - \beta$ for the alternative μ_T/μ_R, $\theta_1 < \mu_T/\mu_R < 1/\theta_1$, in a parallel group design. This total sample size is given by the smallest integer that fulfils the following inequality:

Table 10.3a Crossover design: Total sample sizes n needed to attain a power of 0.80 in the case of an equivalence range $(\theta_1, 1/\theta_1) = (0.80, 1.25)$, $\alpha = 0.025$ and various CV_W and CV_B.

Power	CV_W (%)	CV_B (%)	0.85	0.90	0.95	1.00	1.05	1.10	1.15	1.20
0.80	10	20	60	18	10	8	10	14	26	92
		40	74	22	12	10	10	16	32	114
		60	100	28	14	12	12	20	40	154
		80	134	36	18	14	16	26	54	208
		100	180	48	22	16	20	34	72	280
	15	20	124	34	16	14	16	24	50	192
		40	138	38	18	14	16	26	56	216
		60	164	44	22	16	20	32	66	254
		80	200	52	26	20	22	38	80	310
		100	244	64	30	22	26	44	98	380
	20	20	214	56	26	20	24	40	86	332
		40	228	60	28	22	26	42	92	356
		60	254	66	32	24	28	46	102	396
		80	290	74	36	26	32	52	114	450
		100	334	86	40	30	36	60	132	520
	25	20	330	84	40	30	36	60	130	514
		40	344	88	42	32	38	62	136	538
		60	370	94	44	34	40	66	146	576
		80	406	104	48	36	42	72	160	632
		100	450	114	54	40	48	80	178	702
	30	20	472	120	56	42	50	84	186	734
		40	486	124	58	44	52	86	192	758
		60	512	130	60	46	54	92	202	798
		80	546	138	64	48	58	98	216	852
		100	592	150	70	52	62	106	234	924
	35	20	638	162	74	56	66	114	252	996
		40	654	166	76	58	68	116	258	1020
		60	678	172	80	60	70	120	266	1060
		80	714	180	84	62	74	126	280	1114
		100	760	192	88	66	78	134	298	1184
	40	20	832	210	96	72	86	146	326	1298
		40	846	214	98	74	86	150	332	1322
		60	872	220	100	76	90	154	342	1360
		80	908	228	104	78	92	160	356	1416
		100	952	240	110	82	98	168	374	1486

Table 10.3b Crossover design: Total sample sizes n needed to attain a power of 0.90 in the case of an equivalence range $(\theta_1, 1/\theta_1) = (0.80, 1.25)$, $\alpha = 0.025$ and various CV_W and CV_B.

Power	CV_W (%)	CV_B (%)	μ_T/μ_R 0.85	0.90	0.95	1.00	1.05	1.10	1.15	1.20
0.90	10	20	78	22	12	10	10	16	32	122
		40	98	28	14	10	12	20	40	152
		60	132	36	18	14	16	26	54	206
		80	180	48	22	16	20	34	72	278
		100	240	62	30	20	26	44	96	374
	15	20	164	44	22	16	20	32	66	256
		40	184	48	24	18	20	34	74	288
		60	218	56	28	20	24	40	88	340
		80	266	68	32	24	28	48	106	414
		100	326	84	40	28	34	60	130	508
	20	20	286	74	34	24	30	52	114	444
		40	306	78	36	26	32	56	122	476
		60	340	88	40	30	36	62	134	528
		80	386	98	46	32	40	70	152	602
		100	446	114	52	38	46	80	176	696
	25	20	440	112	52	36	46	78	174	686
		40	460	118	54	38	48	82	182	718
		60	494	126	58	42	52	88	194	770
		80	542	138	62	44	56	96	214	844
		100	602	152	70	50	62	106	236	938
	30	20	630	160	72	52	64	112	248	982
		40	650	164	76	54	66	116	256	1014
		60	684	174	78	56	70	122	268	1066
		80	730	184	84	60	74	130	288	1140
		100	792	200	90	64	80	140	310	1234
	35	20	854	216	98	68	86	150	336	1332
		40	874	220	100	70	88	154	344	1364
		60	908	230	104	72	92	160	356	1416
		80	954	240	108	76	96	168	374	1490
		100	1016	256	116	82	102	178	398	1584
	40	20	1112	280	126	88	112	196	436	1736
		40	1132	286	128	90	114	200	444	1768
		60	1166	294	132	92	116	204	458	1820
		80	1214	306	138	96	122	214	476	1894
		100	1274	320	144	102	128	224	500	1988

Table 10.4a Crossover design: Total sample sizes n needed to attain a power of 0.80 in the case of an equivalence range $(\theta_1, 1/\theta_1) = (0.75, 1.3333)$, $\alpha = 0.025$ and various CV_W and CV_B.

Power	CV_W (%)	CV_B (%)	0.80	0.85	0.90	0.95	1.00	1.05	1.10	1.15	1.20	1.25
							μ_T/μ_R					
0.80	10	20	60	18	10	8	6	6	8	10	18	40
		40	84	24	12	8	8	8	10	14	24	54
		60	122	32	16	10	10	10	14	18	32	80
		80	178	46	22	14	12	14	18	26	46	114
		100	248	64	30	18	16	16	24	36	64	160
	15	20	122	32	16	12	10	10	12	18	32	78
		40	144	38	18	12	10	12	14	22	38	94
		60	184	48	24	14	12	14	18	28	48	118
		80	238	62	30	18	16	16	22	34	62	154
		100	310	80	38	22	18	20	28	44	80	200
	20	20	208	54	26	16	14	16	20	30	54	134
		40	230	60	28	18	16	16	22	34	60	148
		60	270	70	32	20	18	18	24	38	70	174
		80	324	84	38	24	20	22	30	46	84	210
		100	396	102	46	28	24	26	36	54	102	254
	25	20	318	82	38	24	20	22	28	44	82	204
		40	340	88	40	26	22	22	30	48	88	220
		60	380	98	44	28	24	24	34	52	98	244
		80	436	110	52	32	26	28	38	60	112	280
		100	506	128	58	36	30	32	44	70	128	324
	30	20	452	116	52	32	28	30	40	62	116	290
		40	476	122	56	34	28	30	42	66	122	306
		60	516	130	60	36	30	32	44	70	132	330
		80	570	144	66	40	34	36	50	78	144	366
		100	640	162	74	44	36	40	56	88	162	412
	35	20	612	156	70	42	36	38	52	84	156	392
		40	636	162	74	44	36	40	54	86	162	408
		60	674	170	78	46	38	42	58	92	170	434
		80	730	184	84	50	42	46	62	100	184	468
		100	800	202	92	54	46	50	68	108	202	514
	40	20	796	202	92	54	46	50	68	108	202	510
		40	820	208	94	56	46	50	70	110	208	526
		60	858	216	98	58	48	52	72	116	216	550
		80	914	230	104	62	52	56	78	124	230	586
		100	984	248	112	66	56	60	84	132	248	632

Table 10.4b Crossover design: Total sample sizes n needed to attain a power of 0.90 in the case of an equivalence range $(\theta_1, \ 1/\theta_1) = (0.75, \ 1.3333)$, $\alpha = 0.025$ and various CV_W and CV_B.

Power	CV_W (%)	CV_B (%)	0.80	0.85	0.90	0.95	1.00	1.05	1.10	1.15	1.20	1.25
0.90	10	20	80	22	12	8	8	8	10	14	22	52
		40	110	30	16	10	8	10	12	18	30	72
		60	164	44	20	14	12	12	16	24	44	106
		80	236	62	30	18	14	16	22	34	62	152
		100	332	86	40	24	18	22	30	46	86	214
	15	20	162	42	20	14	12	12	16	24	42	104
		40	192	50	24	16	12	14	18	28	50	124
		60	246	64	30	18	16	16	22	36	64	158
		80	318	82	38	24	18	20	28	44	82	206
		100	414	106	48	28	22	26	36	58	106	266
	20	20	276	72	34	20	16	18	26	40	72	178
		40	308	80	36	22	18	20	28	44	80	198
		60	360	92	42	26	20	24	32	50	92	232
		80	434	110	50	30	24	28	38	60	110	278
		100	528	134	62	36	28	32	46	72	134	340
	25	20	424	108	50	30	24	26	38	58	108	272
		40	456	116	54	32	26	28	40	62	116	292
		60	508	130	60	34	28	32	44	70	130	326
		80	582	148	68	40	32	36	50	80	148	374
		100	676	172	78	46	36	40	58	92	172	434
	30	20	604	154	70	42	32	36	52	82	154	388
		40	636	162	74	44	34	38	54	86	162	408
		60	688	174	80	46	36	42	58	94	174	442
		80	762	192	88	50	40	46	64	104	192	490
		100	856	216	98	56	46	50	72	116	216	550
	35	20	818	206	94	54	44	48	70	110	206	524
		40	850	214	98	56	44	50	72	114	214	546
		60	902	228	102	60	48	54	76	122	228	578
		80	976	246	112	64	52	58	82	132	246	626
		100	1070	270	122	70	56	62	90	144	270	686
	40	20	1064	268	120	70	56	62	90	144	268	682
		40	1096	276	124	72	58	64	92	148	276	702
		60	1148	290	130	76	60	68	96	154	290	736
		80	1222	308	138	80	64	72	102	164	308	784
		100	1316	332	148	86	68	76	110	176	332	844

$$n \geq 2(1+\theta_1^2)\left(\frac{CV_R}{\theta_1-1}\right)^2 (t_{1-\alpha,n-2}+t_{1-\beta/2,n-2})^2 \text{ if } \mu_T/\mu_R = 1$$

$$n \geq 2\left(1+\frac{1}{\theta_1^2}\right)\left(\frac{CV_R}{\frac{1}{\theta_1}-\frac{\mu_T}{\mu_R}}\right)^2 (t_{1-\alpha,n-2}+t_{1-\beta,n-2})^2 \text{ if } 1 < \mu_T/\mu_R < 1/\theta_1$$

$$n \geq 2(1+\theta_1^2)\left(\frac{CV_R}{\theta_1-\frac{\mu_T}{\mu_R}}\right)^2 (t_{1-\alpha,n-2}+t_{1-\beta,n-2})^2 \text{ if } \theta_1 < \mu_T/\mu_R < 1.$$

In the case of a two-period, two-sequence crossover design the corresponding formulas can be applied (Kieser and Hauschke, 2000):

$$n \geq \frac{CV_W^2(1+\theta_1^2)+CV_B^2(1-\theta_1)^2}{(\theta_1-1)^2}(t_{1-\alpha,n-2}+t_{1-\beta/2,n-2})^2 \text{ if } \mu_T/\mu_R = 1$$

$$n \geq \frac{CV_W^2\left(1+\frac{1}{\theta_1^2}\right)+CV_B^2\left(1-\frac{1}{\theta_1}\right)^2}{\left(\frac{1}{\theta_1}-\frac{\mu_T}{\mu_R}\right)^2}(t_{1-\alpha,n-2}+t_{1-\beta,n-2})^2 \text{ if } 1 < \mu_T/\mu_R < 1/\theta_1$$

$$n \geq \frac{CV_W^2(1+\theta_1^2)+CV_B^2(1-\theta_1)^2}{\left(\theta_1-\frac{\mu_T}{\mu_R}\right)^2}(t_{1-\alpha,n-2}+t_{1-\beta,n-2})^2 \text{ if } \theta_1 < \mu_T/\mu_R < 1.$$

Investigations of the accuracy (Kieser and Hauschke, 1999, 2000) show that the difference between the sample sizes based on the approximate formulas and the exact ones are only minor. The above approximation formulas can be further simplified without major loss of precision by replacing the quantiles of the t-distribution by the corresponding quantities of the standard normal distribution. Solutions of the resulting formulas need no iterations, and provide a rough estimate of the required sample size. It should be noted that in analogy to the approximate formulas for sample size determination in bioequivalence studies (see Section 5.4), exact calculation is preferred if sample size must be determined for small deviations between test and reference (Kieser and Hauschke, 1999).

10.3.4   Exact power and sample size calculation by nQuery®

The software package nQuery Advisor ® (Elashoff, 2005) can also be used for this application. Two features of this program are power and sample size determination for the proof of equivalence for the ratio of expected means under the assumption of a normal distribution in the parallel group design and in the two-period, two-sequence crossover design, respectively. The method corresponds to the one provided by Hauschke et al. (1999).

For the parallel group design, Table 10.5 gives the sample sizes needed to attain a power of at least 0.80 for values from the alternative $\mu_T/\mu_R = 0.85, \ldots, 1.20$, for the significance level $\alpha = 0.025$, a coefficient of variation $CV_R = 20\%$, and an equivalence range of (0.80, 1.25). It should be noted that the sample sizes are given per group and thus have to be doubled to get the total sample sizes.

Table 10.5 Screenshot from nQuery Advisor®. Power and sample size determination for the proof of equivalence for the ratio of expected means in the parallel group design under the assumption of a normal distribution. Reproduced by permission of Elashoff (2005).

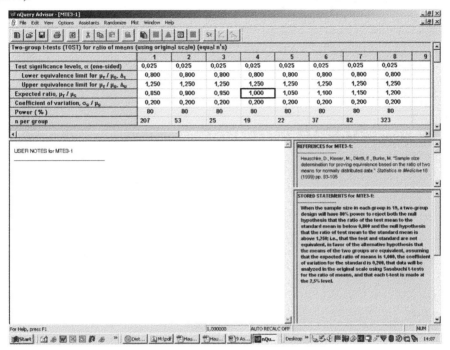

For the two-period, two-sequence crossover design, Table 10.6 gives the sample sizes per sequence needed to attain a power of at least 0.80 for values from the alternative $\mu_T/\mu_R = 0.85, \ldots, 1.20$, for the significance level $\alpha = 0.025$, for within-subject and between-subject coefficients of variation $CV_W = 25\%$ and $CV_B = 20\%$ respectively, and an equivalence range of $(0.80, 1.25)$.

10.4 Conclusions

Planning a study and its statistical analysis are closely linked. In accordance with regulatory requirements, the sample size determination for equivalence trials should be based on the specific methods developed for this type of study.

In this chapter, we considered the case where equivalence is defined in terms of the ratio of population means under the assumption that the untransformed data are normally distributed. This situation also arises when equivalence is defined by the difference of expected means of normally distributed endpoints and when the equivalence acceptance limits are expressed relative to the unknown reference mean.

The methodology of exact sample size calculation for this type of study is presented for the parallel group and for the crossover design. Further information concerning the

Table 10.6 Screenshot from nQuery Advisor®. Power and sample size determination for the proof of equivalence for the ratio of expected means in the crossover design under the assumption of a normal distribution. Reproduced by permission of Elashoff (2005).

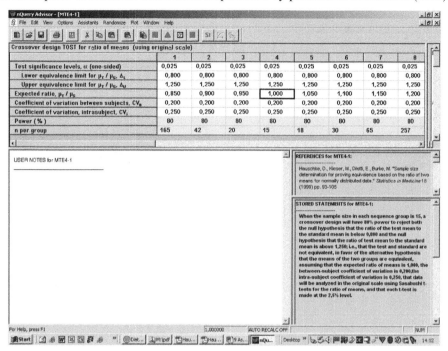

special issues of justification of an equivalence study, choice of the reference treatment, of the primary variable and of the equivalence limits, internal and external validity, double-blindness, intention-to-treat and interim analysis are provided by Jones *et al.* (1996) and Windeler and Trampisch (1996).

Appendix

For the parallel group design, the probability of correctly accepting H_1 is

$$P(T_{\theta_1} > t_{1-\alpha,n-2} \text{ and } T_{\theta_2} < -t_{1-\alpha,n-2} \,|\, \theta_1 < \mu_T/\mu_R < \theta_2 \,, \sigma)$$
$$= Q(\infty, -t_{1-\alpha,n-2}, \Theta_1, \Theta_2, \rho) - Q(t_{1-\alpha,n-2}, -t_{1-\alpha,n-2}, \Theta_1, \Theta_2, \rho),$$

where

$$Q(t_1, t_2, \Theta_1, \Theta_2, \rho) = P(T_{\theta_1} < t_1 \text{ and } T_{\theta_2} < t_2 \,|\, \theta_1 < \mu_T/\mu_R < \theta_2 \,, \sigma)$$

$$= \frac{\sqrt{2\pi}}{\Gamma\left(\frac{n}{2}-1\right)2^{(n/2)-2}} \int_0^{\infty} \Phi_2\left(\frac{t_1 x}{\sqrt{n-2}} - \Theta_1, \frac{t_2 x}{\sqrt{n-2}} - \Theta_2, \rho\right) x^{n-3} \Phi'(x)\,dx,$$

$$\Phi_2(x, y, \rho) = \frac{1}{2\pi\sqrt{1-\rho^2}} \int_{-\infty}^{x} \int_{-\infty}^{y} \exp\left(-\frac{u^2 - 2\rho uv + v^2}{2(1-\rho^2)}\right) dv\,du,$$

$$\Phi'(x) = \frac{1}{\sqrt{2\pi}} \exp\left(-\frac{x^2}{2}\right),$$

$$\Theta_1 = \frac{\frac{\mu_T}{\mu_R} - \theta_1}{CV_R\sqrt{\frac{2(1+\theta_1^2)}{n}}}, \quad \Theta_2 = \frac{\frac{\mu_T}{\mu_R} - \theta_2}{CV_R\sqrt{\frac{2(1+\theta_2^2)}{n}}}$$

$$Corr(T_{\theta_1}, T_{\theta_2}) = \rho = \frac{1 + \theta_1\theta_2}{\sqrt{(1+\theta_1^2)(1+\theta_2^2)}}.$$

By analogy, for the crossover design, the probability of correctly accepting H_1 is

$$P(T_{\theta_1}^* > t_{1-\alpha, n-2} \text{ and } T_{\theta_2}^* < -t_{1-\alpha, n-2} \mid \theta_1 < \mu_T/\mu_R < \theta_2, \sigma_1, \sigma_2)$$
$$= Q(\infty, -t_{1-\alpha, n-2}, \Theta_1^*, \Theta_2^*, \rho^*) - Q(t_{1-\alpha, n-2}, -t_{1-\alpha, n-2}, \Theta_1^*, \Theta_2^*, \rho^*),$$

where

$$\Theta_1^* = \frac{\frac{\mu_T}{\mu_R} - \theta_1}{\sqrt{\frac{CV_W^2(1+\theta_1^2) + CV_B^2(1-\theta_1)^2}{n}}},$$

$$\Theta_2^* = \frac{\frac{\mu_T}{\mu_R} - \theta_2}{\sqrt{\frac{CV_W^2(1+\theta_2^2) + CV_B^2(1-\theta_2)^2}{n}}},$$

$$Corr(T_{\theta_1}^*, T_{\theta_2}^*) = \rho^*$$

$$= \frac{CV_W^2(1+\theta_1\theta_2) + CV_B^2(1+\theta_1\theta_2 - \theta_1 - \theta_2)}{\sqrt{(CV_W^2(1+\theta_1^2) + CV_B^2(1-\theta_1)^2)(CV_W^2(1+\theta_2^2) + CV_B^2(1-\theta_2)^2)}}.$$

References

Committee for Proprietary Medicinal Products (2000) Points to consider on switching between superiority and non-inferiority. EMEA, London.

Committee for Proprietary Medicinal Products (2001) Note for guidance on the investigation of bioavailability and bioequivalence. EMEA, London.

Elashoff, J.D. (2005) nQuery Advisor ® Version 6.0. Los Angeles, CA.

Fieller, E. (1954) Some problems in interval estimation. Journal of the Royal Statistical Society B **16**, 175–85.

Food and Drug Administration (1995) Guidance for industry. Topical dermatologic corticosteroids: in vivo bioequivalence. Center for Drug Evaluation and Research, Rockville, MD.

Food and Drug Administration (2001) *Guidance for industry. Statistical approaches to establishing bioequivalence.* Center for Drug Evaluation and Research, Rockville, MD.

Genz, A. and Bretz (2002) Methods for the computation of multivariate *t*-probabilities. *Journal of Computational and Graphical Statistics*, **11**, 950–71.

Hauschke, D., Kieser, M., Diletti, E. and Burke, M. (1999) Sample size determination for proving equivalence based on the ratio of two means for normally distributed data. *Statistics in Medicine* **18**, 93–105.

Jones, B., Jarvis, P., Lewis, J.A. and Ebbutt, A.F. (1996) Trials to assess equivalence: the importance of rigorous methods. *British MedicalJournal* **313**, 36–9.

Kieser, M. and Hauschke, D. (1999) Approximate sample sizes for testing hypotheses about the ratio and difference of two means. *Journal of Biopharmaceutical Statistics* **9**: 641–50.

Kieser, M. and Hauschke, D. (2000) Statistical methods for demonstrating equivalence in crossover trials based on the ratio of two location parameters. *Drug Information Journal* **34**, 563–8.

Owen, D.B. (1965) A special case of a bivariate non-central *t*-distribution. *Biometrika* **52**, 437–46.

Pigeot, I., Schäfer, J., Röhmel, J. and Hauschke, D. (2003) Assessing non-inferiority of a new treatment in a three-arm clinical trial including placebo. *Statistics in Medicine* **22**, 883–9.

Schuirmann, D.J. (1987) A comparison of the two one-sided tests procedure and the power approach for assessing the equivalence of average bioavailability. *Journal of Pharmacokinetics and Biopharmaceutics* **15**, 657–80.

Schuirmann, D.J. (1989) Confidence intervals for the ratio of two means from a crossover study. *American Statistical Association, Proceedings of the Biopharmaceutical Section*, 121–6.

Senn, S. (1993) *Cross-over Trials in Clinical Research.* John Wiley & Sons Ltd, Chichester.

Steinijans, V.W., Huber, R., Hartmann, M., Zech, K., Bliesath, H., Wurst, W. and Radtke, H.W. (1996) Lack of pantoprazole drug interaction in man: an updated review. *International Journal of Clinical Pharmacology and Therapeutics* **34**, 243–62.

Vuorinen, J. and Tuominen, J. (1994) Fieller's confidence intervals for the ratio of two means in the assessment of average bioequivalence from crossover data. *Statistics in Medicine* **13**, 2531–45.

Windeler, J. and Trampisch, H-J. (1996) Recommendations concerning studies on therapeutic equivalence. *Drug Information Journal* **30**, 195–200.

Index

absorption
  extent 17–19, 178, 190
  rate 24–26, 30–33
absorption, distribution, metabolism and
  excretion (ADME) 175
analysis of variance (ANOVA)
  example 71, 135, 137, 146, 149
  statistical model 80–83, 219, 227, 229,
    232
antihypertensive patch dataset 215–216,
  259–278
area under the curve (AUC)
  composite characteristic 189–194
  excess-AUC 189, 284
  extrapolation to infinity 22–23, 132–133,
    153
  fluctuation 31, 33, 151
  partial 24–25, 33
  single dose 20–23, 33, 187
  steady state 26–27, 33, 187
area under the moment curve ($AUMC$) 23
$AUC/t_{1/2}$ 191–194
auto induction 18
average concentration C_{av} 26, 28

bioavailability
  definition 2
  extent, *see* absorption, extent
  rate, *see* absorption, rate

bioequivalence
  acceptance range
    classical 101–103, 111–112, 134,
      197–199, 284
    modified 101–103, 112–114
  applications 4–5
  average 8–9, 247–249, 253–254
    replicate designs 258–259
  definition 2–3
  individual 11–12, 207, 230–243,
    252–253, 256, 257–258
  population 9–11, 205, 217–230, 249–252,
    255–256
Biopharmaceutics Classification System 4
Blue Ribbon Panel 209

caffeine 180–181, 184–185, 188
carbamazepine 18, 22–23, 179, 181, 188
carryover effect
  estimation of difference
    nonparametric 66
    parametric 59
  graphical illustration 58
  test for difference
    nonparametric 65
    parametric 60, 81
C_{av}, *see* average concentration C_{av}
characteristic, *see* pharmacokinetic
  characteristic

Statistics in Practice

Human and Biological Sciences

Berger – Selection Bias and Covariate Imbalance in Randomized Clinical Trials
Brown and Prescott – Applied Mixed Models in Medicine
Chevret (Ed) – Statistical Methods for Dose-Finding Experiments
Ellenberg, Fleming and DeMets – Data Monitoring Committees in Clinical Trials: A Practical Perspective
Hauschke, Steinijans and Pigeot – Bioequivalence Studies in Drug Development: Methods and Applications
Lawson, Browne and Vidal Rodeiro – Disease Mapping with WinBUGS and MLwiN
Lui – Statistical Estimation of Epidemiological Risk
*Marubini and Valsecchi – Analysing Survival Data from Clinical Trials and Observation Studies
O'Hagan – Uncertain Judgements: Eliciting Experts' Probabilities
Parmigiani – Modeling in Medical Decision Making: A Bayesian Approach
Pintilie – Competing Risks: A Practical Perspective
Senn – Cross-over Trials in Clinical Research, Second Edition
Senn – Statistical Issues in Drug Development
Spiegelhalter, Abrams and Myles – Bayesian Approaches to Clinical Trials and Health-Care Evaluation
Whitehead – Design and Analysis of Sequential Clinical Trials, Revised Second Edition
Whitehead – Meta-Analysis of Controlled Clinical Trials
Willan – Statistical Analysis of Cost-effectiveness Data

Earth and Environmental Sciences

Buck, Cavanagh and Litton – Bayesian Approach to Interpreting Archaeological Data
Glasbey and Horgan – Image Analysis in the Biological Sciences
Helsel – Nondetects and Data Analysis: Statistics for Censored Environmental Data
McBride – Using Statistical Methods for Water Quality Management
Webster and Oliver – Geostatistics for Environmental Scientists

Industry, Commerce and Finance

Aitken and Taroni – Statistics and the Evaluation of Evidence for Forensic Scientists, Second Edition
Balding – Weight-of-evidence for Forensic DNA Profiles
Lehtonen and Pahkinen - Practical Methods for Design and Analysis of Complex Surveys, Second Edition
Ohser and Mücklich – Statistical Analysis of Microstructures in Materials Science
Taroni, Aitken, Garbolino and Biedermann – Bayesian Networks and Probabilistic Inference in Forensic Science

*Now available in paperback

Printed and bound by CPI Group (UK) Ltd, Croydon, CR0 4YY

16/04/2025

14658551-0003